D1035009

FOUNDATIONS OF THE NEURON DOCTRINE

HISTORY OF NEUROSCIENCE

A series of books published by Oxford University Press
in cooperation with Fidia Research Foundation

Editors
Pietro Corsi, D.Phil.
Edward G. Jones, M.D., Ph.D.
Gordon M. Shepherd, M.D., Ph.D.

1. Cajal on the Cerebral Cortex: An Annotated Translation of the Complete Writings
   JAVIER DEFELIPE AND EDWARD G. JONES
2. Disturbances of Lower and Higher Visual Capacities Caused by Occipital Damage
   WALTHER POPPELREUTER, *translated by* J. ZIHL
3. Mind, Brain and Adaptation in the Nineteenth Century: Cerebral Localization and Its Biological Context from Gall to Ferrier
   ROBERT M. YOUNG
4. The Enchanted Loom: Chapters in the History of Neuroscience
   edited by PIETRO CORSI
5. Cajal's Degeneration and Regeneration of the Nervous System
   Edited, with an Introduction and Additional Translations *by*
   JAVIER DEFELIPE AND EDWARD G. JONES, *Translated by* RAOUL M. MAY
6. Foundations of the Neuron Doctrine
   GORDON M. SHEPHERD

FOUNDATIONS OF THE NEURON DOCTRINE

GORDON M. SHEPHERD
Professor of Neuroscience
Yale University School of Medicine

NEW YORK OXFORD
OXFORD UNIVERSITY PRESS
1991

Oxford University Press

Oxford New York Toronto
Delhi Bombay Calcutta Madras Karachi
Petaling Jaya Singapore Hong Kong Tokyo
Nairobi Dar es Salaam Cape Town
Melbourne Auckland

and associated companies in
Berlin Ibadan

Published by Oxford University Press, Inc.,
200 Madison Avenue, New York, New York 10016

Library of Congress Cataloging-in-Publication Data
Shepherd, Gordon M., 1933–
Foundations of the neuron doctrine / by Gordon M. Shepherd.
p. cm.—(History of neuroscience ; no. 6)
Includes bibliographical references.
Includes indexes.
ISBN 0-19-506491-7
1. Neuroanatomy—History. 2. Neurons—History.
I. Title. II. Series.
[DNLM: 1. Neuroanatomy—history.
2. Neurons. W1 HI85J no. 6 / WL 11.1 S548f]
QM451.S47 1991
611′.8′09—dc20
DNLM/DLC
for Library of Congress 90-28814

1 3 5 7 9 8 6 4 2

Printed in the United States of America
on acid-free paper

For Grethe

PREFACE

My interest in this subject began in Oxford in 1959 when my mentors, Charles Phillips and Tom Powell, set me to reading Cajal's account of the organization of the olfactory bulb in preparation for my doctoral work on the electrophysiology of transmission in the olfactory pathway. Immediately intrigued, I committed to memory most of the account of this structure in Cajal's "Studies on the Limbic Cortex," originally published in the 1890s and made available in English in Lisbeth Kraft's fine translation in 1955 (London: Lloyd-Luke). Those images, verbal and graphic, have been the inspiration for my view of nervous organization, as they have been for many of my colleagues in neuroscience. I wish to emphasize this, because the analysis and revisions to which I and others have subjected those images in no way detracts from our indebtedness to Cajal; rather, in the true spirit of science, it is the way we pay homage to him.

Eager for more, I purchased Cajal's great two-volume treatise in French on the histology of the nervous system published in 1911. This not only revealed the full breadth and depth of his understanding of nervous organization but also introduced me to the gallery of other distinguished contributors to the early work on the nerve cell. I began to translate some of the classical papers from the 1880s and 1890s, in order to study more closely the original observations and, following Kraft's example, make them available to English-speaking neuroscientists who would otherwise remain unaware of this basic literature of our field.

The next step along the way involved work with Wilfrid Rall, Tom Reese, and Milton Brightman, which revealed that the cells in the olfactory bulb interact in ways not predicted by classical ideas about the organization of neurons as contained in the "Neuron Doctrine" and the "Law of Dynamic Polarization of the Neuron." This again sent me back to the classical authors, to find out exactly what they had meant when they formulated these concepts. I was surprised and delighted to realize that this was a literature abounding in a ferment of ideas about basic principles of nervous organization, with spirited debates over the terminology of the neuron, structure–function relations at the cellular and circuit level, and rules for the formation of functional pathways and behavioral systems. Several modern authors had begun to reassess the classical doctrine in the light of new findings in the 1950s, and I was stimulated by these contributions to do the same for our own new findings, publishing several articles on the subject, which have appeared over the past two decades.

All this while I knew that the centennial of the promulgation of the neuron doctrine would fall in 1991, and that this would be an appropriate time to bring together translations of the classical papers with a critical commentary, in order to give a modern perspective to this subject and make it more immediate and accessible to everyone with an interest in the nervous system. This book is the result.

For an experimentalist like myself the prospect of writing a historical account has been a daunting one. My initial strategy was to regard this literature as an extension of the literature one would include in a review of the background for one's current research. This meant that historical issues would be considered only as they have had enduring relevance for current research interests. While keeping to that goal, I also discovered that the interplay of the personalities of the main contributors was crucial to the development of the ideas; furthermore, the ideas themselves, involving as they do the basis for our cognitive capacities, have a much broader interest than is generally appreciated. Hence the proposal that the neuron doctrine deserves attention as a case study in the history of ideas. Within that context, the present volume is a small but, I hope, useful beginning.

My first debts in writing this book are to Javier DeFelipe, Carol Hightower, Grethe Shepherd, Tali Zulman, Juliana Vanucchi, and Lisbeth Shepherd, who have provided most of the translations of the original documents into English. I am particularly grateful to Javier DeFelipe for obtaining the early papers of Cajal, and for translating them and discussing them with me. Each translation has been gone over word by word, and any errors of interpretation are solely mine. I have resisted the temptation to make the documents more readable by too much smoothing over of awkward phraseology or by using modern terms. The manner in which a result or an idea was expressed, in the then current terminology, is critical to understanding the way the field was evolving and the issues at stake at any particular time. Full acknowledgment for the translations of documents from the different languages is made in the Comments on Sources.

Tali Zulman and Margaret Schwartz have been outstanding assistants in tracking down original books and articles, typing parts of the manuscript, assembling the bibliography, and generally making the whole project possible. The Yale Medical Historical Library has been a wonderful source of the original materials for this project, and I am grateful to Janice Braun, Ferenc Gyorgey, and the entire staff for their unfailing assistance. Barbara Frank has provided expert typing; Vladim Shkolnikoff has assisted with the bibliography. For preparation of the illustrations I am grateful to the Yale Medical Illustration Department and to Sarah Whitaker. Pasquale Graziadei and Pasko Rakic have generously provided photographs from their collections.

I am grateful to Jeffrey House at Oxford University Press and to my colleagues Ted Jones and Pietro Corsi for encouraging me to undertake this project, and for sustaining me during the writing. The Fidia Foundation has been most generous in its support. Walle Nauta particularly encouraged me to emphasize the relevance of the historical period to current research interests. Special gratitude goes to Javier DeFelipe for extensive discussions of Cajal, Jan Jansen, Jr., for stimulating my interest in Nansen, Robert Byck for discussions of Freud's early years, and Frederic L. Holmes for reading the manuscript and making many suggestions for improvements. In the fall semester of 1990 I gave an undergraduate course at Yale on "Historical Foundations of the Neuron Doctrine," using the manuscript of this book as the text; my thanks to those students, both science and nonscience majors, for many stimulating discussions and suggestions to make various subjects clearer. The material has also been the basis for a lecture at Yale to The Beaumont Medical Club of Connecticut entitled "Perspectives on the Neuron Doctrine: 1891–1991" in January, 1991, and a lecture entitled "Foundations of the Neuron Doctrine" on the occasion of the centennial celebrations of the University of Texas Medical Branch in February, 1991. My thanks to these organizations for their interest in this topic and the opportunity to develop further the ideas in this book.

Finally, I dedicate this book to my wife, Grethe, who has lived with these materials for over three decades, and is responsible for seeing this project through to a long-awaited completion.

Hamden, Conn. G. M. S.
March 1991

CONTENTS

FOUNDATIONS OF THE NEURON DOCTRINE

1
Introduction

For a century, the "neuron doctrine" has been the basis for our concepts of the organization of the nervous system. Formulated in 1891, it finally ended a debate that had lasted for half a century, and demonstrated that the cell theory applies to the cells of the nervous system. Ramón y Cajal was the main architect of the neuron doctrine, but in fact it was the culmination of intensive studies of the nervous system by many European scientists during the nineteenth century. Its introduction stimulated a vigorous debate that fashioned most of the basic terminology of the neuron that we use today. Furthermore, the neuron doctrine became the core around which concepts of the functional organization of the brain have been developed to the present time.

Despite this importance, the neuron doctrine remains little known, certainly one of the least understood and appreciated among the major concepts of modern science. Most textbooks of neurobiology, neurology, and neuropsychology acknowledge its importance without examining it critically. In a recent article commemorating all the centenary achievements of science to be celebrated in 1991, the neuron doctrine is not even mentioned (Bynum and Heilbron, 1991). Thus, it is not surprising that this theory has not received a systematic reevaluation in the light of modern research. There is little current awareness of the issues that were at stake in its formulation, or of the unresolved issues that carry forward to the present. It seems obvious that a theory of this central importance to the field of neuroscience, and to an understanding of brain function, merits close and constant review. The aim of this book is to provide such a review.

The Classical Period

In order to orient the reader to the issues involved in establishing the neuron doctrine, it will be useful to begin with a brief overview of the work as it evolved during the nineteenth century. The theory in fact emerged through a series of stages.

The cell theory, enunciated by Theodor Schwann in 1839, stated that all tissues in the body are composed of individual cells. The theory gained immediate acceptance for all organs except the nervous system, where two basic problems were encountered. One was the difficulty, with the microscopical methods then available, to determine whether all nerve fibers arise directly from nerve cells, or whether some might exist independently of the cells. The other problem was that it could not be seen whether the long and thin branches arising from nerve cells and nerve fibers have definite terminations, or whether they run together with neighboring thin branches to form a continuous network. A great deal was at stake in this controversy, not only the cellular basis of nervous organization but also whether that basis differed fundamentally from the way all other organs of the body were constructed.

The difficulties in establishing the relations between nerve cells, nerve fibers, and terminal branches delayed the application of the cell theory to the nervous system for half a century. This early work, though limited by the available methods, introduced some of our basic ideas about the neuron and its parts. Furthermore, two fundamentally different views of the organization of neurons arose, one holding that individual neurons are connected in chains to form specific pathways, the other that their thin branches form continuous diffuse networks.

The key technological advance that led to the resolution of most of these uncertainties came in the 1870s with the introduction by Camillo Golgi of a new method of staining individual nerve cells; however, it was largely ignored for more than a decade. Then came five exciting years, starting in 1886, during which studies in several laboratories pointed directly toward a new theory. In 1887, Santiago Ramón y Cajal stumbled on the Golgi stain and began an intense study of neuronal morphology throughout the nervous system; his clear-minded interpretations of Golgi-stained cells essentially solved the problem of neuronal form and neuronal interconnections. This stimulated a wave of studies culminating in Wilhelm Waldeyer's review of 1891, in which he summarized the new findings in a coherent theory, which stated that *the nerve cell is the anatomical, physiological, metabolic, and genetic unit of the nervous system.* To emphasize the newly recognized character of the nerve cell, Waldeyer bestowed on it a new name, the *neu-*

ron. This formulation of the cell theory in terms of the specific types of cells found in the nervous system came to be called the *neuron theory*, or *neuron doctrine*.

In the period following 1891, different views regarding terminology of the neuron were aired, as well as opposition from the remaining partisans of the reticular theory of neural organization, including Golgi himself. The introduction of the concept of the *synapse*, by Charles Sherrington in 1897, provided an anatomical and functional explanation for the mechanism by which the individual neuronal units could communicate with each other. The general acceptance of the neuron doctrine, by anatomists, physiologists, neurologists, and psychologists, was manifest by several exhaustive reviews in the years around 1900, and the authoritative textbook of Ramón y Cajal in 1909.

Reassessing the Classical Neuron Doctrine

This outline of the history of the work surrounding the neruon doctrine is well understood. The most complete account to date may be found in Clarke and O'Malley's volume on *The Brain and Spinal Cord* (1968), which contains translations and commentary on a range of topics in the history of research on the nervous system, including an extensive section on "The Neuron." Different perspectives on the topic are provided in Liddell's *The History of Reflexes* (1960), Meyer's *Historical Aspects of Cerebral Anatomy* (1971), and, for the early period, van der Loos' article on "The history of the neuron" (1967). Critical comments are given in Peters, Palay, and Webster's definitive textbook on *The Fine Structure of the Nervous System* (1990), and by Nauta and Feirtag in their *Fundamental Neuroanatomy* (1986).

The motivation for my interest in this topic came from research in the 1960s suggesting that some of the tenets of the classical doctrine would have to be revised. It seemed that a thorough review of the classical literature would be necessary in order to provide the soundest possible basis for a reevaluation. The present book is the result of that reevaluation. It builds on previous accounts in several ways. Perhaps most important, its main aim is to assess in depth the relevance of the classical doctrine for research in modern neuroscience on the neuron and on brain function. Second, it is written from the perspective of physiology as well as anatomy, with particular emphasis on modern issues concerning the functional organization of neurons in relation to information processing in the brain. Finally, it gathers together a more complete series of the classical papers on the subject than has hitherto been available.

The reevaluation has shown that the evolution of the classical doctrine followed a more complex course, involving issues that are deeper and broader than is generally realized. The main issues that have emerged, and have guided the preparation of this book, may be summarized as follows.

Which Were the Essential Contributions?

The original intention was to identify, present, and evaluate the key papers that established the neuron doctrine. That aim has remained, and those papers are at the core of this book. However, even with that narrow focus, the number of papers has grown considerably beyond the commonly accepted corpus. Thus, in addition to Golgi, His, Forel, Kölliker, and Cajal, who are recognized by all authors on the subject, the present account gives considerable attention to Leydig, Freud, Nansen, Retzius, van Gehuchten, and von Lenhossek, none of whom is covered by Clarke and O'Malley (1968) or most of the other accounts, yet whose contributions were widely recognized at the time. Consideration of this wider range of contributors gives a much more accurate idea whence came each brick in the conceptual edifice. It shows that the theory was much more a collective enterprise than formerly thought, while at the same time giving added lustre to Cajal's role as chief mason.

In asessing this enlarged series of studies of the classical authors, the emphasis here is on the earliest and most seminal papers. This is particularly the case for the central figures of Golgi and Cajal. Despite the old adage *Nihil simul inventum est et perfectum* (Nothing is invented and perfected at the same time), the earlier papers are crucial in showing more vividly the new ideas struggling for expression, much as do Michelangelo's half-finished figures in the Accademia struggling to free themselves from the granite. Moreover, it will be better appreciated how both Golgi and Cajal, virtually from the beginning, had their basic view of what they considered to be the essential aspects of the neuron. Very little attention is given here to later more polemical writings.

An important aspect of the task of studying these classical papers is the variety of languages in which they were written: German, Italian, Spanish, French, and English. One may hazard the guess that few major scientific concepts—indeed, few other major intellectual endeavors of any kind—have engaged as many key contributors writing in as many different languages. This undoubtedly is the main reason why the origins of this concept have remained largely inaccessible, especially to English-speaking scholars. Special efforts have therfore been given to making translations of the key articles into English. The assistance of a number of colleagues in this large undertaking is gratefully acknowledged (see Comment on Sources). In addition to extracts from a large number of different authors, the full texts of Cajal's earliest experimental and conceptual papers are provided in English, for the first time to my knowledge, as well as the full text of Waldeyer's review article in 1891.

Conceptual Issues Surrounding the Neuron and Brain Function

The authors considered here in the classical period were mostly neuroanatomists actively engaged in carrying out microscopical studies of nerve cells. The immediate problems confronting these investigators therefore concerned the validity of the methods and the interpretation of the results. However, the larger issues at stake were conceptual.

The most obvious issue was whether the nerve cell is a bounded structure, like all other body cells, or whether its finest branches are continuous with each other. The first view led to the neuron doctrine, the second to the reticular, or network, theory. The first required the additional postulate that neurons interact at sites of contact, whereas the second view postulated that activity can spread in continuous fashion through the network of branches. The neuron theory was enunciated when the evidence seemed overwhelming that neurons are indeed cellular units like other cells, and interact, as Cajal insisted, by contact.

A second main conceptual issue centered on what kind of a unit this was. The cardinal, yet most enigmatic, feature of nerve cells as revealed by the Golgi stain was the fantastic variety of their branching patterns. There was a strong tendency by most investigators to try to reduce this variety to a simple underlying pattern that would apply to all nerve cells. The debates on this issue yielded the terminology we now use for the two main types of branches, axons and dendrites. Cajal carried this process of reduction the furthest with the "Law of Dynamic Polarization," in which every neuron is conceived of as a unit that receives input in its dendrites and sends output in its axon. A law like this seemed absolutely essential if the structure and function of the brain were to be understood on the basis of first principles. This idea of the neuron as a relatively simple input-output unit has been a strong legacy from classical times.

Following the enunciation of the neuron doctrine in 1891, the dispute over networks seemed settled; Golgi's persistent defense of this idea was a nuisance to most of his contemporaries, and has seemed futile in retrospect. However, a closer reading of his original articles suggests a new perspective on this issue. Both Golgi and Cajal were concerned not only with the nature of the nerve cell as a cell but also with the ways that nerve cell populations could mediate brain functions. The neuron doctrine became the basis for understanding how nerve cells and their connections form specific pathways and systems in the brain. However, the idea that nerve fibers and their branches form a complex network in the brain may also be considered as a valid attempt to address the issue of the neural basis of brain function. Thus, whereas Golgi's views on the precise anatomy of nerve cell connections have not survived, our discussion will present the case that his concerns with the holistic aspects of brain function have a more enduring interest.

Significance of Personal and Cultural Factors

Like most scientific and intellectural endeavors, the neuron doctrine did not emerge in a vacuum. Analysis of the documents and the issues has suggested that progress in this field of inquiry depended especially on a complex interplay of three main factors: personalities, technology, and institutions.

Personalities played an important role at virtually every step of the way. The balanced judgment of Kölliker, the conceptual fixity of Golgi, the seething experimental and intellectual intensity of Cajal, the youthful energies of Nansen, the studious offerings of Freud—it is impossible not be impressed by these personal qualities in studying the work. I have therefore included sufficient biographical material to give the reader a clear idea of the life and times of the main contributors, in order to give a better understanding of their personalities as factors that motivated their work, shaped their ideas, and either facilitated or hindered their interactions with their colleagues.

A second important factor was the way that progress depended on technical developments. If Ludwig's dictum—*Teknik ist Alles* (Technology is everything)—were true, it might be supposed that this should be the first and only factor to consider. In line with that view, the present account emphasizes the critical roles played by improvements in microscopical optics and by the rise of the chemical industry in central Europe for the introduction of new cell stains. And, of course, the unique selective properties of the Golgi stain were the key that opened the door onto the neuron doctrine. However, the moral of the present story is more complex. The path to the neuron doctrine is replete with cautionary tales regarding techniques. Instances will be cited, starting with the introduction of the microscope itself, in which a technical advance is of little value, and may even be discredited, if all the parts have not come together; or, as in the case of general cell stains, continued refinement of one methodology may lead a whole field into a cul-de-sac. The means out of that cul-de-sac, the Golgi stain, was itself an instance of a method discredited for over a decade as unreliable; in the end, it was an example of an advance that promised more in apparently resolving an issue than it could actually deliver. Our study will thus provide numerous examples of the way that the successful use of a technique depends on experimental acumen and the right ideas conjoining at the right time.

The third factor that has seemed worth emphasizing is the role of institutions. There is a tendency in studying previous work to assume that it took place in an environment of university, departmental, and laboratory support bearing some similarity to that which we have today. In fact, this academic structure did not exist before the early nineteenth century, and its growth was contemporaneous with the development of microscopical work on the nerve cell. And we shall see that the work in this field was one of the driving forces behind institutional growth; the institutions in turn were crucial both for supporting the work and for training new students. Many of the participants took special notice of the leading role played by central European, particularly German, institutions, in this regard. I have let this theme emerge in their writings in order to highlight how much some of the early pioneers had to struggle without this support, the role it came to play in the work under review, and how important it was as the model for the eventual emergence of modern academic institution.

The Neuron Doctrine as a Case Study in Nineteenth Century Intellectual Thought

An unexpected outcome of this study has been the realization that the work on the neuron reached deeper into the fabric of nineteenth century life and thought than is generally appreciated. This manifested itself in several ways. During the nineteenth century most of the modern academic disciplines in the sciences were established. Many of the contributors to the neuron theory played key roles in this process, particularly in the rise of the fields of histology, embryology, cytology, neurology, neuropathology, anatomy, and physiology. These disciplines, in turn, provided the seed bed for the eventual emergence of neuroscience as a multidisciplinary field for study in all aspects of the nervous system. Some, like Helmholtz, made contributions of equal magnitude to physics and chemistry. Not only were these among the greatest scientists of the dawn of the modern era, but they included remarkable individuals who made significant contributions to society in other ways, as Freud, the founder psychoanalysis, and Nansen, Arctic explorer and Nobel Peace laureate.

Of broader interest is the potential significance of the neuron doctrine as one of the great ideas of modern thought. One thinks here for comparison of such great achievements of the human intellect as quantum theory and relativity in physics; the periodic table and the chemical bond in chemistry; the cell theory, evolution, and the gene in biology. Notably missing from this register is a theory for explaining how the brain makes these accomplishments and all other human activity possible. The pioneers of the neuron doctrine believed that they were laying the foundation upon which such a theory had to be built. Descartes had set the philosophical agenda for the mind-body problem some 300 years previously, but these scientists were the first to come face to face with the cells and their connections where that problem will likely have its resolution. We are accustomed to thinking of Darwinian evolution as the dominating contribution of nineteenth century biology to modern thought; is it not reasonable to suppose that a theory that accounts for human brain function will be of equal stature? When that theory is constructed, it is likely that it will rest on the principles contained within the neuron doctrine.

The Modern Era

Adequate means to test the tenets of the neuron doctrine awaited the modern era of neuroscience research, ushered in by the advent of the electron-microscope in anatomy and the intracellular microelectrode in physiology in the early 1950s

The electronmicroscopical studies of neuronal fine structure and the microelectrode recordings of the axonal impulse in the 1950s appeared to provide resounding confirmation of the theory. However, further work during the 1950s and 1960s revealed that the relation between structure and function in different parts of the neuron is more complicated than previously envisioned. This has been newly emphasized by recent evidence for many different types of intrinsic membrane properties. The current explosion of techniques of molecular neurobiology is revealing molecular properties of the neuron that make the need for review and revision all the more acute. A profusion of neuromodulator substances is severely straining our simple concepts of how neurons interact. Analysis of developmental mechanisms is providing new insights into the ways that neurons arise and interact during the different stages in the life of the organism. Finally, the new field of computational neural networks is forcing us for the first time to define precisely the information processing properties of real neurons and relate them to the computational operations of both real and artificial networks.

The discussion of this modern work will be organized in relation to the anatomical, genetic, metabolic, and physiological tenets of the classical doctrine. This format helps one see more clearly which parts of the doctrine have been confirmed and which stand in need of revision. In addition, we will introduce a fifth tenet, the neuron as a unit for information processing, in order to characterize the functions of neurons in computational networks. There is an irony in this latest development, because in some respects the present generation of neural networks can be regarded as an intellectual descendent of the reticular theory of neural organization. What is needed are network representations of brain systems that are based on the real properties of synapses and neurons, as expressed in the neuron doctrine, a challenge that is already being taken up. We will discuss some of the new directions for incorporating modern work on these five tenets into a revised set of principles that can provide the basis for a more accurate and comprehensive understanding of the neuronal basis of brain function.

2
From the Beginnings to the Cell Theory

Earliest Microscopy

The struggle to understand the neuron as a cell began with the earliest microscopical investigations of body tissues. As always in science, the state of knowledge depended on the state of development of the instruments. The first microscope was a mechanical device with a compound lens and an eyepiece, which Robert Hooke of London in 1665 used to observe the outlines of cells in slices of cork. The earliest applications to animal tissue were by Anton von Leeuwenhoek of Delft in Holland in 1674. His best efforts in the nervous system came very late in his career; in 1718, at the age of 84, he published longitudinal and transverse views of a peripheral nerve of a cow, which he claimed showed that the nerve was composed of many individual hollow tubes, which he called "very minute vessels" (Leeuwenhoek, 1719; 1817; see also van der Loos, 1967). These were the first views of large myelinated axons. Conceptually this had important implications, for it was taken to confirm the classical idea, first held by the ancients and elaborated in the seventeenth century by René Descartes, that the nerves were tubes containing fluids ("spirits") that actually moved from the sensory organs to the brain to carry sensations, and from the spinal cord to the muscles to bring about movement.

During the eighteenth century, interest in the microscope waned, with only intermittent observations by isolated individuals. One may well ask why this was so, if the microscope was such an important technical advance. The main problem was that the compound lens refracts light of different wave lengths by different amounts, so that at higher magnifications the image is increasingly obscured by "chromatic aberrations". The solution lay in the development of better kinds of glass and improvements in lens making, which had to await the early nineteenth century. A second problem involved the methods of tissue preparation. Generally, a small piece of tissue was mashed up in water and pressed between a glass slide and a coverslip. Small wonder, then, that there were reports of fibers with fanciful shapes, and "granules" and "globules" of every description, all candidates for what we would now call artifacts. So low, in fact, had estimation of the microscope sunk that Marie-Francois Bichat, in Paris, whose *Anatomie Générale* in 1801 came to be regarded as the founding work of the field of histology, could write, "The microscope is a kind of agent from which physiology or anatomy never appear to me to derive much help" (see Liddell, 1960).

A New Age

A new dawn was breaking, however, and when we arrive at the 1820s, we find ourselves in a period of tumultuous advances in science and engineering that are akin to our own. Let us briefly set the scene. Fulton's steamboat in 1807 ushered in the new era of steam-powered transportation; the first railroad was laid in 1825. In 1820, Hans Christian Oersted, professor of physics in Copenhagen, reported the magnetic effect of electric current, which unleashed the power of electricity. Lest we think that events move swiftly only in our day, it is recorded that when Michael Faraday reviewed the publications in electromagnetism that had appeared in just the eight months following Oersted's discovery, it took "great labor and fatigue . . . to go through systematically . . . everything that had appeared in journals and elsewhere" (Meyer née Bjerrum, 1932). In 1825, Leopoldo Nobili, professor of physics in Florence, invented the astatic galvanometer, making it possible to detect and measure small electric currents, a necessary step in harnessing electricity for the development of electrical motors and instruments. This also was the crude beginning of the electrophysiological measurement of biological activity, soon to give rise to the new field of neurophysiology.

Socially, the early part of the nineteenth century was a time of considerable upheaval. During the Napoleonic period, armies swept back and forth across central Europe, blowing away by war and by decree much of the social infrastructure persisting from feudal times. There was considerable unrest, some on a large scale, such as the uprisings in 1830 and 1848, and much on a smaller scale in many locations. Nationalism was in the air. The loosening of social bonds and increased linking by rail encouraged travel and communication, which, in the case of science, helped to foster an increasing awareness of the international community of scientists. However, this tendency was opposed by the shouts in the streets and the incipient rigidities of nineteenth century social mores and the expression of national, racial, gender, and ethnic prejudices. Although these tensions affected the careers of many of those who worked on the nervous system, as in other areas of academic life, one of the most heartening themes is the way young scientists sought training from the best minds no matter where they were, and senior scientists increasingly interacted as colleagues across these artificial borders.

From Nerve Globules to the Cell Theory

The achromatic microscope was introduced in the mid-1820s. Many of the earliest instruments were not of sufficient quality to dispel the disrepute still hanging over microscopy as a science. Such were the observations of Christian Ehrenberg, professor of medicine, in Berlin, in 1833. Ehrenberg has been regarded by some as the discoverer of the nerve cell (cf. Clarke and O'Malley, 1968; Meyer, 1971). His published views of nerve cell bodies and nerve fibers were certainly suggestive, but they were replete with water-induced artifacts. His interpretations included the idea that peripheral nerve fibers are "direct extensions of . . . brain fibers," and that "the cerebrum can . . . be compared to a *capillary vascular system for the nerve fibers*" (Clarke and O'Malley, 1968). This could conceivably be regarded as the first salvo fired for the network cause. Certainly the continuity of the arterial and venous systems through a capillary network provided microscopists and physiologists with an undeniable example of an anatomical and functional reticulum of anastomosing conduits.

The first studies that afforded reasonably accurate views of nerve cells and nerve fibers by modern standards were carried out in the laboratory of Jan Purkinje (Purkyně), and aimed straight at the cell theory. Purkinje was professor of physiology at the University of Breslau (the present day Wroclaw in Poland; see below). In 1825, he applied to the university for one of the new achromatic microscopes; seven years later, after much persistence, he got an excellent instrument built by Ploessel, in Vienna (the cost was 220 gulden = 110 dollars) (John, 1959). Since he lacked adequate space in the university, Purkinje set up the instrument in his home and threw himself into work on the new worlds that opened up. He taught his students as well, assigning different dissertations to different tissues, so that from his laboratory came a series of papers that provided a comprehensive new look at the cellular composition of the body. These studies appeared only under the students' names (see John, 1959), belying the myth of the autocratic *herr geheimratt*, and serving as an example of the generosity displayed by many professors within the rigid framework of nineteenth century academic institutions in central Europe.

Gabriel Valentin

One of the students assigned to the nervous system was Gabriel Valentin (1810–1883), a German born and raised in Breslau. Still working with tissue prepared in water, he nonetheless obtained views of small *Kugeln* ("globules"), which are clearly nerve cells (Valentin, 1836). Kölliker (see below) called this paper "epoch-making, and the first good description of the nervous system elements"; according to Clarke and O'Malley (1968), the illustration shown in Figure 1 "is the first of its kind in the biological literature." As can be seen, the globule has a sharp outline (i.e., the cell membrane), and an interior substance he called *parenchymasse* ("parenchyma") filled with a viscous fluid containing numerous granules. Inside this is a "nucleus," and inside this is a small *corpuscle* (our "nucleolus"). Here, at a stroke, are the basic structures of the nerve cell body, and the terminology, that we recognize today.

In describing the cell body, Valentin noted that it often gave rise to a tail-like appendage, raising the possibility of continuity with an individual nerve fiber. However, he also thought he saw a sheath around each cell and

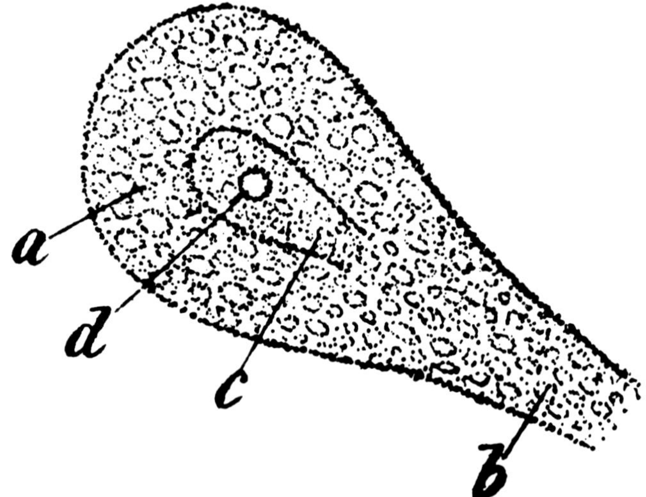

Fig. 1. The first clear microscopic image of a nerve cell (called a globule, *Kugeln*, by Valentin); probably a Purkinje cell, from the human cerebellum. a, cell body; b, appendage (probably the dendritic trunk); c, nucleus; d, small internal corpuscle (probably the nucleolus). (Valentin, 1836)

fiber element, and therefore concluded that the two were separate, and that the sheath "affects the degree of influence of each . . . part upon the other" (Clarke and O'Malley, 1968). Thus, Valentin missed the critical point that the nerve fiber arises from the nerve cell; on the other hand, he appears to have been the first to introduce the idea that a nerve fiber ends on a nerve cell without being continuous with it (cf. Liddell, 1960).

Jan Purkinje

Purkinje was born in 1787 in the Czech town of Libochovice, just north of Prague. After gymnasium, he became a novitiate in the Piarist Order, but left in 1807 to pursue his love for science. He began studies in philosophy in Prague, then entered the medical school, finishing in 1818. Prague, the capital of Bohemia, was then predominantly German, so Purkinje's prospects were bleak, and his applications for positions were rejected. But his doctoral studies of vision, including the phenomenon that came to be called the Purkinje shift, made him well known, and finally, through the intervention of friends, he obtained the chair of physiology in Breslau in 1823. This city was then mostly Polish, but under Prussian rule (a poignant example of the twists of nationalism). Here the Czech Purkinje settled down to his scientific studies, despite only reluctant support from the university during his 27 years there (John, 1959).

Purkinje was one of those towering figures, like Ramón y Cajal later, who illuminate broad landscapes of their science and our history. His contributions were numerous. His research in vision made him a founder of clinical ophthalmology and retinoscopy, including his instrument that has been regarded as the first ophthalmoscope. He constructed a forerunner of the microtome for cutting thin sections of tissue for microscopical examination, treated tissue with staining and mounting materials, devised one of the first micromanipulators, and made the first "stroboscope." From his laboratory came the first description of cilia and ciliary movement, "Purkinje" fibers in the heart, the germinal vesicle in the hen's ovary, the sweat glands, the structure of teeth and of many other cells and tissues. He founded the first physiological institute, occupying a building of its own, in 1839. Thus, in addition to being regarded as the founder of histology (John, 1959), he has also been regarded as the founder of experimental physiology. His institute was a model for the establishment of similar institutes that made Germany preeminent in this field in the nineteenth century.

Purkinje's own contribution to knowledge of the nerve cell was made mainly in a talk to the Congress of German Physicians and Naturalists held in Prague in 1837. His description of the large ganglion cells in the cere-

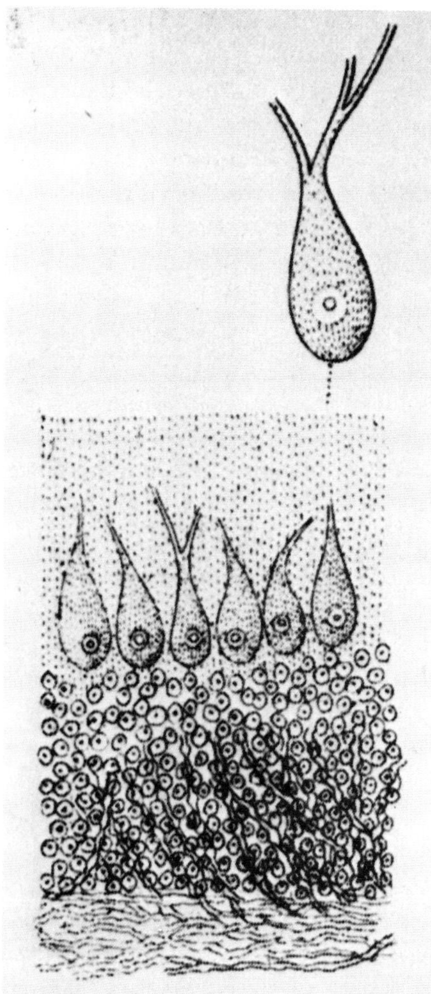

Fig. 2. The first identified nerve cell in the nervous system: the large corpuscles of the cerebellum, which became known as Purkinje cells after their discoverer. This was also the first published view of the cellular composition of the histological layers within a brain region. From below: fibers, granules, large corpuscles (Purkinje cells), molecular layer. (Purkinje, 1837)

bellar cortex (Fig. 2) earned them immediately the name "Purkinje cells" (Purkinje, 1838; modified from Clarke and O'Malley, 1968):

> Each of these corpuscles faces the inside [of the organ], with the blunt, roundish endings towards the yellow substance [the granule layer], and it displays distinctly in its body the central nucleus . . . ; the tail-like ending [the dendritic trunk] faces the outside and, by means of two processes [dendritic branches], mostly disappears into the gray matter [of the overlying molecular layer] which extends close to the outer surface which is surrounded by the pia mater.

In this account we have a clearer picture of the "processes" that will ultimately be called "dendrites," and the first distinction between them and a single, different process that will ultimately be called the "axon." Still crucially lacking is a demonstration of the relation of the nerve cell to the nerve fibers. Purkinje provided clear illustrations of individual fibers, but stated that "nothing definite could be ascertained about the connection between the ganglion corpuscles and the elementary brain and nerve fibres"; however, he speculated that the ganglionic corpuscles "may be related to the elementary brain and nerve fibres the same way as centers of force are related to conduction pathways of force" (Clarke and O'Malley, 1968).

The illustration in Figure 2 is also important as one of the first representations of populations of neurons differentiated from each other and located in their appropriate layers within a part of the brain. It thus marks the beginning of the histological investigation of specific regions of the brain. It took many years for investigators to realize that the differentiation of neurons into specific types, and the development of their interconnections within the constraints placed by the laminar arrangements of cell bodies and processes, were critical for understanding how brains mediate behavior.

Further work on nerve fibers from Purkinje's laboratory appeared in the dissertation of another of his students, J. F. Rosenthal, in 1839. Here was introduced the term *Achsencylinder* ("axis cylinder"), which was to become the prevalent mode of referring to the long fibers of the nervous system for the rest of the nineteenth century, until replaced around 1900 by "axon." Another term to come from his laboratory in 1839 was "protoplasm" (cf. Haymaker 1953), which was universally adopted and applied to the living substance of cells until the modern era.

It remains to note that in his review of 1837, Purkinje included comparisons with plant cells. He emphasized that animal tissues and organs are composed of "three fundamental structures: fluids (blood plasma and lymph), fibers (. . . connective tissue . . . tendons and fasciae) and granules (*Körner*) which subsequently came to be called cells" (John, 1959). He stated his belief "that by a closer recognition of the nature of . . . the granules" it would be possible to learn also the basis for life itself. He saw the future progress of science "in the physical and chemical research of the substance of living beings" (John, 1959). Thus, in all but name, did he state much of the essence of the cell theory enunciated by Schwann two years later (see below).

Robert Remak

Before arriving at the cell theory, we must take note of the contributions of Robert Remak on the nature of the nerve fiber. Remak was born in 1815 in Poland. He took his medical training at the University of Berlin, studying under Johannes Müller (1801–1858), one of the leading physiologists of that time.

His earliest work, published as papers in 1836 and 1837 and a thesis in 1838, made an immediate impression by establishing several new features of nerves. First, he reported that peripheral nerves consisted of a "primitive band" within a thin-walled "primitive tube." Most observers have surmised that these were the axon and the myelin sheath, respectively. For much of the rest of the nineteenth century, there were frequent references to the "band of Remak," synonymous with the axis cylinder or axon. Second, he described for the first time, within the sympathetic nerves, fine fibers that lack the tubular covering. These he termed "organic fibers" or "primitive fibers." They were subsequently referred to as the "fiber of Remak," and are the unmyelinated axon as we know it today.

A third contribution in these early papers concerned the relation between the nerve cell and the nerve fiber. Remak stated it unequivocally: "The organic (non-myelinated) fibers arise from the very substance of the nucleated globules (nerve cells)" (Clarke and O'Malley, 1968). It is in fact not at all clear that Remak actually proved this point, for the processes that can be seen to be arising from the cell bodies, and that are claimed to be the origins of the fibers, are variously quite thick or very thin; to what extent, one must ask, were these differences due to the fact that at this time tissue was still prepared for observation in water, and therefore subject to uncontrolled swelling or shrinkage? Remak went out of his way to emphasize that his findings ran counter to the conclusion of the "celebrated Valentin." Remak was impulsive and contentious (Meyer, 1971), while Valentin was arrogant (Papez, 1953b), so the two protagonists indulged themselves in an acrimonious debate. Remak encountered a good deal of opposition in his career, which has been attributed by modern observers both to anti-Semitism, ever present in European culture, and to his volatile nature (cf. Meyer, 1971).

His gifts, however, outweighed these factors and were widely recognized. In 1844, he provided the first description of "neurofibrils," the finest thread-like structures visible under the light microscope in nerve cells. In 1855, amplifying a suggestion of Benedict Stilling, he proposed that (Remak, 1855; cited by Meyer, 1971):

> 1) Each multipolar anterior horn cell connects with *one* motor root fibre.
> 2) The other processes of the cells are (physically and chemically) different from that fibre.

This was the first statement of the principle that a nerve cell characteristically gives rise to one process, different from the rest, which extends out to become the single axon from that cell. As we shall see, it was recognized as a critical advance by later workers (see Deiters below).

In his subsequent career, Remak turned his interest to the development of the nervous system. Karl Ernst von Baer (1792–1876) had described the ovum in 1827, and subsequently founded the field of embryology by showing that cleavage of the fertilized ovum gives rise to leaf-like cell layers, and that these layers roll up into tubes to form the organs of the body. Von Baer had postulated four primordial layers, an outer and an inner leaflet, each of which gave rise to an additional inner leaflet. Remak, in 1845, proposed that the two inner leaflets form a single layer. Thus arose the concept of three germ layers—ectoderm, endoderm and mesoderm—which has been one of the main tenets of developmental biology ever since.

Remak's students included Wilhelm His and Albrecht von Kölliker (Papez, 1953b) who were to figure so prominently in the development of the neuron doctrine and who acknowledged their indebtedness to him. Among his other contributions, Remak supported the idea that the cerebral cortex has six histological layers.

Theodor Schwann

After the tremendous advances by giants like Valentin, Purkinje, and Remak, Theodor Schwann's contribution at first glance seems almost an anticlimax. Born in 1810, he studied medicine in Berlin and was one of those who came under Müller's beneficent influence. During the late 1830s, Schwann worked there on a variety of microscopic studies. In 1839 he published his historic work entitled *Mikroskopische Untersuchungen über die Übereinstimmung in der Struktur und dem Wachsthum der Thiere und Pflanzen*, translated into English in 1847 under the title *Microscopical Researches into the Accordance in the Structure and Growth of Animals and Plants*. Of interest about the nervous system was his clear description of the cells that accompany and ensheath the myelinated nerve fibers of peripheral nerves. These have been known as "Schwann cells" ever since.

Of far broader significance to biology was the implication carried in the book's title. Schwann's interest in generalizing the findings regarding cells across all plants and animals had been piqued by Matthias Schleiden (1804–1881). Schleiden was an unusual character who trained as a lawyer but went back to study medicine and eventually became a botanist. He got intrigued by the question of how a plant cell originates, and came up with the idea that the nucleus is a "cytoblast" located in the cell wall, and that a new cell arises from this cytoblast rather than by cell division. Despite these flawed notions, Schleiden's paper in 1838 contained the essential idea that a basic cellular structure applied to all plants.

Schwann was a friend of Schleiden, and heard of these ideas one evening over dinner in October, 1838. As the story goes (Locy, 1908):

> Schwann was immediately struck with the similarity between the observations of Schleiden and certain of his own upon *animal* tissues. Together they went to his laboratory and examined the sections of the dorsal [spinal] cord, the particular structure upon which Schwann had been working. Schleiden at once recognized the nuclei in this structure as being similar to those which he had observed in plants, and thus aided Schwann to come to the conclusion that the elements in animal tissues were practically identical with those in plant tissues.

The fact that these two misunderstood the cell wall, the cell nucleus, and the mechanism of development of the cell would seem to be an unpromising foundation for any useful contribution to biology. Despite this muddle, the conclusion that Schwann drew and states in his book rang clear (Schwann, 1839; English translation: Schwann, 1847; 1869):

> The elementary parts of all tissues are formed of cells in an analogous, though very diversified manner, so that it may be asserted, *that there is one universal priniciple of development for the elementary parts of organisms, however different, and that this principle is the formation of cells.* This is the chief result of the foregoing observations.
>
> The same process of development and transformation of cells within a structureless substance is repeated in the formation of all the organs of an organism, as well as in the formation of new organisms; and the fundamental phenomenon attending exertion of productive power in organic nature is accordingly as follows: *a structureless substance is present in the first instance, which lies either around or in the interior of cells already existing: and cells are formed in it in accordance with certain laws, which cells become developed in various ways into the elementary parts of organisms.*

Note that the theory did not simply propose a way of relating the structures of cells in different organs, but it phrased the problem in terms of how they might develop; this was a crucial step in the unification of biology. Schwann not only proposed his theory but gave it a name:

> The development of the proposition, that there exists one general principle for the formation of all organic productions, and that this principle is the formation of cells, as well as the conclusions which may be drawn from this proposition, may be comprised under the term *cell-theory*, using it in its more extended signification, whilst in a more limited sense, by theory of the cells we understand whatever may be inferred from this proposition with respect to the powers from which these phenomena result.

Thus, although the idea of the "cell" was prevalent among biologists at that time, and far-sighted workers such as Purkinje understood its general implications, it was the light touch of Schwann's verbal sword that ennobled the concept so that it could gain universal acceptance. Such is the power of the word.

3

Do Nerve Cells Belong in the Cell Theory?

Although biologists quickly accepted Schwann's formulation of the cell theory as a general proposition, there was plenty of room for exceptions to the rule. Foremost among these appeared to be the nervous system. The cell theory held that all cellular structures are formed from cells. Although Purkinje had suggested that the nerve fiber has its origin in the cell body, and Remak had asserted that this is so, it still remained to be demonstrated conclusively and in a variety of cells and species.

Scrutinizing the Nerve Cell and Nerve Fiber

This challenge was taken up with vigor by anatomists in the 1840s. Almost every conceivable relation between nerve cell and nerve fiber had its proponent. We may recall that Valentin denied a direct connection between a cell and a fiber. Perhaps the nerve fiber was secreted by the cell. Perhaps it was formed by coalescence of several elongated cells.

Hermann von Helmholtz

In attempting to solve this problem, anatomists studied different species in which the relations might be clearer. One of these observers was Hermann von Helmholtz (1821–1894), who studied medicine at Berlin, and was yet another to come under the helpful hand of Johannes Müller. Helmholtz's medical thesis in 1842 (when he was just 21 years of age) covered his studies of the structure of invertebrate nervous systems. He could report that, at least in some cases, nerve fibers ("fibrillae nervae": he does not use the vernacular terms then current) could be seen to arise from cell bodies. He marks a step forward in the development of histological procedures by routinely employing wine alcohol (first introduced for this purpose in 1809) for hardening the tissue. In his use of such species as crayfish, leeches, insects, and spiders (Liddell, 1960), he was among the first to suggest invertebrates as model systems. This was not a trivial step in the search for general biological principles, because at that time most research on animal tissue was carried out by research workers who were medically trained and studied mainly human tissue. Helmholtz went on to make other outstanding contributions to studies of the nervous system (see below) as well as in physics, and became one of the greatest scientists of the nineteenth century.

Adolph Hannover

Connections between nerve cell bodies and nerve fibers were soon confirmed by several others. Adolph Hannover (1814–1894) was a Dane who studied first in Copenhagen under Ludwig Jacobsen (the discoverer of the vomeronasal organ), then in Berlin under Müller, where he also knew Remak. During his early studies in the 1830's, Hannover began using chromic acid to fix and harden tissue. This substance not only preserved the tissue against water-induced distortions but also made it easier to cut thin sections for viewing under the microscope. In his thesis (published in Danish in 1843 and in French in 1844), he clearly illustrated nerve cells giving rise to a single large process ("nerve fiber"), thus supporting Remak's suggestion. He also differentiated between the nerve fiber (i.e., axon) and other processes (i.e., dendrites). However, the situation was not yet clear, because some nerve cells in his drawings appear not to give rise to any fibers (undoubtedly shorn off during tissue preparation), and some nerve cells appear to give rise to more than one nerve fiber. Hannover was also interested in cellular pathology; in the year of his thesis, he also published a dissertation in competition for a professorship in Copenhagen, entitled *Hvad er Cancer?* (*What is Cancer?*), indicating the range of interests of these early pioneers.

Rudolph Wagner

A third contribution to the problem of relating nerve cell and nerve fiber came from Rudolph Wagner (1805–1864). While professor of physiology at Göttingen, he carried out a combined anatomical and physiological study of the brain of the electric fish *Torpedo*, especially that part related to the electric organ. He reported that in cells with several processes emanating from the cell body there is characteristically one that is different from the rest, and it is this one that appears to elongate into a nerve fiber (*Nervenfaser*) (Wagner, 1847). This was one of the earliest clear statements that if a nerve cell gives rise to a nerve fiber (i.e., axon) it gives rise to only one, and that at its origin this fiber is different from all the other processes (i.e., dendrites) emanating from the cell body. At the same time, he also believed that in many cases the cell body was merely a bulbous dilatation of the nerve fiber (Liddell, 1960), so again there was a muddle of ideas.

Kölliker Enters the Scene

The preceding discussion indicates that during the 1840s, despite continuing problems with flawed tissue preparations, there was a growing consensus that nerve cells tend to give rise to several processes, and that in many cases one of these, different in structure from the rest, gives rise to a long process that presumably becomes the nerve fiber of the long tracts within the brain or of the peripheral motor nerves. The time seemed ripe for someone to review this work and enunciate the principles that would allow the nerve cell to be incorporated into the cell theory.

Just such a person appeared to be Albrecht von Kölliker. He provided authoritative pronouncements on the early work in the 1840s, and continued to play this role at virtually every step along the way over the next half century. In the 1890s, he served as the final arbitrator of the work that established the neuron doctrine. He was the only person to play a significant role in all these phases of the work, and the only one of the early pioneers of the cell theory to live into the twentieth century.

Kölliker was born in Zürich in 1817, and began medical studies there in 1836. During 1840–41 he studied in Berlin, where he came under the influence of both Müller and Remak. For his doctoral thesis, in 1841, he demonstrated the cellular nature of invertebrate sperm, and for his medical thesis, in 1845, he studied the development of the larva of the fly. Thus, from the start, he was focused on the structure of cells and tissues, and problems revolving about the cell theory.

After securing a position back in Zürich, Kölliker launched his career with a series of studies between 1844 and 1846 in which he introduced the term "Pacinian corpuscle" for these sensory structures, observed the early stages in the formation of red blood cells in the liver, and published the first description of smooth muscle cells. During this time, he also began his work on the nervous system with an investigation, "On the independence and dependence of sympathetic nervous systems" (1844). Here he reported (without illustrations) that in sympathetic ganglia, "thin nerve fibers take their origin from the ganglionic corpuscles" (Meyer, 1971), although he also noted that some corpuscles are "independent" and do not give rise to fibers. As we have seen, this general proposition was very much current at that time.

In 1849, Kölliker returned to this subject in a review entitled *Neurologische Bemerkungen* (*Neurological Observations*), in which he published a number of figures of nerve cells giving rise to a "pale process" that, in turn, gives rise to a "dark-bordered" (i.e., myelinated) fiber (Fig. 3*A*). In modern terms, the "pale process" corresponds to the initial axonal segment. Meyer (1971) notes that these illustrations "surpass those of his predecessors in instructiveness," and they became the basis for the frequent later reference to Kölliker as the first to have proven that nerve fibers arise from nerve cells. Certainly Kölliker believed it; he states unequivocally that "in 1845 I was the first to reveal the connection of genuine nerve fibers with the pale process of the ganglion globule in vertebrates" (Clarke and O'Malley, 1968). This seems unfair to Remak, who had previously made this claim for himself. Since Kölliker became known as a paragon of impartiality, this slight seems out of character, and has puzzled subsequent writers (cf. Clarke and O'Malley, 1960; Meyer, 1971). There are, I think, several explanations: (1) Remak's claims lacked sufficient documentation by illustrations; (2) Kölliker, ever the arbitrator, was sensitive to Valentin's objection that the "fiber of Remak" was not a true nerve fiber but rather the connective tissue around the nerve fiber; (3) Kölliker had his own objections that the "nucleated fibers" of Remak were not true nerve fibers (Kölliker, 1854), and (4) the further objection that the "primitive band" of Remak was a coagulation artifact (Kölliker, 1854); (5) finally, there was the possible intrusion of the personality and ethnic factors that made Remak's career so difficult (see above). In sum, although Kölliker recognized Remak as the discoverer of the axis cylinder, he did not recognize his evidence regarding the nature of the process through which a nerve cell was linked to it.

In 1852, Kölliker published his *Handbuch der Gewebelehre des Menschen*, which was immediately translated into English, in 1853, as the *Manual of Human Histology* by George Bush and Thomas Henry Huxley. Kölliker's masterly work summarized the new knowledge of body tissues and organs in terms of the cell theory. Bichat had founded the field of histology by

Fig. 3. Examples of different types of nerve cells in Kölliker's 1853 textbook. *A.* "Nerve-cell(s) with the origin of a fibre [from the acoustic (VIII) nerve] of the Ox; a, membrane of the cell; b, contents; c, pigment; d, nucleus; e, continuation of the sheath region of the nerve-fibre; f, nerve-fibre . . ." *B.* "Large nerve-cells with processes from the anterior cornua (horn) of the spinal cord in man." *C.* "Large cells [Purkinje cells] of the grey layer of the cortical substance of the human cerebellum." *D.* "Nerve-cells of the *Thalamus opticus* of man—three of them having their processes torn off." *E.* "From the internal convolutions of the grey layer of the convolutions of the human cerebrum. . . . Nerve cells; a, larger; b, smaller; c, nerye-fibres with axis-cylinder." (Kölliker, 1853)

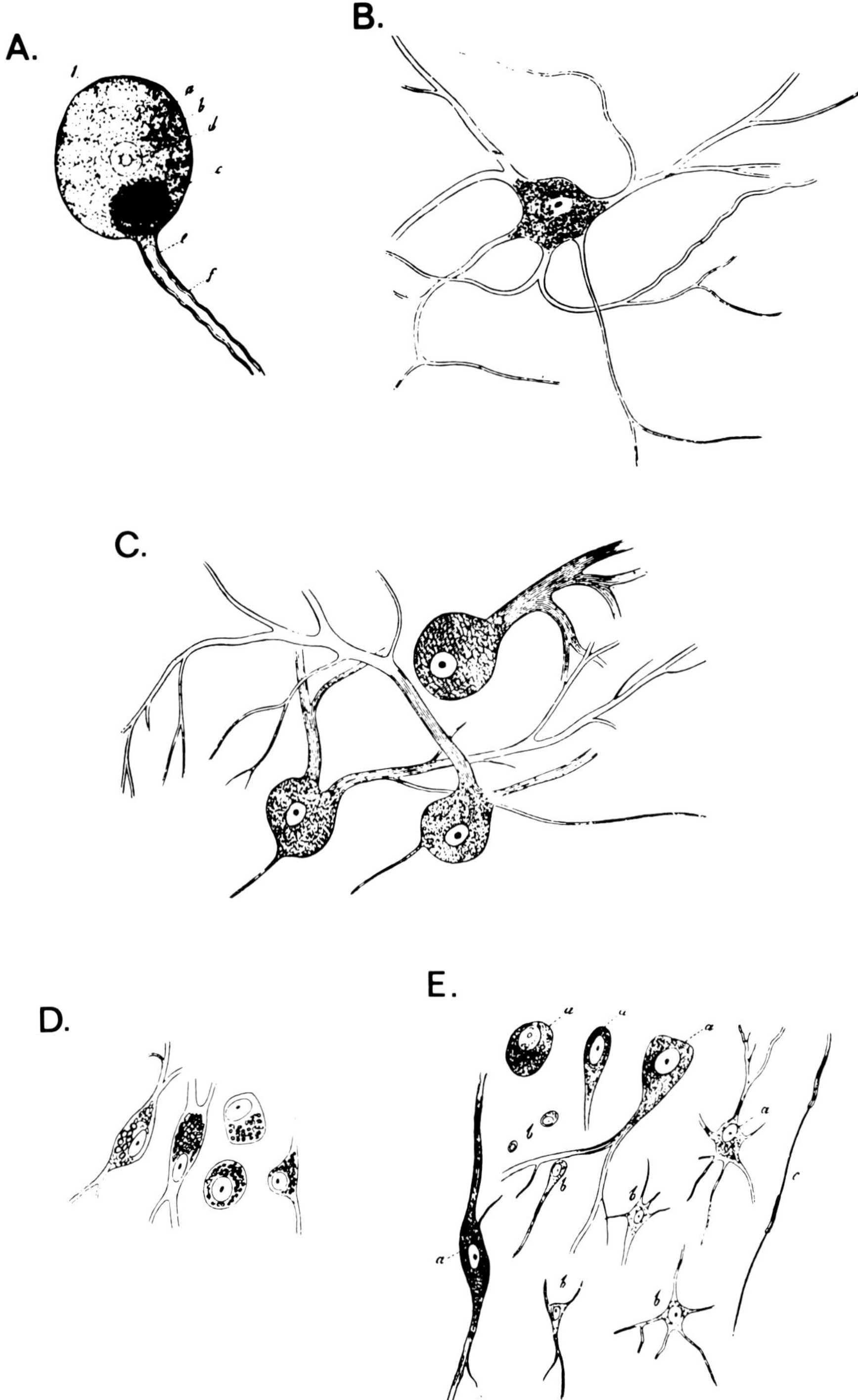
A.
B.
C.
D.
E.

showing, without resort to the microscope, that organs are composed of tissues; Kölliker took the next step, half a century later, by summarizing the microscopic evidence of how the tissues are composed of cells.

It may be noted that his translator, Huxley (1825–1895) began his career as a naturalist and comparative anatomist. His early studies on the jelly fish *Medusae* suggested the class *Hydrozoa*, based on the presence of only two germ layers, ectoderm and endoderm, in all the species within this group. He thus had a professional interest in Kölliker's attempt to synthesize knowledge about cells into a new systematic framework. After Darwin published his *On the Origin of Species*, in 1859, Huxley became the great champion of the new ideas. It would be interesting to analyze more closely the influence of Kölliker's thinking about the cellular composition of the body on Huxley's contribution to Darwinian thought.

In his textbook, Kölliker began by observing that progress since Schwann's fundamental insight in 1839 "has not amounted to a step so greatly in advance as to constitute a new epoch." That would only come, he felt, when "the molecules which constitute cell membranes, muscular fibers, axile fibre of nerves, etc., should be discovered"; then "a new era will commence for Histology," based on a "*molecular theory*" and a "*law of cell genes.*"

This is an important statement, for it indicates that the idea of a "molecular biology" based on "genetic laws" appeared very early in the rise of modern biology, though, of course, those terms lacked any of the precision they have today. In order to appreciate why Kölliker placed so much emphasis on discovering molecular-based laws for the organization of cells, we need to consider briefly the parallel emergence of experimental physiology during the 1840s.

Reducing Physiology to Physics

The astatic galvanometer invented by Nobili in 1825 not only opened the way to accurate measurements of electric currents with broad applications in industry but also provided the means for measuring with adequate sensitivity the very small currents generated by nerve fibers. Following the first attempts by Nobili, Carlo Matteuci (1811–1868), in Italy, reported the first clear evidence in 1840 that a steady current could be recorded between the surface of a muscle fiber and its cut end; this was called a "demarcation current." It is due, as we now know, to the discharge of the resting membrane potential of the cell membrane through the cut ends of the fiber, but at the time there was no clear idea of its mechanism. Johannes Müller showed Matteuci's paper to one of his students, Emil du Bois-Reymond (1818–1896), who took up the problem and carried out an exhaustive series of experiments. His most significant early finding was that the "current of rest" ("demarcation current") was reduced during repetitive (tetanic) stimulation of the muscle; he called this reduction the "negative variation"; it was the first evidence of what we know as the muscle "impulse," or "action potential" (du Bois-Reymond, 1843; see Liddell, 1960; Clarke and O'Malley, 1968). He soon extended these observations to peripheral nerve fibers, and published his results in 1848 in a massive tome entitled *Untersuchungen über thierische Electricität* (*Investigations of Animal Electricity*). This work did much to found the new field of electrophysiology.

Du Bois-Reymond's experiments convinced him that the electrical currents recorded from muscle and nerves provided the means to free physiology from romantic and idealistic ideas, as embodied in *naturphilosophie*, and put it on an entirely new and scientific basis. In the preface to his book he wrote, "The true method . . . lies . . . in the effort to determine the basic connections of the natural phenomena beneath the mathematical structure of their relationships. . . . It cannot fail that . . . physiology . . . will dissolve into organic physics and chemistry." (cited in Cranefield, 1957).

In order to work toward this goal, du Bois-Reymond joined in a pact of four young physiologists in 1847. The second member was Ernst von Brucke (1819–1892), who had been a student with du Bois-Reymond under Müller. Brucke worked on a variety of problems during his career, such as the striations in skeletal muscle and the biochemical composition of the urine. He is best remembered as the person under whom Sigmund Freud obtained his early training in neuroanatomy and carried out studies of nerve cells (see Chapter 7). The third was Helmholtz, also a former student of Müller. Following the histological studies mentioned above, Helmholtz, in 1850, demonstrated that the nerve impulse has a finite conduction velocity. This put an end to the notion, embedded in *naturphilosophie*, that the nerve impulse represented a mystical "nerve force" spreading with infinite velocity throughout the nerves and brain. The fourth member of the quartet was Carl Ludwig (1816–1895). Ludwig was the quintessential physiologist, ranking with Claude Bernard (1813–1878) in laying the foundations of modern physiology. Among his many contributions he introduced the kymograph, a rotating smoked drum for recording physiological measurements; this was the basic recording instrument in most physiological laboratories until it was replaced by chart recorders and cathode ray oscilloscopes in the 1960s.

In their pact, as Ludwig recalled later, "We four imagined that we should constitute physiology on a chemico-physical foundation, and give it equal scientific rank with physics" (quoted by Burdon-Sanderson, 1911; see Cranefield, 1957). This attempt to make physiology into a science governed by physical laws has become a case study in the history of science (see Temkin, 1946; Cranefield, 1957, 1966). By their own admission, the four fell far short of their philosophical goal. In practical terms this did not much matter, being far outweighed by the fact that they helped to establish physiology as an experimental science. Nonetheless, it is important in considering Kölliker's comprehensive book establishing histology as a new field to realize that at the time he was writing, in the early 1850s, the idea of basing biology on mathematical, chemical and physical laws was a strong motivation for a number of young scientists coming into the field.

Toward a Science of Histology

Kölliker was in fact very much alive to the new ideas expressed by his colleagues in physiology. In his book (Kölliker, 1853), he discussed at some length the nature of the task lying ahead if the same kinds of goals were to be realized for histology:

> If Histology is to attain the rank of a science, its first need is to have as broad and certain an objective basis as possible. . . . When the morphological elements have been perfectly made out, the next object is to discover the laws according to which they arise . . . here as in the experimental sciences generally, continual observation separates . . . the occasional from the constant . . . till at last a series of more and more general expressions of the facts arises, from which, in the end, mathematical expressions or formulae proceed, and thus the laws are enunciated.
>
> As regards the general propositions of Histology, the science has made no important progress since Schwann, however much has been attained by the confirmation of the broad outlines of his doctrines. The position that all the higher animals at one time consist wholly of cells and develope [sic] from these their higher elementary parts, stands firm, though it must not be understood as if cells, or their derivatives, were the sole possible or existing elements of animals. In the same way, Schwann's conception of the genesis of cells, though considerably modified and extended, has not been essentially changed, since the cell nucleus still remains as the principal factor of cell development and of cell multiplication. Least advance has been made in the laws which regulate the origin of cells and of the higher elements, and our acquaintance with the elementary processes which take place during the formation of organs must be regarded as very slight. Yet the right track in clearing up these points has been entered upon; and a logical investigation of the chemical relations of the elementary parts and their molecular forces . . . combined with a more profound microscopical examination of them, such as has already taken place with regard to the muscles and nerves [and] a histological treatment of embryology . . . will assuredly raise the veil, and bring us, step by step, nearer the desired though perhaps never to be reached, goal.

The reader is left in no doubt that this is a man who takes the long view. There is the same hope of deriving laws as expressed by the physiologists, but there is less in the way of actual physical measurements with which to advance toward this goal. The book in its six editions wielded great authority over the study of cellular anatomy for the next half century. We consider it further here because it gives the opportunity to assess what was then known about the nerve cell in the light of the new cell theory. Kölliker's judgments on this issue provided much of the framework for thinking about this problem over the following 40 years.

Almost Seeing the Nerve Cell

In his systematic framework for the structure of the body, Kölliker considered that cells were the *simple elementary parts. Higher elementary parts*, he went on to state, "correspond, genetically, to a whole series of the single ones." Among these were networks of connective and elastic tissue, capillary plexuses, tracheae in the lung, and muscle fibers. Here he also placed "the networks of the nerve cells in the brain of the Torpedo (Wagner)" and, in a separate entry, "the nerve-fibers and nerve-fibre networks." The single and higher elementary parts "are united according to determinate [but still unknown] laws, into the so-called *tissues* and *organs*. . . . When several organs . . . are united into a higher unity, this is called a *system*" [italics added]. Here we have an early expression of what we now call levels of organization, and the idea that they constitute a hierarchy (see Chapter 20).

In his introduction to the general structure of cells, Kölliker chooses as his first illustration some nerve cells from the optic thalamus (lateral geniculate body) of the human (Figure 3*D*). This seems a revealing point. It suggests that there was widespread agreement at the time that the nerve cell is a cell and is covered in a general way by the cell theory, because it was used in this definitive textbook as the prime example to illustrate that theory.

Kölliker describes the composition of cells: the membrane (consisting of a "nitrogenous" protein), nucleus, nucleolus, and intracellular fluid (a "nitrogenous, mucus-like substance"; he says little of its possible composition or of the granules it contains). He then goes on to discuss at length the various properties of cells. These include development by cell division, growth, absorption (including endosmosis), metabolism (a term introduced by Schwann for the "chemical metamorphoses" that occur in cells), and excretion. These "vital phenomena" are common to all cells; nowhere does he single out nerve cells as exceptions.

These considerations indicate that there was no doubt in Kölliker's mind that the nerve cell is a cell. It is when he comes to the detailed description of the nerve cell that the doubt arises as to just what kind of a cell it is. First he takes up the axis cylinder, "undisputably the most difficult of investigation, and the least known portion of the nerves". There is a controversy, he notes, on whether it even exists as an entity: a few (including Hannover and Müller) support Remak's and Purkinje's view of "the axis-cylinder as a constant element in recent [i.e., fresh] nerve, while most observers have adopted the views of Valentin . . . and Henle . . . who regard it as not always present, but rather as a secondary formation, which does not exist during life." His own studies, he states, confirm that the axis cylinder "is an essential constituent of the living nerves"; it is a solid protein core distinct from the surrounding medullary sheath. He reiterates his view that "the dark-bordered nerve fibres were in direct connection on the one side through the axis-cylinder, with the pale processes [i.e. initial segments] of the nerve cells . . . and on the other, that they passed into the pale terminal nerves [i.e., unmedullated terminal branches]." However, this clear statement is followed by a tedious discussion on whether the medullary sheath is derived from the "nerve contents," which throws the whole subject of the relation between the nerve cell and nerve fiber in some doubt.

The nerve cell, according to Kölliker, consists of a "coagulated although soft protein-compound, which appears to correspond very closely with that of the axis-fibers." They have "one, two or several pale processes . . . which are frequently ramified; and the former [i.e., single process] in many situations, continuous with dark-bordered nerve fibers, and even having the nature of non-medullated nerve-fibers." Kölliker cannot say for sure whether a membrane surrounds the nerve cells in the brain and spinal cord: "In this case, as in that of the finest nerve tubes, we must for the present abstain from any definite opinion."

Taking up nerve cells in specific parts of the nervous system, Kölliker illustrates anterior horn cells of the spinal cord, which most probably are motor neurons (Figure 3*B*). These he calls "many-rayed cells," in the jargon of the day, referring to the numerous branching "pale processes" that appear to constitute "the bulk of the central grey substance." We have here, even with these primitive methods, a clear appreciation of the large size and multiple dendrites of a motor neuron. Lacking, however, is the differentiation of one process, different from the rest, into the initial segment of the axon, as well any evidence about how the processes terminate. These limitations are even more apparent in the cerebellum, where the large cells discovered by Purkinje (not yet termed "Purkinje cells") are clearly illustrated (see Fig. 3*C*). However, there is little evidence of the extensive dendritic tree and its planar geometry, nor is there an appreciation of the origin of the axon, even though the thin pale process arising from the deeper aspect of two of the cells is most likely an initial segment (here, as elsewhere, the occasional observance of a cell whose axon had been broken off complicates the interpretation).

In the cerebrum, Kölliker divides the cortex into six layers, and describes a variety of cell forms; one may note that there is little evidence of the pyramidal type among these (Fig. 3*E*). In the human, he reports that nerve cells in the inner layers display "pigmentary" contents, particularly in older people; one may speculate that these might be lipofuscin granules. He expends great efforts in identifying the origins of nerve fibers from the nerve cells in the cortex. His description of these efforts is worth quoting at length (it is contained in a single paragraph extending over three pages, which I have edited slightly and arranged in several paragraphs for easier reading):

> With respect to the *origin of the nerve-fibres* in the brain . . . it is several years since I first observed the origin of dark-bordered fine fibres from the processes of the nerve-cells in the spinal cord of the Frog. . . . In *man* I have not as yet been so fortunate as to perceive anything of the sort with certainty, though I do not myself doubt that similar conditions obtain. . . . In fact, R. Wagner and Leuckart think they have seen, in man, the processes of the many-rayed cells in the *substantia ferruginea*, passing into nerve-tubes . . . as has Prof. Domrich, in the cortical substance of the cerebellum. . . . R. Wagner . . . has . . . also found in the electric lobes of the Ray, that from the many rayed ganglion-globules or nerve-cells, one, or more rarely two, unbranched processes are continued into dark-bordered fibres. He now explains this transition, in the same way as before, saying that the processes were continued as axis-cylinders into the dark-bordered tubes, in which Leydig, who has observed the same transition in the *cerebellum* of the "Hammer-headed Shark," agrees with him. . . . Nevertheless, it is still not quite evident to me, that any condition should exist in this case, different from that which obtains in the ganglia, where the processes of the nerve-cells are not simply axis-cylinders, but also have a coat, which investing the medullary matter of the nerve, is continuous with the sheath of the dark-bordered tubes; although, seeing that the presence of tunics on the nerve corpuscles . . . and their processes, in general, is still a disputed point, I am prepared to admit that the fact may be otherwise.
>
> These researches have opened the way . . . and I have no doubt . . . that in time we shall succeed in demonstrating the origin of dark-bordered tubes [i.e., axons] in many other situations in the central organs, in man, and other animals. On the other hand, however, supported by repeated investigation of the human brain, I must assert, *that it is in the highest degree probable that in many places it will be altogether impossible to demonstrate the origin of fibres from nerve-cells* [italics added], because very many nerve-tubes, particularly those of the

cortical substance of the *cerebellum* and *cerebrum*, ultimately become so pale and slender, as not to allow of their being distinguished from the processes of nerve-cells.

Whether the loops which distinctly exist in the convolutions of the *cerebrum*, and which I have also seen in the *corpora striata*, are terminations, or whether free prolongations of nerve-tubes exist, we know not, and the less so because it cannot even be asserted that certain fibres really do terminate. It may fairly be assumed that the fibres of the *corpus callosum* and the commissural fibres in general, commence in the one hemisphere in connection with cells and terminate in the other, and that the fibres which proceed from the surface of the convolutions to the *optic thalami* and corpora striata terminate in the latter, but to assert, that it is so, is impossible, notwithstanding the visible loops, for it may be that these latter are not terminations at all, and that the fibres in question are all in the one place and the other in connection with nerve-cells. *That nerve-fibres should originate independently of any connection with cells would be contrary to all analogy, but in such an obscure subject we must always be prepared for much that is new* [italics added] and be careful not wholly to reject any possibility, simply from *a priori* considerations.

Several authors have noticed divisions of the nerve-tubes [i.e., axonal branching] in the central organs [most recently] in the brain of various vertebrate animals, especially at the junction of the white and grey substance. I am not inclined to doubt these statements, especially the latter, but I cannot avoid the remark, that in the human brain, I have, hitherto, in vain sought for divisions of this kind and have had many hundreds of fibres from the grey substance before me, under the most favorable circumstances, which presented no indications of the sort, whilst I have invariably found such divisions in the spinal cord. . . .

The many-rayed nerve-cells with branched processes [i.e., dendrites] are not as yet fully known in all their relations. I have described their processes, (as will be universally allowed, correctly,) as a sort of pale, non-medullated nerve-tubes, and have isolated them occasionally to the extent of 1/5 and 1/4‴, without being able to notice anything more with regard to their termination, than the fact of their ultimately assuming an exteme degree of fineness. R. Wagner states, that *those processes*, which do not pass into dark-bordered nerve-tubes, *serve to connect the separate nerve-cells together* [italics added], but in so doing he manifestly says more than actual observation warrants, as he has, hitherto, seen such a connection only in the electric lobes of the Ray.

In the present state of neural Anatomy [note the new term] *there is nothing which should be more carefully avoided than the general application of isolated observations* [italics added], and I am therefore of the opinion that this question must as yet be regarded as an open one. It may indeed be very consonant with physiological considerations, to explain the reflex and alternating actions of separate sections of nerves by such connections between the cells, but it is precisely for that reason, that we should be the more careful, and the more so because less obvious theories explain the conditions just as well. I conclude therefore, from the observations hitherto made, only this much, that *nerve-cells may anastomose* [italics added], leaving to future inquiries to decide,

> whether they do so universally and with all their processes, or whether in certain situations the latter do not stretch out *without any attachment, exerting a mutual influence and affecting the nerve-fibres simply by juxta-position* [italics added], as appears to be the case in the large nerve-cells of the cord and the roots of the spinal nerves.

These passages mark the limits of knowledge about the nerve cell reached with the methods then available; at this furthermost salient one has to admit that the battle cannot yet be won; nay, perhaps, in the inhospitable terrain of the brain, it will be lost. Perhaps it will turn out to be impossible to demonstrate the origins of some nerve fibers; perhaps—awful thought—some nerve fibers may originate in some manner independently of cells; perhaps the branching unmedullated processes (dendrites) are connected together through anastomoses; perhaps, on the other hand, nerve fibers and nerve processes may influence each other not through attachments but through "juxtapositions" (possibly the earliest intimation of the "synapse"?).

Here were expressed all the frustrations of those histologists due to lack of adequate methods and stains. Here also were the clouds of doubt that were to hang over the nerve cell for most of the rest of the century. Were they justified? Is it true that Kölliker "had all the data of the neurone theory, whose birth he might have advanced by as much as fifty years" (Meyer, 1971; cf. also von Bonin, 1953; Clarke and O'Malley, 1968)? Given his role as arbiter of scientific evidence, one would have to conclude, with him, that the methods simply were not yet up to it. Even if his imagination had leapt ahead to the right conclusions, it would most likely have added yet more speculations to the already overcrowded arena. On balance, it seems that this was as far as the field could go toward a clear view of the nerve cell as a cell at that time; Kölliker's insistence on hard evidence would at least set high standards for judging future studies, and for the final resolution.

4
Nerve Cells or Nerve Nets?

By the middle of the nineteenth century, the task of understanding the nerve cell as a cellular unit depended on answering several questions: (1) how do axis cylinders arise from nerve cells? (2) what is the extent and significance of the pale branched processes of nerve cells? (3) how are nerve cells connected with each other? The main mode of connection that could be imagined at that time was by anastomoses of the branched processes (i.e., dendrites), which left the connections of nerve fibers (i.e. axons) and the ways they exert their influence pretty much up in the air.

Answers to these questions obviously required better visualization of the nerve cell and the finer nerve processes and terminals. Progress toward this goal in the 1850s and 1860s was slow and incremental. Various agents were tried for hardening the tissue and treating it with stains. By the 1860s most of the basic steps we use today for routine histology were emerging, though the chemical agents were still limited; chromic acid was a popular fixative, for example. Staining compounds did not become prevalent until the introduction of carmine by Joseph von Gerlach in 1858, indigo in 1859, and aniline dyes in 1862; after that, the German chemical industry became a source of a widening variety of dyestuffs (see Clarke and O'Malley, 1968).

Deiters: The Keats of the Nerve Cell

Advances during this period were made by histologists experimenting with different agents and combinations of agents and applying their imaginations to what they saw. Such a person was Otto Deiters. Deiters was born in 1834 in Bonn. After medical training there, he studied under Rudolf Virchow, who had recently moved to Berlin from Würzburg. Virchow

(1821–1902) was a renowned pathologist, who had, among other things, extended the cell theory to apply to pathology and disease, and therefore was one of the founders of modern medicine. He also was the discoverer of "neuroglia", the nonnervous type of cell that is an important constituent of the brain. After working with Virchow, Deiters returned to Bonn and launched into microscopical studies of nerve cells in the early 1860s under the tutelage of Max Schultze (1825–1874), himself a prominent histologist who made a number of fundamental contributions to knowledge of cellular structure.

There is unfortunately little more to tell of Deiters' life, because he died of typhus in 1863 at the age of 29. He left an unfinished manuscript covering his studies, which Schultze undertook to prepare for publication. The task lasted two years, and resulted in a monograph of over 300 pages and six plates, the latter consisting of 16 lithographs of nerve cells of surpassing beauty. The monograph was entitled *Untersuchungen über Gehirn und Rückenmark des Menschen und der Säugethiere* (*Investigations on the Brain and Spinal Cord of Man and Mammals*). If, as it appears, Deiters was working his way up the neuraxis, we can only lament the loss of his views of higher structures, much as we regret the early deaths of a Keats or a Schubert. The volume in my hand bears inscriptions by Helmholtz and Dusser de Barenne. I strongly recommend that the reader view the illustrations in the original monograph, as a reproduction does not do justice to the delicacy of line or the insightful ways in which Deiters conceived of the cellular organization of the spinal cord and brainstem.

Schultze was a leader in developing histological methods, and Deiters made good use of them (Liddell, 1960). His methods included fixing the tissue in chromic acid or potassium bichromate, staining with carmine, and preparing the tissue for microscopical examination by serial sections or by microdissection with thin needles to tease out individual nerve cells and their fibers. After a description of these methods, the monograph has introductory chapters on the *Bindesubstanz* ("connecting subtance," "ground substance") of the central nervous system, the central ganglion cell, and the nerve fiber, before taking up in sequence the cellular organization of the spinal cord, medulla oblongata, pyramidals, olivary nuclei, pons, and cerebellar peduncles. Included in the later chapters is a clear description of the lateral nucleus of the vestibular complex, which has come to be known as "Deiters' nucleus."

The illustration in Figure 4 from Deiters' work has often been reproduced, and is usually taken to represent his main contribution to the development of concepts of the nerve cell. In it we see a large motor neuron of the anterior horn of the spinal cord. Deiters differentiated two main

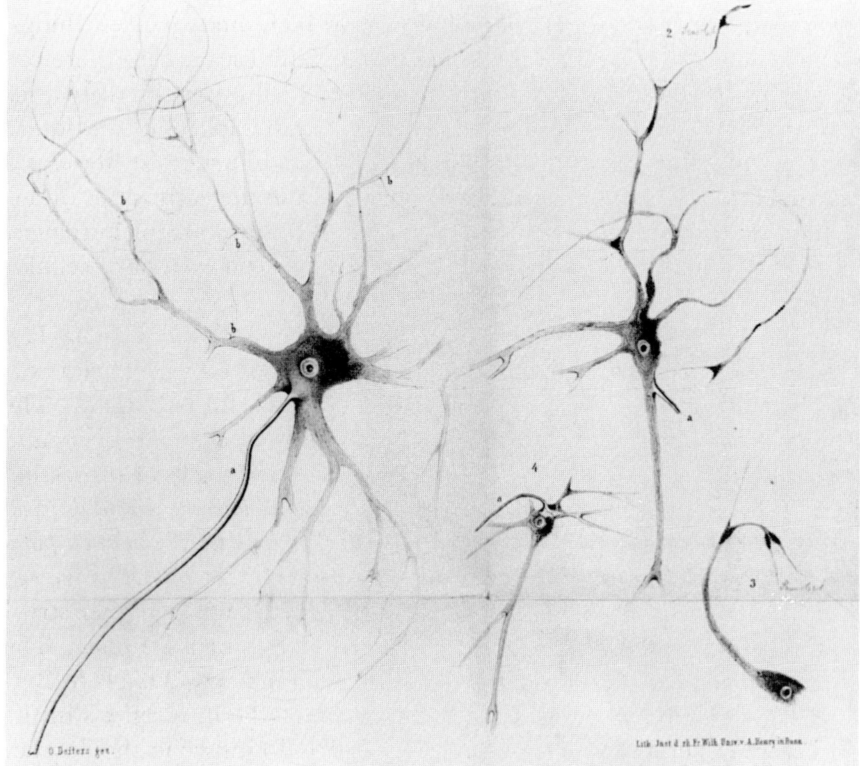

Fig. 4. Illustrations of nerve cells by Deiters. "Isolated ganglion cells from the grey matter of the spinal cord, enlarged 300–400 times. Fig. 1. A large ganglion cell from the anterior horn with possibly completely retained extensions. In the cell substance dark yellow pigment is deposited. a, the main axis cylinder extension. b, b, b the fine axis cylinder extensions coming from the protoplasmic extensions. . . . Fig. 2. A medium-sized ganglion cell with much yellow pigment in the cell body and in the branched protoplasmic extensions. a, the main axis cylinder extension which arises from the base of a broad protoplasma extension in a manner that is characteristic for the cells of the posterior horns (sensory cells). Fig. 3. Part of a presumably similar sensory cell with pigment in the extension. Fig. 4. Smaller ganglion cell with manifold branched extensions and yellow pigment in the cell body. a, the main axis cylinder extension." (Deiters, 1865)

kinds of process that arise from the cell body. Since this is the first clear distinction between what we now call dendrites and axon, it is worth quoting his text. First, with respect to dendrites (Deiters, 1865; modified from Clarke and O'Malley, 1968):

> The cell body is continuous with a variable number of processes which frequently branch but have long *unbranched* stretches. . . . The granular, fre-

> quently even pigmented, protoplasm can be readily followed into them. . . . These ultimately become extremely thin and disappear in the spongy ground substance. . . . These processes which, even in their ultimate, invariable branches, must not be considered to be the source of axis cylinders or to have a nerve fibre growing from them, will hereafter be called, for the sake of convenience, *protoplasmic processes* [dendrites].

The important point is that the body of the cell passes uninterruptedly into the processes; thus, the initial trunks of the processes are indistinguishable in their internal composition from the protoplasm of the cell body. For this reason, they soon came to be called "protoplasmic processes" or "protoplasmic prolongations."

Deiters then goes on to differentiate a second type of process (Deiters, 1865; modified from Clarke and O'Malley, 1968):

> A prominent, single process which originates either in the body of the cell or in one of the largest protoplasmic processes, immediately at its origin from the cell, is distinguishable from these [the protoplasmic prolongations] at a glance. . . . However, at its point of origin, we can still recognize in this single nerve fibre or axis cylinder the granules of the protoplasm in which [the base of the process] loses itself, for there is no easily recognizable break. But, as soon as it leaves the cell it appears at once as a rigid, hyaline mass, much more resistant to reagents, and on the whole with a different reaction to them; and, from the start, *it does not branch* [italics added]. *Shortly after leaving the cell this process becomes thinner* [see (a) in Fig. 4] . . . *and as a rule it simultaneously snaps off because of the angle which usually occurs here.* But such torn-off pieces are also characteristic and easily and distinctly recognizable among the small cells in well-preserved areas. They are characteristic enough for a cell to be identified as a nerve cell. They are sufficient for anyone who does not wish to take the time to explore the direct transition [of a cell] into a dark-bordered nerve fibre which is found only by chance, but is always a possibility, as will be asserted in the subsequent discussion. This characteristic is not peculiar merely to the large motor cells in which Remak has already partly recognized it, *but also to the sensory ones, to those of the olive, the pons, and, on the whole, to all which could so far be examined thoroughly; indeed, if I am not mistaken, it is also peculiar to the cells of the cerebrum.*

There are several important points here. First is the recognition that the origin of the axis cylinder (axon) is different from the origin of the other processes. The cone of origin later came to be called the "axon hillock." This distinction between axon and dendrite has continued to the present day. The second point is that each nerve cell gives off only one such axis cylinder. It is an important rule about nerve cells, that if they have an axon they have only one (see Chapters 12, 15). We still do not know the developmental mechanisms that determine this, or what may be its significance for the input-output functions of the nerve cell in processing information. Third, Deiters notes that the axis cylinder becomes thinner soon after its origin from the cell body, as shown clearly in his diagram in Figure 4. This may be regarded as the first description of the "initial segment" of the axon. A fourth interesting point is the claim that the axis cylinder is unbranched; this, of course, put severe limitations on the connections a nerve cell could have with its neighbors (see below). A final point is the implication that the presence of an axon is the identifying characteristic of a nerve cell. This turns out not to be an adequate criterion for defining a cell as a nerve cell, because certain types of nerve cells lack an axon (see Chapters 15, 20).

Deiters' observations thus provided evidence that the basic structure of a nerve cell was made up of a cell body, protoplasmic prolongations (dendrites), and a single axis cylinder (axon). This helped to define the nerve cell as a unit, but the definition was incomplete without dealing with the problem of how nerve cells are connected. We have seen that Kölliker had promulgated his *belief* that each nerve cell is an independent unit, like cells elsewhere, but neither he nor anyone at the time could provide an explanation for how the independent nerve cells could interact through their protoplasmic processes or their axis cylinders, nor could they prove that the finest processes might not be continuous with each other in some instances. Thus, the door had to be left open a crack.

Scientists faced with uncertainty such as this tend to divide into two camps; most suspend judgment and get along with incomplete theories until the data are clear, but there are always a few whose imaginations cannot resist the temptation to put together an underconstrained theory. The latter squeezed through the crack in this door, mainly espousing the idea that the nerve processes must anastomose. As we shall see in the next chapter, this idea was becoming increasingly prevalent in the 1860s, despite the earlier resistance against it by Kölliker and others.

Deiters was well aware of this problem, and discussed it at length in the book. His conclusion was unequivocal. Schultze prepares the reader for it in his introduction to Deiters' book:

> Many will find surprising the pronouncement of Deiters that, in hundreds of successful preparations, from all parts of the central nervous system, and despite the most direct attention given to this point, a definite anastomosis between neighboring ganglion cells was never encountered. As is well known, this result concurs with what Kölliker has taught on the subject of anastomoses between ganglion cells, against the contrary results of other researchers.

Deiters summarized his results thusly:

> To the discussion above, I add a question which has often been "aired", often alluded to, and has been answered by different authors in quite different ways: I mean the question of the so-called anastomoses of ganglion cells. Several researchers have made this an established fact; in particular, Schröder van der Kolb has ascribed the most importance to anastomoses and drawn the most extensive physical conclusions from that. In the most diverse places in the central organs, systems of connected ganglion cells thus originate to which a "nimble mind" could easily ascribe a common function. The question has been especially cultivated by those researchers who see the presence of such connections as a physiological necessity. According to these researchers, including Mauthner, Jacobovitch etc., working under Funke the physiologist, there are nearly everywhere the most diverse connections, situated either near ganglion masses or much further away, whose long branches [should] join together. It must have made a certain impression and would have made many researchers alarmed whenever the advocates of this view treated the observation of the anastomoses as being simple, convenient and frequently appearing, whereas Kölliker, who had no desire to dispute this knowledge and expertise of observation, asserted that he had never seen any such. In fact, from the very first to the present, Kölliker has been opposed to this kind of thinking, and I think every modest, sensible working researcher without pre-conceived notions must come to the same conviction. In my own experience I am of necessity drawn to the view that all data to date which draw upon such connections are based upon deception.

Having convinced himself of the lack of anastomoses, Deiters had to come up with another way by which nerve cells could communicate with each other, and he thought he had found it (Deiters, 1865; modified from Clarke and O'Malley, 1968):

> If one checks the various protoplasmic processes [i.e., dendrites], one becomes aware . . . that . . . a number of very fine, easily destroyed fibres proceed from them, which do not appear as simple branches since, for the most part, they rest laterally on a triangular base [see (b) in Fig. 4] . . . These processes are very delicate and can be preserved intact only in certain solutions; they show no marked difference from the axis cylinder of the finest nerve fibres with which they share a somewhat irregular appearance [because of] a slight varicosity and the same physicochemical behavior. [Note that Deiters calls them "axis cylinders" in the legend to the figure.] Sometimes they branch. I very rarely succeeded in identifying a dark-bordered outline [i.e., as found in large myelinated axis cylinders] in any of these processes, and I do not hesitate to consider them as a second system of efferent axis cylinders which seem to be altogether different from the large ones just mentioned.
>
> Thus the ganglion cells which I have examined so far appear to be central points for two systems of genuine nerve fibres; a system of mostly large, always simple, and undivided fibres, and a second extensive system of the smallest fibres, which are attached to the protoplasmic processes.

How does this type of fiber relate to the large single axis cylinder? In order to answer this question, Deiters began to construct a theoretical framework for the organization of the individual nerve cell. The starting point was Remak: "I find the outline of a theory of central nerve cells in Remak's (1855) statement that each cell is in contact with only one motor root fibre, and that this fibre is chemically and physically different from all other processes" (Deiters, 1865, cited in Meyer, 1971). With regard to the fine fibers, Deiters tried to conceive of their significance in relation to the "local physiological arrangement of the individual ganglion cell"; he surmised that "the cell, as a central point, appears to be of different significance for the two fibre systems" (Deiters, 1865, cited in Clarke and O'Malley, 1968). This was one of the first attempts to conceive of the nerve cell as an anatomical and physiological unit in relation to its output functions (see the "Law of Dynamic Polarization," Chapter 15). But speculation about the significance of the two fiber systems was frustrated by the lack of evidence, as is obvious in the following passage (Deiters, 1865; modified from Clarke and O'Malley, 1968):

> Theory demands a connection between tracts of different functions, and it demands the influence of different organs upon one point; as is known, the reflex phenomena particularly demand such an arrangement. *Since cells are not connected by means of the protoplasmic processes* [italics added] and since a simple union of different fibres without the intervention of cells is hardly sufficient for the theory, it follows that *one necessarily falls back upon the fine nerve fibres* [italics added] i.e., [the second set of fibres arising from the dendrites] which ramify *and therefore may well unite* [italics added]. One is not only justified but, it seems to me, one has the duty of considering such possibilities because, if the arrangement does not take place in the assumed manner, we are dealing with a fact which in all likelihood will always exceed the limits of anatomical research.

The ending of this passage echoes Kölliker's earlier counsel of despair.

Despite this pessimistic note, Deiters nonetheless realized that behavior such as "reflex phenomena" depended on populations of neurons and interconnections between them. The monograph includes several impressive illustrations of his conceptions of the cellular organization of the spinal cord and brainstem; the drawing of the spinal cord is shown in Figure 5. Here the anterior horn (above) is seen containing numerous large cells corresponding to motor neurons and giving rise to the ventral roots. Although there is a strong implication that the axis cylinders of the anterior horn cells enter the anterior roots (and proceed to become the motor nerves to the muscles), the diagram is curiously vague in depicting this connection. Similarly, the second set of fine fibers is nowhere depicted precisely; it

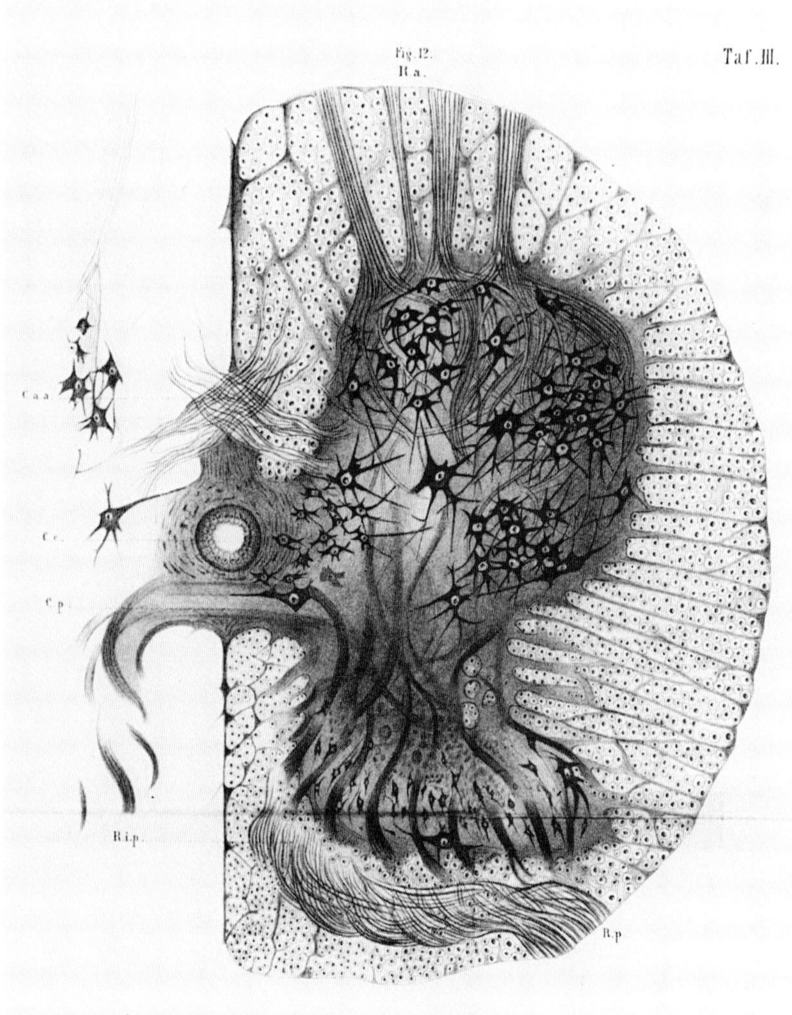

Fig. 5. Cellular organization of the spinal cord as depicted by Deiters. "Transection of a half of the lower end of the human spinal cord. Probably beginning of the conus medullaris. *R. a.* anterior root cluster arising from the anterior horn inside which the medullated nerve fibers are seen between the large ganglion cells; *R. p.* posterior root arising from the posterior horn whose ganglion cells (except for a few) are paler and much smaller than those from the anterior horns; *R. i. p.* inner part of the posterior root . . . ; *C. c.* Central canal with its lining of ciliated epithelium, surrounded by connective (cohesive) substance. *C. p.* posterior grey commissure; *C.a.a.* anterior white commissure. Surrounding the grey matter horns the transections of the different areas show various thick medullated nerve fibers with axis cylinders." (Deiters, 1865)

seems to be present only in a background of fine lines crisscrossing here and there.

We are left to conclude that the imprecision in these otherwise beautiful diagrams reflects Deiters' own reservations on the adequacy of his data regarding the two key questions: (1) how do the fibers arise? and (2) how do they exert their influence over other cells or fibers? Despite the clarity of Figure 4, there is little attempt in Figure 5 to depict clearly the origin of an axis cylinder (axon) in any of the populations of neurons. With regard to the fine fibers, his doubts were well justified. Later work by Held (1866–1942) was to show that incoming fibers end in rounded end bulbs, or *boutons terminaux*, on the dendrites (see Chapter 17). Indeed, the triangular bases of Deiters' fine fibers on the protoplasmic prolongations have very much the appearance of boutons. Barker, writing in 1899, observed, "These finer axis cylinder processes have recently proved by the delicate histological methods of Held to be the terminals of axis-cylinder processes of other cells thus ending on, not arising from, the cell with which they seem to be connected." Later, van der Loos (1967) arrived at the same conclusion: "I am convinced that Deiters in describing his second system axons [sic] has given us an accurate portrayal of *boutons terminaux* and their pre-terminals." Thus, without being aware of it, Deiters provided the first description of axon terminals on dendrites.

On the problem of how fibers terminate, Deiters could get no further than the passage cited above. The large fibers enter the nerve tracts, and a tract may have an influence "either simple or complicated," but there was no idea of how that influence was communicated. One problem was that the axis cylinder (axon) at its origin appeared unbranched, so that it was hard to conceive of how its influence could be distributed among a target population; there was no evidence for branches or terminals of the axis cylinders. The small fibers, on the other hand, appeared to be numerous and diffusely organized. Since Deiters denied anastomoses between the protoplasmic prolongations, the small fibers seemed an ideal means for interconnecting the populations of nerve cells in a central region, because one could conceive that they "ramify and therefore may well unite." So, like Kölliker, he leaves the door open.

It is ironic that by his clear observations on dendrites and on the single axon Deiters had placed himself on a direct path to the neuron doctrine and indeed to modern times, but by the introduction of his second set of fine fibers he at the same time contributed to the reticular theory.

5
Kölliker Gives In

Liddell (1960), in his account of the history of this period, refers to Deiters as the "forgotten histologist." This might have been true of his person, because of his early death, but it seems not to have applied to his work. Not only did Schultze ensure the publication of the monograph, but Kölliker was there, keeping a watchful eye on the field. During the 1850s and 1860s, his *Histology* went through five editions, charting the development of the new discipline at a rate of better than a new edition every four years.

The fifth edition appeared in 1867, giving plenty of time to include the results contained in Deiters' monograph. The early section on the basic structure of nerve tissue is a disappointment: the same views of nerve fibers and of a typical nerve cell are shown that appeared in the first edition some 15 years earlier, with no mention of Deiters. However, the section on the spinal cord is radically revised, giving clear evidence that Kölliker had read Deiters' monograph closely and had carefully weighed its results and implications. The two issues in his lengthy account that concern us most are the description of the nerve cell, and the mode of interconnection between nerve cells.

Description of the Nerve Cell

In the main body of the text (Section 107), Kölliker introduces "the newest investigations of Deiters," referring briefly to the "axis cylinder extension," the "protoplasma extensions" (whose endings are undetermined), and the finest fibers arising from them. However, he is cautious as always, and the illustration accompanying this text is the same as in the first edition (see

Fig. 3*A* above). It is only in a subsequent section (Section 109) that he goes into these matters in detail. The following text is translated from the subsection entitled "Relations of the nerve cells to each other and to the nerve fibers":

> It seems that recently some real progress has been made in this difficult subject by Deiters' research. This prudent and careful worker, who unfortunately died much too early in the cause of science, believes, with regard to the relationships between cells and fibers in the central organ, to have discovered a specific principle, from which, as already mentioned in Section 107 above, he draws a double inference. On the one hand, each central cell gives rise to an extension which, single and undivided, passes into a dark-bordered nerve fiber surrounded by a medullated sheath. These *nerve fibers*, or *axis cylinder extensions* [i.e., axons], are described as rigid, hyaline, more resistant to reagents, and darker and sharper in contour. Opposed to these are the branched cell extensions of Deiters which he calls *protoplasma extensions* [i.e., dendrites], which arise out of the same fibrillar nuclear structure as the cell: they are fainter, not sharp-edged, and more delicate. According to Deiters, the protoplasma extensions, in their final ramifications, are definitely not to be considered as the direct source of axis cylinders; on the contrary, there are on them, arising laterally, the finest delicate type of small fiber, like the finest real axis cylinders; in these, Deiters believes he has found a transition to fine dark-bordered nerve fibers. Thus, each nerve cell in this double fashion is connected with nerve fibers.
>
> Undivided extensions of multipolar central cells passing into nerve fibers were already described in 1851 by Wagner in the electric eel *Torpedo* . . . where he usually saw one, rarely two, nerve fibers arise from one cell. More recently, Remak (1855) reported, for the large cells of the anterior horn, that each cell sends only a single, chemically and physically specific, extension into the motor root. Also, Clarke, Dean and I reported undivided extensions continuing into nerve fibers . . . [that proceed] . . . partly into the root fibers of the anterior horns and partly into the lateral tracts, but we did not succeed in exploring this condition as far as Deiters was able to do.
>
> Recently I have taken up this question again, and can in the main confirm, together with Schultze [ed.: see preface to Deiters' monograph cited above] and Boddaert, . . . Deiters' statements concerning the single nerve fiber extensions. In the multipolar cells of the anterior horn of human, calf and ox, I also observe regularly a single special extension, different from the others, though I do not find these quite as striking in this regard as did Deiters. . . . *I cannot better compare these nerve extensions than to a genuine axis cylinder.* . . . In the accompanying woodcut [see Fig. 6] the peculiarities of the two kinds of extensions cannot quite be rendered. . . . I have not yet been able to observe transitions of nerve fiber extensions into dark-bordered fibers, but it seems to me there can be no further doubt about this . . . [in view of the findings cited above].
>
> As fortunate as Deiters was in this concern, as unsatisfactory were his studies regarding the so-called *protoplasma extensions, which name I, like Max Schultze,*

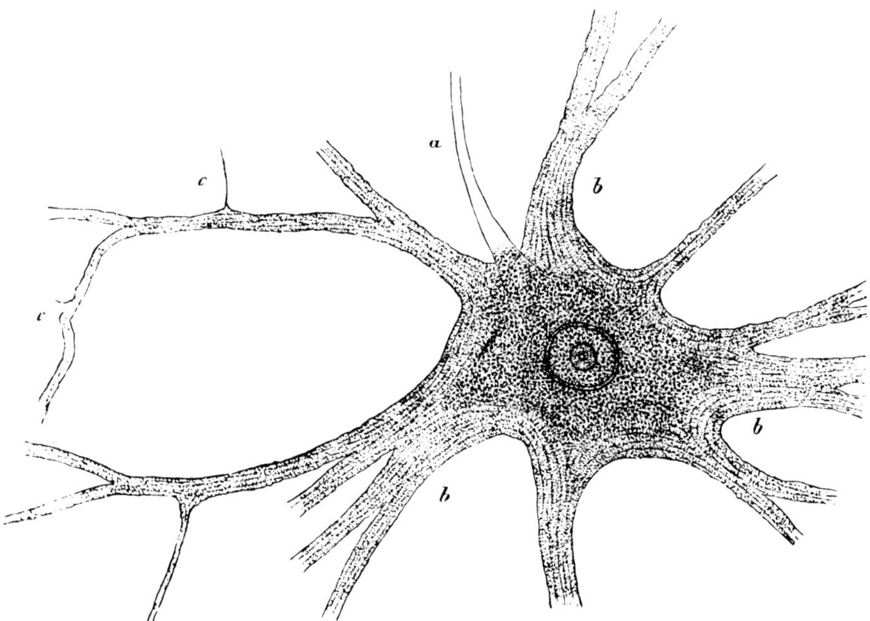

Fig. 6. Kölliker's drawing of a large nerve cell from the anterior horn of the spinal cord, showing the difference between the origin of the single axis cylinder and the multiple protoplasmic extensions. Labels: a, origin of axis cylinder [axon]; b, origins of protoplasmic prolongations [dendrites]; c, fine fibers, believed by Deiters to arise from the protoplasmic prolongations, but most likely terminal fragments of axons making connections onto the dendrites (see text). (Kölliker, 1867)

> *find unsuitable* [italics added]. . . . Deiters omits any discussion of the terminations of the branches of these extensions, which, together with his hypothesis about the fine nerve fibers that extend laterally from the terminal branches, all gives the impression of an unfinished study. That such fine threads are found on the branched extensions is certain, and I myself have for several years represented them in various illustrations. . . . However, I cannot in any way see that these differ from the other processes of these extensions except by their fragility. . . . I will not deny that these continue into dark-bordered nerve fibers, but, first, Deiters did not prove this for certain . . . and second, it has not in any way been shown that *the branched extensions do not terminate in the same way*. Under these circumstances, Deiters' hypothesis regarding the double significance of the terminations of the branched extensions is not sufficiently supported.
>
> To complete this picture of our knowledge of central nerve cells, it should be stressed that, until more evidence is forthcoming, one may assume that all nerve cells follow the schema of Deiters.

In summary, Remak's idea that the nerve cell gives rise to a single large unbranched process that continues into the axis cylinder is confirmed and pronounced to be a general rule. That there are other, protoplasmic extensions emanating from the cell body (which we now call dendrites), is also clear, but what to call them is undecided and, most important, how they terminate is completely unknown. Least satisfactory is the status of the very fine lateral threads hanging off the branched extensions; Kölliker seems eager to claim partial credit for their discovery, and is willing to consider the possibility that they are continuous with fine axis cylinders, but he hedges by recognizing that there is no direct evidence for this.

The Problem of Anastomoses

The uncertainties about the finest branches of the protoplasmic extensions raised the vexed question of the possibility of anastomoses. As we have seen, Kölliker had led the fight against them in the early years. But his resolve was giving way:

> I am moreover not inclined to deny anastomoses through shorter, stronger extensions, and I am willing to admit that some of the findings up to this point, such as for example those of R. Wagner and of Buser, among others, are based on quite good observations. At this point it may be remembered that similar anastomoses of multipolar cells were already observed long ago by Corti and myself in the retina. One may note, however, that connections of this kind are, to a large extent, perhaps nothing but developmental stages of cells, as dividing nerve cells with short anastomoses have been seen by Remak, Valentin, Schäffner and myself in the ganglia of young animals, and Blake also sees what he calls anastomoses in similar preparations. Besides these connections of nerve cells there may be others between the finest extensions of their branches; we have as yet no evidence on this point, and for now can therefore only justify such an assumption in the name of an acceptable hypothetical claim from the standpoint of physiology.

A Hypothesis of Nerve Connections

Notwithstanding the various uncertainties, Kölliker felt the time had come to suggest a hypothesis about how nerve cell extensions and fibers are related to each other in forming pathways for nervous conduction. He was not alone; others had put forth partial, tentative views, but this was the most ambitious, comprehensive attempt to pull together the anatomical findings and try to give them a physiological interpretation; it was also a rare instance for that time in which the hypothesis was illustrated with a specific diagram of the postulated relations.

> If one uses the available facts to attempt to portray the fiber pathways in the spinal cord the resulting picture is incomplete, and it must appear very daring

to complete it by means of hypotheses. I have previously preached caution in this matter, an admonition heeded by the researcher [Deiters] who most recently has worked on the structure of the spinal gray matter. In assessing the implications of this work, I restrict myself to the following remarks . . .

a) The nerve fiber continuations of the cells pass in part into sensory and motor root fibers and in part into the fibers of the longitudinal tracts. The latter tenet is doubted by Deiters, but I have followed certain single cell extensions far into the lateral tracts, which I cannot interpret in any other way.

b) Some of the fibers of the tracts of the cord appear to pass immediately into root fibers, whereas some are only connected with them through nerve cells. At present there is no evidence that the branched cell extensions [dendrites] pass directly into root fibers.

c) The branched cell extensions are by no means all connected in a simple way with tract fibers, such that each terminal branch of a cell extension would continue into a single dark-bordered tract fiber [axon], considering that the number of terminal branches exceeds by far the number of tract fibers. In addition to the possibility that an extension passes directly into a tract fiber, it may be that many extensions from one or several cells could be joined to a single tract fiber [i.e., to an axis cylinder]. In favor of the latter possibility might be mentioned the divisions of axis cylinders and nerve tracts of the cord, though these occur only rarely.

d) Connections between the branched cell extensions [dendrites] of the various cells cannot be demonstrated, but they are to a high degree probable; it seems to me such an assumption offers the simplest solution to the enigma of these extremely numerous extensions, and also the best explanation for the large conduction capacity of the grey matter and the reflexes. The cell connections could in part be made through the pale extensions themselves and in part through the dark-bordered tubes [axons] as intermediaries (in the retina Corti saw cells connected through various optic fibers similar to these extensions). The latter possibility might explain the large number of fine tubes in the grey substance.

e) Crossings of nerve fibers and cell extensions from one half of the spinal cord to the other can be found extensively in both commissures; however, the actual trajectories of the crossing fibers have nowhere been precisely determined.

After laying this foundation, Kölliker then sets forth his hypothesis, illustrated by the diagram in Figure 7.

The simplest hypothesis that can be supported by the points discussed above concerning the fiber pathways in the spinal cord is the following:

1) The fibers of the motor and sensory roots have their origins [endings] partly in the spinal cord and partly in the brain, including the *medulla oblongata*.

2) The root fibers originating from the spinal cord come from nerve fiber extensions of specific motor and sensory cells.

3) In each half of the spinal cord *all cells of one type are connected through their branched extensions* [*dendrites*], *which form a net* [italics added] arranged,

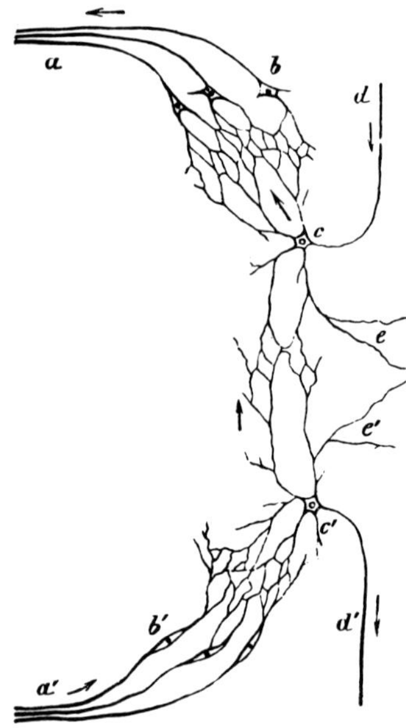

Fig. 7. "Scheme of the connections of cells and nerve fibers in the spinal cord. a, motor root fibers, b, motor cells of the anterior horns, c, motor conduction cells, e, extension connecting with the other side of the spinal cord. All cells are interconnected through the nets of their branched extensions. The corresponding sensory parts are described with a–e." (Kölliker, 1867)

however, into a certain number of compartments (nuclei), which in each case are related to the number of roots, but may be more numerous.

4) In the same way, the sensory and motor cells, and the cells of the right and left halves of the spinal cord, are also *linked by anastomoses* [italics added].

5) The correctness of the assumption of such anastomoses seems as likely as that connections between nerve cells are formed through the unchanged branched cell extensions, or that, in part or everywhere, these take on the nature of dark-bordered fibers.

6) The cells that constitute the origin and termination of the root fibers are connected through specific conducting fibers with the brain, which fibers probably all course through the white matter tracts.

7) As the number of these conducting fibers appears to be smaller than that of the root fibers, it is possible that a conducting fiber always corresponds to a group of nerve cells and root fibers.

8) The conduction fibers, like the root fibers, are in all probability continuations of the nerve fiber extensions of the cells. If this is so, then, since no cell gives off two nerve fiber extensions [axons], it follows that specific cells must be employed for the conduction fibers; to these, the remarks regarding anastomoses under point 4 above must apply. . . . Besides this, there may also be many cells which serve as connecting elements, and are not connected directly with either the root fibers or the conduction fibers.

Since physiology and pathology have such a great interest in an understanding of the construction of the spinal cord, I allow myself to illustrate this hypothesis with the schema [of Fig. 7], in which, however, interrupted fibers are not represented.

Figure 7 is the first appearance in the general literature of a specific schema for the cellular organization of the spinal cord, and possibly for any region of the nervous system. It depicts inputs and outputs by specific pathways. It provides for the combining of two different input pathways in the cells of a given center, and thus lays the foundation for concepts of the integration of inputs at the cellular level. But it also assumes that nervous activity can travel in the reverse direction along the axis cylinder (axon) into the cell body; shows communication within a center by means of anastomoses between the distal processes of branched nerve extensions (dendrites); and even shows these branches giving off long distance fibers to the other half of the spinal cord.

All these assumptions are wrong. Thus, when Kölliker finally committed himself, the result was deeply flawed. Far from aiding the attempt to incorporate nerve cells into the cell theory, he in fact went in the other direction, introducing in his principles the term "net" (principle 3 above), using the idea of anastomoses (principle 4) and depicting these concepts in an explicit diagram (Fig. 7). Kölliker's fifth edition lasted for almost 30 years. It bestowed a legitimacy on the attempt to persuade, by speculation if not by evidence, that the nervous system is constructed of diffuse networks of fibers, in which the significance of the nerve cell as a cellular entity is subsidiary to the role of the fiber network.

6

Support Builds for Networks

Kölliker was not alone in gravitating toward the concept of nerve networks. The idea is commonly ascribed to von Gerlach, but in fact it was born in the early 1850s and by the 1880s had acquired many fathers. We will chart its rise briefly in this chapter in order to understand the microscopical evidence on which it was based, to gauge its depth of support, and to gain an appreciation of how it set a rather hostile tone to the intellectual environment from which the neuron doctrine emerged. In subsequent chapters, we will see that the network idea came into direct opposition with the idea of the nerve cell as a cell. From this perspective it has been regarded as the major conceptual hurdle facing the founders of the neuron doctrine. However, we will see that, independently of this issue, the idea needs to be viewed from another perspective as well, as an attempt to address some broader questions about the structural basis for more holistic functions of the brain. From this perspective it left a legacy for concepts of brain organization that has resurfaced in recent years in the form of neural networks (see Chapter 20).

The "Dotted Substance" of Leydig

Most of the work we have discussed thus far was carried out in mammals, a substantial amount on the brains of large species; one is surprised to read a figure legend referring to some nerve cell from an ox, a horse, or even an elephant. Human brains were also frequently studied. When tissue preparation was so primitive, the larger the brain, the better the chance to observe the larger nerve cells contained therein.

On the other hand, there was also active interest in the nervous systems of invertebrate species. We have seen that the ranks of these investigators included Kölliker and Helmholtz. Franz Leydig (1821–1908) was one of the main workers in this area. His papers between 1849 and 1862 covered an extensive series of studies on the anatomy of many invertebrate species: Hirudineen, Artemia and Paranchipus, Corethra larvae and Lacinularia, Coccus, Rotifers, Arthropoda, and Annelids. Close on the heels of Kölliker he published his own textbook of histology (1857), followed in 1864 by *Vom Bau des thierischen Körpers* (*On the Structure of the Insect Body*), which helped to establish insect histology as a distinct subfield of investigation.

The central nervous systems of most invertebrate species consist of accumulations of cells called "ganglia," interconnected by nerve fiber tracts called "connectives." In his studies of different species Leydig discerned nerve cell bodies and nerve fibers that resembled their counterparts in the vertebrate nerve system. Invertebrate ganglia are characteristically arranged with cell bodies surrounding a central core, where, we now know, the nerve fibers and nerve branches (the dendrites, or, in more general terms, the "neurites") interconnect through their terminal processes. In the primitive preparations of that time these processes, like their vertebrate counterparts, could not be seen; instead, the core appeared to have a consistency that was variously described as "grainy" or faintly fibrillary. In the early 1850s, Leydig began to refer to this as a *Molekularmassen* (molecular mass), *Punktmasse* (dotted mass), or *Punktsubstanz*, (which is most nearly rendered into English as dotted substance). He was the first to describe this type of nervous region, and was in no doubt that it was important (1857): "The essential substance of the nerve centers consists of the molecular mass, in which smaller and larger cellular elements are embedded."

Speculations on the "Dotted Substance"

Over the following three decades, speculation was vigorous on the nature of the "dotted substance." Leydig's view was succinctly summarized by Fridtjof Nansen (1887):

> Leydig is the first writer to give a somewhat detailed description of the central mass of the ganglia. He calls it "Punktsubstanz" [dotted substance] and characterises it as a "netzförmig gestrickte Gewirr feinster Fäserchen" [net-like knitted tangle of the finest fibrils]. This "Punktsubstanz" receives on one side the branching processes [dendrites] of the ganglion cells (these lose themselves in the fibrous substance), and on the other side it gives origin to the peripheral nerve-tubes [axons].
>
> This not very detailed description by Leydig has been supplemented by

> very few scientists. Most writers seem to be satisfied with it, they use the name without entering more closely upon this difficult subject, and do not try to define the structure of the central mass more exactly.

Nansen, in his thesis, which we will examine in some detail in Chapter 9, gives an exhaustive account of the succession of noble knights who tilted at this particular windmill. It is worth summarizing this pursuit in order to illustrate the frustrations of anatomists before the advent of the Golgi stain.

Generally, as Nansen observes, the authorities divided into three main camps: the majority who favored the view that there is an immediate connection between nerve cells and nerve tubes, a minority who believed that the nerve tubes have an "indirect origin" from the "granula-fibrous mass" of the dotted substance, and a small group who felt that both were possible. The structure of the dotted substance can thus be seen as a crucial question for interpreting the relations between nerve fibers (axons) and nerve cell bodies.

Within these main groups were various shadings of interpretation concerning this question. Let us consider several examples.

Bucholz (1863), according to Nansen, calls the dotted substance "that *finest fiber system*, which is spread out everywhere within the nerve centers." He reports that "the broad axis cylinders become narrower by giving off . . . (the) finest small twigs . . . from these an extraordinarily large number of immeasurably fine fibers arises, which present manifold criss-crossing everywhere within the interiors of the nerve centers."

Waldeyer (1863) believes that the "molecular central stratum" consists of "a kind of braid-work," formed of "fine extensions of the large cells, small cells, and their finest extensions." Nansen believes that Waldeyer is confused between his small cells and neuroglia. He quotes a passage in which Waldeyer expresses an opinion that opposes the direct origin of nerve tubes (axons) from ganglion cells. This is a most interesting opinion coming from this source, because it dramatically illustrates the long distance Waldeyer will have to travel in order to arrive at the concept of the neuron 28 years later (see Chapter 14).

Hermann (1875) carried out the most detailed study of the "central fibrous mass of the invertebrate nervous system" and finds it "to be formed by fibrillae, and by a granulous, viscous, 'Zwischensubstanz' [interstitial substance]." He believes that the nerve tubes (i.e., axons) do not arise directly from nerve cell bodies but rather arise indirectly from fibrillae that have three origins: from "nodal points" (*Knotenpunkte*) formed by the confluence of fibrils within the grey matter; and from fibrils of the longitudinal commissures, which may end in "nodal points" or pass directly into fibrils giving rise to nerve tubes (i.e., axons). Here perhaps is one of the first applications of the term "node" to nervous organization.

It seems like some kind of fated progression, from the crisscrossing fibers of Bucholz to the formation of nodal points at the crisscrossings. How ironic, even perverse, to confer on the imagined nodal point the all-important site of origin of the nerve fibers (i.e., axons), rather than to the obvious cell body. However, it expresses a theme that has persisted even to modern times, that nervous function resides primarily in nerve fibers (axons), with nerve cell bodies and dendrites relegated to subsidiary roles such as nutritional maintenance.

By 1876, Dietl was referring to a "network" of the finest fibrils, which would suggest that networks and nodal points were fast becoming established as the common way to think about nervous organization at the cellular level. Floegel's (1878) paper on the insect brain refers to a "netlike knitted substance." In his study of the cockroach brain, Newton (1879) believes that nerve fibers anastomose with each other, that networks extend between ganglion cells, and that "connective tissue combines with nervous tissue" in some preparations observed under the microscope. Nansen (1887) notes the likelihood that some of these early observers may have been misinterpreting the fibrous extensions of neuroglial cells for those of nerve cells. In this regard, Kölliker (1867) discussed at great length the reticulum formed by cells lining the ventricles of the brain, distinguishing it from the network of nerve extensions he described in the spinal cord (see Chapter 5).

More support for the network concept came from Krieger (1880) in his study of *Astacus*: "The dotted substance is a network or perhaps more correctly a blanket of the finest fibers," from which the nerve tubes (i.e., axons) arise. Bellonci (1881) uses the French term *substance grenue-reticulée* (granular-reticular substance) to refer to the "central fibrous mass" of invertebrate ganglia. He distinguishes a connective tissue stroma and a nervous network (*réseau nerveux*), but has not, Nansen surmises, succeeded "in finding the real relation between these two substances." Nerve tubes arise from both the reseau and the cell bodies. Another worker, Lang (1881), believes "that the spongy looking 'reticulation' in the dotted substance of the brain, as also in the nerves, is produced by a 'stutzgewebe' or, as I call it, *neuroglia*, which in reality forms tubes; an opinion in which I do quite agree with him" (Nansen, 1887).

Another neuroanatomist noted by Nansen is Sigmund Freud:

> Freud (1882) does not seem to have paid any special attention to the structure of the dotted substance. The relation of the ganglion cells to the nerve-tubes,

> he supposes to be the same in invertebrates as in vertebrates, and he believes, to a certain extent at all events, in a direct origin. He expresses himself, however, very indistinctly on this subject.

We will consider Freud's contributions to studies of the nerve cell further in the next chapter.

Summary

We may conclude from this review that, from the early 1850s, the view gained acceptance among anatomists that nerve cells give off branches (dendrites), one of which is different from the rest and becomes a nerve cylinder (axon). The terminal divisions of the branches were too small to resolve with the microscope, so it was natural to assume that the finest processes were joined to form a network. This network was conceived to be the means for nervous conduction within a region. Whether or not the network could also give rise to nerve cylinders (axons) was a matter of debate.

We have also seen that this view tended to emphasize the importance of the network as a system that functioned largely independently of the nerve cell bodies and larger branches. Thus, the special properties of the nervous system—its ability to conduct activity, and mediate sensation, reflexes, and other brain functions—were assumed to require the special fibrous constituents of nerve cells—the long axis cylinders (axons) and the network of thin anastomosing fibers—whereas the cell body with its immediate protoplasmic extensions resembled other cells in the body, and could well be imagined to share with them more general nutritive and supportive functions.

The Network of Gerlach

The preceding account should make it clear that the idea of a nerve network was a consensus view to which many workers contributed, both in terms of their microscopical observations and their attempts to conceptualize the form of the network and its relations to nerve cells and axis cylinders. Later writers, however, have given almost sole credit for the idea to Joseph von Gerlach. Now that we have obtained a broader perspective for understanding the development of this idea, let us examine Gerlach's contribution to it.

Gerlach was born in Mainz, near Frankfurt, Germany, in 1820. He obtained his M.D. at Würzburg in 1841, with further studies in Munich, Berlin, Paris, Vienna, and London. He then settled in Mainz to practice medicine, but continued to carry out microscopical studies; these led to his appointment as professor of anatomy and physiology at Erlangen in 1850.

Networks in the Human Cerebrum.

Gerlach soon became well known for his introduction of carmine for staining nerve cells. Carmine was one of the first of the aniline dyes to be used for this purpose. As noted above, the German chemical industry produced an increasing number of these and related substances that, together with better reagents for fixation, yielded better visualization of nerve processes, though, alas, not of the finest branches.

Another improvement came with the introduction of metallic reagents, and here too Gerlach was a pioneer. The application of gold chloride solutions to nerve tissue gave especially clear views, and in 1872 came a short paper entitled "Über die Structur der grauen Substanz des menschlichen Grosshirns. Vorläufige Mittheilung" which follows in its entirety (Gerlach, 1872; partially in Clarke and O'Malley, 1968):

> **ON THE STRUCTURE OF THE GREY MATTER IN THE HUMAN CEREBRUM. PRELIMINARY COMMUNICATION**
>
> Yesterday Prof. Rindfleisch kindly sent me a short printed communication concerning the nerve endings in the cerebral cortex of the rabbit; this has occasioned me to announce briefly the main results of a study of the grey matter of the human cerebral convolutions that I have undertaken this winter, and also because in the main we both have arrived at the same results though working with different methods.
>
> Rindfleisch used osmic acid and glycerin as hardening and solution reagents, and showed that the medullated nerve fibers originate in a double manner in the grey matter, on the one hand through the nerve extension of Deiters which becomes the axis cylinder [axon], and secondly, from netlike, very fine origins which, as Rindfleisch expresses it, show an extremely delicate transition from the "thread-like" to the "granular", like the ramified extensions [dendrites] of the ganglion cells.
>
> I used the gold method, which served me so well in the spinal cord, to study the grey matter of the cerebrum, and so far have specifically limited my study to the central convolutions of the human brain.
>
> The results of my investigations now follow briefly:
>
> 1) In addition to the already long known medullated nerve fibers [axons] extending from the white into the grey matter, where they course radially arranged in bundles almost to the surface of the cerebrum, there are numerous nerve fibers which are also medullated but horizontally-coursing; these are especially clearly seen in the interstitial spaces between the radial bundles where groups of ganglion cells also are mainly found; [these cells] are interconnected with each other as well as connected with the radial bundle, whereby a coarsely meshed network of medullated fibers is produced which can already be seen at 60-times-magnification.

2) In the spaces of this coarse network of medullated fibers lies, beside the ganglion cells, a second, extremely finely-meshed network of the finest, no longer medullated, fibers, which like the network generally, can only be visualized by means of the strongest immersion system. Sharing in the formation of this second network are, on the one hand, the finest extensions of the protoplasmic prolongations [dendrites] of the nerve cells; on the other hand, this network gives rise to fibers that are larer and become myelinated, and enter the first wide-meshed network of medullated fibers. Whereas Rindfleisch believes that between the origins of the second, very fine network and the endings of the protoplasmic prolongations of the nerve cells a fine grained substance is interpolated, *I have been able to show with the gold method the continuity of the network with the protoplasmic prolongations* [*dendrites*] *of the nerve cells.*

3) At the nerve cells themselves is the nervous extension [axon] of Deiters which, without ramification, directly becomes the axis cylinder of a medullated tube which then joins a bundle of radial fibers. Whether or not all nerve cells of the cortex are supplied with a nervous extension, I must leave unanswered. Until now I have only several times seen evident nervous extensions, and then only from those larger nerve cells which send a thicker and often very long branched protoplasmic prolongation [apical dendrite?] to the brain surface and numerous finer ones outwards. The nervous extension [axon] is always among the latter.

4) In the grey matter of the convolutions of the human cerebrum there is thus a double mode of origin of medullated nerve fibers, one directly from cells and one from the network.

In the spinal cord where we also have both kinds of origins, as I showed earlier, the two fiber groups are differentiated, in that those coming directly from cells leave the spinal cord in the pathways of the anterior roots, whereas those of network origin leave in the posterior roots; I hardly need emphasize the significance of this interpretation for the double origin of the nerve fibers in the grey matter of the cerebral cortex.*

*Herr Gerlach was kind enough to show me gold preparations by which the two networks could be seen most clearly. J. Rosenthal.

Although this view does not appear to differ significantly from those of many others, as we noted in our previous review, it achieved much wider currency because Gerlach included a summary of it, together with an illustration, in the chapter that he wrote (*Von dem Rückenmark*) (*On the spinal cord*) for the widely read textbook of histology edited by Salomon Stricker in 1869–1872. The following extract is from the American translation of 1870–1873 (also in Clarke and O'Malley, 1968):

Deiters thinks that these ultimate endings of the protoplasmic processes do not differ from the axis cylinders of the finest nerve fibrils and that they form a system of nerve pathways connected with the ganglion cells. If Deiters had taken a step further, he would have discovered the fine nerve fibre plexus;

but as he did not use ammonium carminate in his preparations, and as the gold [chloride] method was unknown to him, the nerve fibre plexus remained hidden from him. I can confirm those observations of Deiters that have been cited, but, in addition, the finest branches of the protoplasmic processes ultimately take part in the formation of the fine nerve fibre network which I consider to be an essential constituent of the gray matter of the spinal cord [see Fig. 8]. The finest divisions of the protoplasmic processes which are surrounded by a dark-edged, double contour are none other than the beginning of this nerve fibre net. The cells of the gray matter, which are provided with nerve processes [axons] and protoplasmic processes [dendrites], are therefore *doubly* connected with the nerve fibre elements of the spinal cord: on the one hand *by means of the nerve process which becomes the axis fibre of the tubules of the anterior roots, and on the other through the finest branches of the protoplasmic processes which become a part of the fine nerve fibre net of the gray matter.*

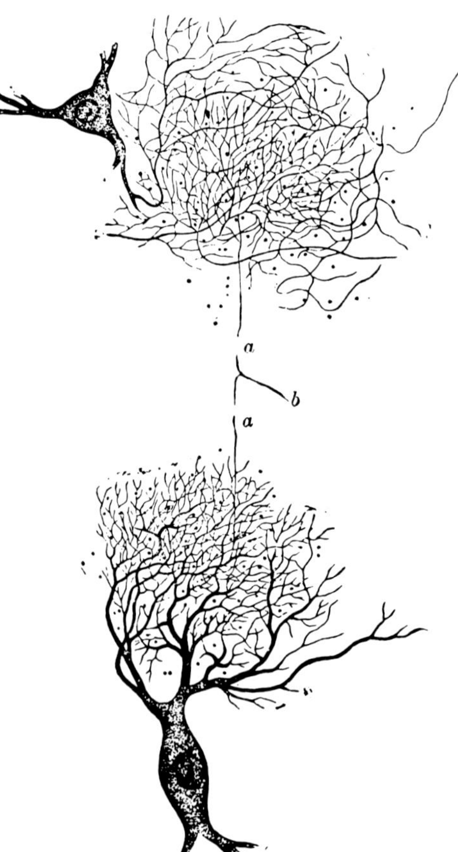

Fig. 8. Gerlach's theory of the nerve network and the origin of nerve fibers. "A nerve fibre is here seen to divide, and the two branches to communicate with the plexus of nerve fibres that are in connection with two nerve cells. Prepared with carmine and ammonia. From the spinal cord of the Ox." (Gerlach, 1872)

Conclusion

Clarke and O'Malley (1968) have expressed the common opinion that "Gerlach must . . . be considered the originator of the net theory of neuron tissue." As Barker (1899) described it, "Gerlach's view was that the axis cylinders of motor nerve fibres represent nervous processes coming off directly from nerve cells, while the sensory fibres of the dorsal roots are to be looked upon as nerve fibres arising from nerve cells only indirectly through the intervention of a diffuse nerve network made up of their protoplasmic processes. Thus, according to his scheme, with which Roll and Haller essentially agreed, the whole nervous system represents a protoplasmic *continuum*—a veritable *rete mirabile*." But this view seems to fall into the category we have already discussed. It does not differ very much from Kölliker's scheme. It was shared by those who believed in the "double origin" theory, that axis cylinders arise either directly as single extensions from the nerve cell body, or indirectly from the network of fine anastomosing branches of the protoplasmic extensions; in fact, some conceived of there being nodes in the network from which fibers could arise.

Why did Gerlach come to be regarded as the sole representative of this view and all its shadings and variations? A number of explanations can be offered:

1. The line of work we followed in the previous section was in invertebrates. By contrast, Gerlach worked on vertebrates; some of his studies were specifically in the human; some of them were in the human cerebral cortex. Since most biological scientists of the time were medically trained, it was natural to feel that important principles need to be validated in humans. Moreover, a principle elucidated in the human cerebral cortex obviously has the most direct relevance to concepts of human brain function.

2. The improvements in staining introduced by Gerlach gave added weight to his conclusions; Barker (1899), for example, states that "Gerlach, by means of methods of isolation and treatment with chloride of gold, obtained pictures surpassing by far, in extent and delicacy, any obtainable with the older methods, and affording an entirely new concept of the complexity of the structure of the gray matter of the spinal cord and brain. In addition to the bodies of the nerve cells and their main processes, protoplasmic and nervous, the new method revealed the most intricate and involved appearances, which led Gerlach to believe that he had discovered a most extensive and delicate diffuse network within the gray matter."

Be that as it may, visualization of the thinnest branches was still not achieved: the methods were still inadequate to the task.

3. There is a tendency for subsequent generations of workers to fix on

one person as representative of a previous body of work. Thus, in modern times, it is common, when referring to classical studies of the neuron, simply to cite Cajal's textbook of 1909–1911, even though the original work on a particular cell may have been done by someone else. A similar tendency may have been at work to fix all credit (or disrepute!) on Gerlach.

4. There may have been a tendency, conscious or not, to downplay the roles of some workers who later rejected the network idea. We will have a chance to assess this possibility in later chapters.

5. A picture (like Fig. 8) is always worth a thousand words!

7

The Nerve Cell Studies of Freud

Although Gerlach gave a new level of credibility to the reticular idea, there were many microscopists in the 1870s who were relatively unswayed by such theoretical considerations, and simply pushed forward in the attempt to see more clearly the nerve cell and its relation to nerve fibers. As noted in the previous chapter, one of these was Sigmund Freud. His neuroanatomical work early in his career is of particular interest because of the claim by several of his biographers that it led him to the brink of the neuron doctrine (Brun, 1936; Jelliffe, 1937; Jones, 1953). These studies are also of interest because they were the first step in the scientific career pursued by Freud before he began the work that led to his theories of psychoanalysis. We will briefly review the aspects of his early work that directly concern the structure and organization of nerve cells (see Jelliffe, 1937; Bernfeld, 1944; 1947; 1950; 1951; Jones, 1953; Amacher, 1965).

The Young Student

Freud, the son of a wool merchant, was born in 1856 in Freiberg, now Pribor, Czechoslovakia. The family moved to Vienna in 1860, where Freud grew up in rather straitened circumstances. Being Jewish, of a nonacademic family, and impecunious were considerable obstacles to an academic career in nineteenth century Europe. However, there was always a chance for a youth if he had talent, ambition, and persistence (recall Remak, Chapter 2). Freud entered medical school in Vienna in 1873. Drawn toward biology, he spent the summer of 1876 in the new Zoological Station in Trieste on the Adriatic. He engaged in several attempts at anatomical research, with little satisfaction, and his studies were moving at a desultory pace until he met Professor Ernst Brucke.

When last we encountered Brucke he was one of the four zealous young students in Germany in the 1840s determined to rebuild the field of physiology on the laws of chemistry and physics (see Chapter 3). He had come to Vienna in 1849 as professor of physiology (his friends teased him that he was their "ambassador to the Orient"). As mentioned previously, he had broad interests in a range of physiological processes. Unlike many physiologists, he found it quite natural to pursue microscopical studies as well. Over the years his Institute of Physiology gained considerable fame; however, as with others we have met (Purkinje, Chapter 2), or will meet (Meynert, Chapter 9), the institute was poorly equipped (Jones, 1953):

> The Institute was miserably housed in the ground floor and basement of a dark and smelly old gun factory. It consisted of a large room where the students kept their microscopes and listened to lectures, and two smaller ones, one of which was Brucke's sanctum. There were also on both floors a few small cubicles, some without windows, that served as chemical, electrophysiological, and optical laboratories. There was no water supply, no gas, and of course no electricity. All heating had to be done over a spirit lamp, and the water was brought up from a well in the yard where also a shed housed the animals experimented on. Nevertheless this Institute was the pride of the medical school on account of the number and distinction of its foreign visitors and students.

In his *Autobiographical Study,* Freud's description of how he began his neuroanatomical studies under Brucke is succinct to the point of perfunctory (Freud, 1935/1952):

> At length in Ernst Brucke's physiological laboratory, I found rest and satisfaction—and men, too, whom I could respect and take as my models: the great Brucke himself, and his assistants Sigmund Exner and Ernst von Fleischl-Marxow. Brucke gave me a problem to work out in the histology of the nervous system; I succeeded in solving it to his satisfaction and in carrying the work further on my own account.

This cryptic passage has suggested that Freud came to his studies of nerve cells with no great passion for them, but simply with the resolve to "work out" the problem set for him by the great master. It was not that he did not enjoy the work, for he looked back on these years as the happiest of his life.

Nerve Cells and Fibers in a Primitive Fish

The problem Brucke gave to Freud was to clarify the structure of a particular large type of nerve cell, discovered by Reissner, that is situated in the spinal cord of a fish, Petromyzon, belonging to the cyclostomata. This is a primitive vertebrate species, and therefore has always been of interest for the insights it can give into early vertebrate evolution. Within a few weeks (Jones, 1953), Freud reported to Brucke that he could not only trace peripheral sensory nerves to their origins from Reissner's cells, but he could also see fibers in the dorsal (sensory) roots that arose from these same cells and passed centrally into the spinal cord. This led to his first scientific papers (Freud, 1877, 1878), in which he concluded that Reissner's cells "are nothing else than spinal ganglion cells which, in those low vertebrates, where the migration of the embryonic neural tube to the periphery is not yet completed, remain within the spinal cord."

Although he subsequently found in searching the literature that this had been described by a Russian investigator some years before, it was nonetheless a significant study. His further observations led him to an even more interesting conclusion:

> The spinal ganglion cells of the fish have long been known to be bipolar . . . while those of the higher vertebrata are unipolar. . . . The nerve cells of the Petromyzon show all transitions from uni- to bipolarity.

In other words, the observations in Petromyzon enabled one to construct an evolutionary sequence for dorsal root ganglion cells, from the bipolar form, to transitional forms that are either bipolar or unipolar, to strictly unipolar forms as seen in the higher vertebrates. We do not know how much of this synthesis came from Freud and how much from his three mentors, but it is likely that Freud drew both inspiration and ideas from Brucke, who had a very broad view of anatomical structure and physiological processes. We will see that the unipolar form of the dorsal root ganglion cell posed a difficult problem for later workers seeking to embrace all nerve cells in one functional framework (see Chapter 15).

Nerve Cells and Fibers in Crayfish

Freud next took up, "on his own account," according to his autobiography, a study of nerve cells in the crayfish. This was published in 1882 as an article entitled "Über den Bau der Nervenfasen und Hervenzellen beim

Flusskrebs" (On the structure of nerve fibers and nerve cells of the crayfish"). It consisted of 37 pages, accompanied by a plate of five illustrations carefully drawn by himself (Fig. 9). We will quote at some length from this article, because it represents Freud's most mature work on the microscopic structure of nerve cells. The first paragraph introduces the subject and the reasons for selecting the crayfish:

> The observations presented here were started in the summer months of 1879 and 1881 in the hope of advancing the understanding of the finer structure of nervous tissue by studying, where possible, fresher surviving elements. As . . . this task encounters far too great difficulties in the vertebrates, I have put my confidence in the general significance of results obtained in invertebrates, and chose from these, being most accessible to me, the crayfish, in which animal the size and the looser connections of elementary parts, as well as the generous presence of an apparently protective supplementary fluidity in the blood, promised to ease the research.

After a thorough presentation of his observations, Freud drew his conclusions concerning the internal structure of the nerve cells:

> The results of my observations of the nerve cells of the crayfish may be summarized as follows: *The nerve cells in the brain and in the stomatic ganglionic chain consist of two substances, of which one, arranged in a netlike fashion, extends into the fibrils of the nerve fibers, whereas the other goes into the ground substance. . . . The nucleus of the nerve cell consists of a homogeneous mass, not sharply defined at the boundary with the cell body, in which formations of various shapes and durability are visible. These nuclear bodies show changes in shape and location which reflect the conditions of survival of the cell.*

This conclusion is entirely consistent with Deiters' description of the origin of the axis cylinder from the nerve cell body (Chapter 4). The paper ends with a more general discussion of the significance of these findings:

> *The nerve cell up to this point does not show any unique structural aspects; its function is consistent with the general structure of the animal cell as far as this can be determined (Brucke, 1861).* However, this does not permit any conclusion to be drawn as to a higher or lower physiological dignity of the nerve cell.
>
> I remind you that there is no reason to assume that the relationship of the nerve cell to the nerve fiber is any different in the invertebrates from that in the vertebrates. Waldeyer has stated that the extensions of the large central nerve cells of invertebrates never become peripheral nerve fibers, but instead go into the central substance of the ganglion where they dissolve into fine

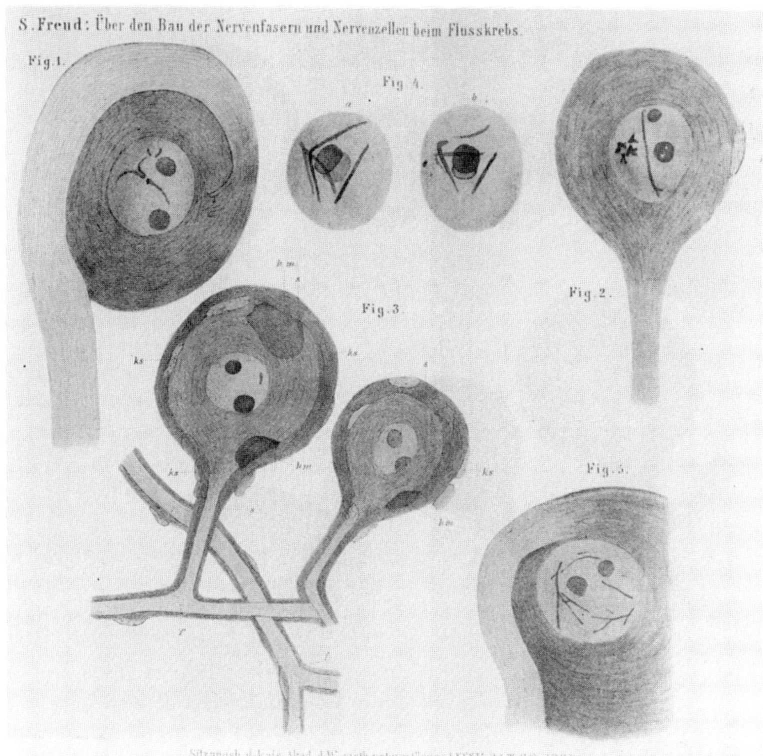

Fig. 9. Illustrations of nerve cells by Sigmund Freud.
"Fig. 1. Nerve cell from the tail ganglion of the crayfish which (joins with) the cell peripherally. In the nucleus, besides the roundish nuclear bodies are several short thick small rods and a nuclear figure consisting of two parts. Drawn by Hartnack 3/8. Magnification of the drawing 360.
Fig. 2. Surviving nerve cell from an abdominal ganglion with cone shaped arising extension. In the nucleus, which does not have a nuclear membrane, are four multi-pointed small clusters and one long rod bent and forked at one end. At *k* is a nucleus of the covering sheath. The same magnification.
Fig. 3. Border section from the spindle shaped stomatogastric ganglion of the crayfish. Two unipolar nerve cells with their extensions of which one undergoes a T-shaped division. The smaller cell is indicated by a focus near the surface.

s The thick, concentric layered cell sheath.

ks The nucleus itself.

hm Strong, shiny homogeneous mass at the edge of the cell, yet situated inside the covering sheath.

f A fiber coming from another cell. The same magnification.

Fig. 4. The nucleus of a large nerve cell which showed suggestions of movement on both kinds of nuclear bodies. *b* is drawn five minutes later than *a*. Hartnack 3/x. Magnification of the drawing 400.
Fig. 5. A portion of a cell with extension as in Fig. 1. In the nucleus a large number of neatly forked and bent (small) rods. The same magnification as in Fig. 4." (Freud, 1882)

fibrils and that on the other side the peripheral nerve fibers originate by the coming together of fibrils of the central substance. It was obvious to add a further assumption to this, that in an invertebrate nerve fiber, fibrils belonging to different nerve cells come together.

Leydig's . . . view differs from that of Waldeyer's, in that he sees a direct transition of extensions of central nerve cells into nerve fibers, which would do away with the stated difference by Waldeyer between the nerve tissue of invertebrates and vertebrates. In the vertebrates, as we know, the direct transition of cell extensions in peripheral nerve fibers has been shown for the cells of the central organ, and Deiters himself has indicated signs by which the axis cylinder, already at its origin from the nerve cells, is recognizable. However, it has not been ascertained throughout in the vertebrates that all nerve fibers are interconnected with nerve cells in the same way. It is moreover possible that here, too, nerve fibers originate from a central fiber mass and that a peripheral fiber contains fibrils of different origins and significance. This relationship has neither been proven for the invertebrates nor disproven for the vertebrates.

Several findings moreover support an even deeper agreement of the nerve tissue of the two large animal classes on this point. In the Phrominides, a family of water flea, Claus, in experiments on the stomatic ganglionic chain, has found in longitudinal sections that the extensions of the large nerve cells pass directly into the fibers of the nerve trunk—indeed, mostly into those crossed, with some on the same side. Claus goes so far as to assume that most of the large cells of the stomatic ganglionic chain are multipolar.

A number of multipolar cells are now known with certainty to be present in the central nervous sytems of crustacea, as it appears in Claus' pictures and from my isolated preparations. Moreover, the multipolar cells which I have presented in the crayfish show, as already indicated, each of the characteristics in their extensions which Deiters set forth to differentiate between axis cylinder—and protoplasma—continuations. Concerning the low number of cells of Deiters in the crayfish, it must be remembered that in the vertebrates as well, presumably only certain groups of cells are constructed according to Deiters' schema.

Final Thoughts on Nerve Cells

Within the year after the crayfish paper appeared, Freud delivered a lecture to the local Psychiatric Society, which was published in 1884 under the title "The structure of the elements of the nervous system." His views on the general question of the relation between nerve structure and nerve functions are summed up in the following passage (cited in Jones, 1953):

If we assume that the fibrils of the nerve have the significance of isolated paths of conduction, then we should have to say that *the pathways which in the*

> *nerve are separate are confluent in the nerve cell:* then the nerve cell becomes the "beginning" of all those nerve fibers anatomically connected with it. . . . I do not know if the existing material suffices to decide the problem, so important for physiology. If this assumption could be established it would take us a good step further in the physiology of the nerve elements: we could imagine that a stimulus of a certain strength might break down the isolation of the fibrils so that the nerve as a unit conducts the excitation, and so on.

This was an interesting conclusion. Freud here was emphasizing the possible role of the neurofibrils within the nerve fibers in conducting nervous activity. This was an erroneous view, kept alive by anatomists; physiologists by that time knew pretty well that the nerve impulse was a membrane property, that is, the impulse spreads along the outer membrane of the nerve, without any involvement of internal structures beyond their providing a pathway for intracellular current. On the other hand, the idea of pathways becoming confluent in the cell body was an echo of Deiters (Chapter 4), and anticipated Sherrington's concept of the nerve cell as a final common path (see Chapter 17). It is interesting in this regard that Sherrington himself was much influenced by Exner (see Sherrington, 1906), who was one of Freud's mentors in Brucke's laboratory. Freud's reference to "the nerve as a unit" in the conduction of activity is also an echo of Deiters, and is an early instance of that phrase in the literature. It suggests that he, and perhaps his colleagues, were beginning to think in general terms of the nerve cell as an anatomical and functional unit. Unfortunately, the specific kinds of mechanisms that might be mediated by this unit are contained in the final phrase "and so on"!

The Significance of Freud's Microscopical Studies

Several of Freud's biographers have suggested that his work made a direct contribution to the neuron doctrine. Thus, according to Jelliffe (1937):

> Freud maintained the essential similarities of the nervous tissues and functions in invertebrates and in vertebrates which in his day was not the generally held opinion. Thus he may correctly be said to have grasped the significance of the neuron theory net work, from his studies on the living tissues of the fresh water crab [sic].

The generalization of results between invertebrates and vertebrates was a valid contribution, but it was neither new nor unique; we have seen that the idea that invertebrates were useful in this respect began with Helmholtz and Kölliker in the 1840s and Leydig in the 1850s. Just what is meant by the "neuron theory net work" is not at all clear. Jelliffe translates *Flusskrebs* as "fresh water crab." The dictionary translation is "river crayfish," and most authors have translated it as "crayfish" (cf. Amacher, 1965; Jones, 1953).

A more persuasive case is made by Ernest Jones. This is perhaps not surprising, given that Jones was chairman of the "Committee" that during Freud's lifetime passed judgment on the purity of doctrine in the psychoanalytic movement; he was in addition the author of the first comprehensive biography of Freud (Jones, 1953). With regard to Freud's observations on the continuity of nerve cell body and axis cylinder, he states that Freud was the first to demonstrate that axis cylinders "are without exception fibrillary in structure" (Jones, 1953). We have seen that many workers had been intrigued by the fibrils contained in nerve fibers. This became a frequent topic of investigation around 1880 as new stains and improved microscopic techniques allowed better visualization of the internal structure of nerve cells (see Chapter 14). Freud certainly made a solid contribution in that progress toward the new field of cytology.

With regard to the significance of Freud's work for the neuron doctrine, Jones sums up his judgment as follows:

> With this paper [on the crayfish] and the two preceding ones [on Petromyzon] Freud had done his share to pave the way for the neurone theory. One might safely go even a little further and claim, as have Brun (1936) and Jelliffe (1937), that Freud had early and clearly conceived the nerve cells and fibrils to be one morphological and physiological unit—the later neurone. . . .

After discussing Freud's final overview in 1884, quoted above, Jones further comments:

> This unitary conception of the nerve cell and processes—the essence of the future neurone theory—seems to have been Freud's own and quite independent of his teachers at the Institute. There is certainly in his few sentences a boldness of thought and a cautiousness in presentation; he makes no real claim. But two comments seem in place. The lecture containing those remarks was delivered four or five years after he had conducted the researches on which they were based, so that the period of rumination was a long one. Then, after so much time for reflection, one would have thought that a little of the free and bold imagination he was so often to display in later years would have carried him the small step further, for he was trembling on the very brink of the important neurone theory, the basis of modern neurology.

In the endeavor to acquire "discipline" he had not yet perceived that in original scientific work there is an equally important place for imagination.

Actually no notice was taken of these precious sentences, so that Freud's name is not mentioned among the pioneers of the neurone theory. . . . It was not the only time that Freud narrowly missed world fame in early life through not daring to pursue his thoughts to their logical—and not far-off—conclusion.

From Nerve Cells to Neurology

Freud received his M.D. degree in Vienna in 1881. Although he appeared to be ready for a career of laboratory investigation on the histology of nerve cells, his prospects for an academic position were poor because Brucke had not just one but two heirs-apparent, Exner and von Fleishl-Marxow, both relatively young and very able. In 1882, Brucke advised Freud, in view of Freud's "bad financial position," to "abandon his theoretical career" (Freud, 1935/1952). Freud seems to have accepted this advice without discussion, and forthwith became a junior resident physician in the main General Hospital in Vienna. Here he began specialization in neurological disorders; also, under Meynert, he pursued microscopical studies of nerve tracts in the human brain, especially the hind brain (medulla oblongata).

In 1885, Freud submitted his application for the position of *Privatdozent*, which was essential for continuing his professional and academic career. The research accomplishments that he included in the application rested on his microscopical studies of nerve cells under Brucke and of nerve tracts in the medulla under Meynert, and clinical studies of a case of cerebral hemorrhage (see Jones, 1953). He had also initiated experiments on the behavioral effects of cocaine (see Byck, 1974). He was successful in his application, and successful as well in obtaining in the same year a travel grant to study under the great neurologist, Charcot, in Paris. With his professional future at last assured, he married in 1886 (Fig. 10).

For the next several years he was absorbed in his work in clinical neurology. His earlier microscopical work, especially on the origin of dorsal root fibers, was usually referenced by the later workers whose studies led to the neuron doctrine (see Chapters 9–14). In 1891, the same year in which the neuron doctrine was promulgated, he published a book on aphasia. From that time he moved step by step toward his theory of psychoanalysis, through the studies of hysteria (1895), dreams (1899), and sexuality (1905).

It might be assumed that during this period he had turned his back on the studies of the nerve cell; for example, the subject of the neuron doctrine receives no mention in his *Autobiography*. But the influence of his early

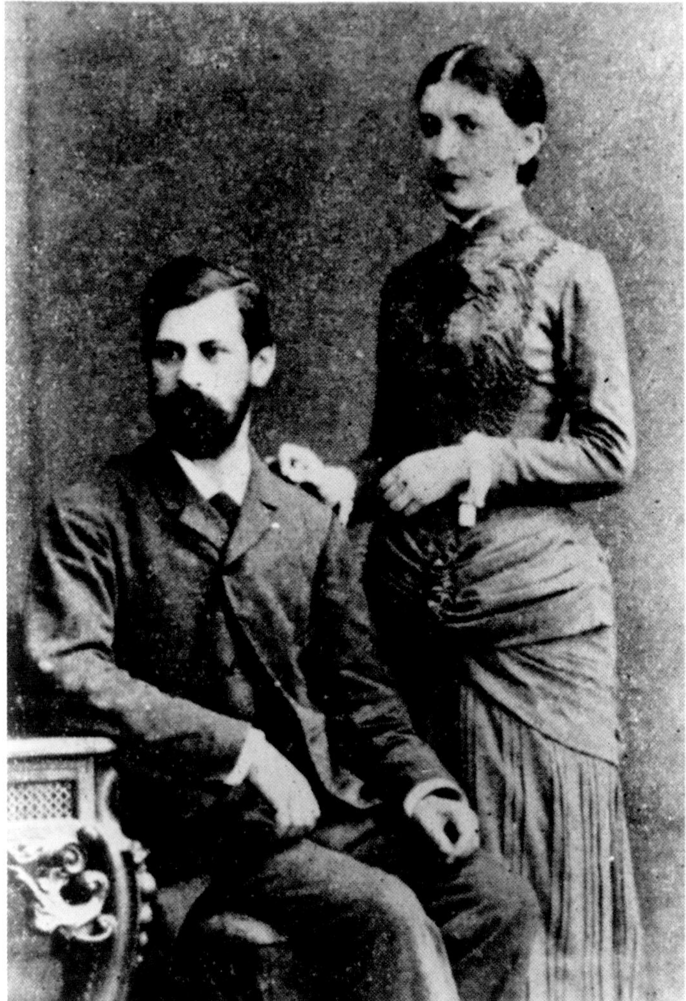

Fig. 10. Sigmund Freud and Martha Bernays, in 1885, the year before they were married. (From Jones, 1953)

neuroanatomical training was not to be shaken so easily. In 1895 Freud tried to put his emerging psychological concepts on a mechanistic basis by writing "Project for a Scientific Psychology," drawing on everything he had learned about nerve cells and brain structure from Brucke and Meynert, as well as from keeping up on the work leading to the neuron doctrine. His hope, which would seem to have gone straight back to Brucke's early vow in the 1840s, was to define how nerve cells and their mechanistic states of energy could generate quantitatively determined psychical processes. After several months of feverish effort he gave up the project in despair; it was not published in his lifetime. However, according to his most recent biographer (Gay, 1989), "he never abandoned his ambition to found a scientific psychology." Previous scholars have analyzed many aspects of his early scientific training (cf. Brun, 1936; Bernfeld, 1951; Amacher, 1965). It would appear that there is a rich field here for analyzing more specifically how Freud's studies of nerve cells found their way—consciously and unconsciously—into his concepts of normal and pathological mental processes.

8

The Revolutionary Method of Golgi

The studies described thus far, from Purkinje's first glimpse of nerve cells to Gerlach's networks, were largely carried out in central Europe, by academic researchers trained and working in the main university centers. Indeed, we can contain most of them within an area bounded by Berlin in the north, Bern in the south, Bonn in the west, and Breslau in the east—an area falling within a circle of diameter of no more than 700 kilometers (see map, Fig. 11). This reflects the leading role that German universities played in the rise of modern science during the nineteenth century. Not that the traditional great universities of Paris, London, Cambridge, Oxford, and Edinburgh did not contribute, but it was less institutional and more in terms of individuals, such as Augustus Waller of London, who described nerve degeneration in 1850 (see Chapter 9), and Louis-Antoine Ranvier of Paris, discoverer of the nodes in myelinated nerves, in 1871. Progress in microscopical science depended, as we have pointed out, on technical advances in optics and chemicals, and on institutes of anatomy and physiology that could provide stable environments for training and research with the new methods.

Despite this concentration of authorities, the attempt to define the nerve cell and all its processes had, as we have seen, slowed to a creeping pace, if not a virtual halt. The debate over the existence and nature of the unseen terminal branches grew more and more polarized and sterile. As Barker (1899) observed, Gerlach's hypotheses "were responsible for an immense amount of polemical writing during the fifteen years which followed their introduction." Resolution of the conflicting views seemed increasingly unlikely. The methods depended on a common set of reagents. Improvements were made by trying different combinations of reagents at different

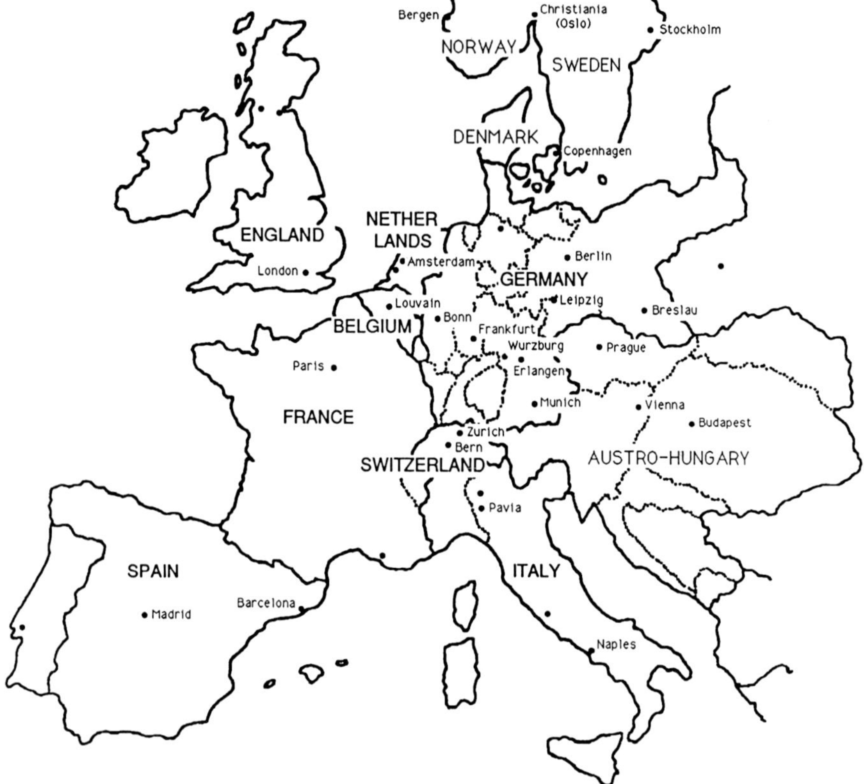

Fig. 11. Map of central Europe, showing political boundaries from 1871 to 1914. Broken lines indicate local and regional boundaries. Cities and universities where the main microscopical work on nerve cells was carried out are indicated.

concentrations. But progress was increasingly marginal. Perhaps Kölliker had been right, that the thinnest nerve processes might defy even the experts, and never be seen. The thought that the problem would not be solved by one of the "experts" probably never occurred to anyone.

Camillo Golgi

Camillo Golgi was born in 1843 in a small village nestled in a valley of the southern Alps, north and east of Milan, in the then city-state of Lombardy. His father was a doctor, who moved the family to another village near Pavia, south of Milan, where Golgi grew up. Golgi studied medicine at the University of Pavia, receiving his degree in 1865 at the age of 22.

Three factors were important in these formative years. First was growing up as the son of a medical practitioner. Golgi was to become one himself, and he retained the outlook of applying laboratory studies to practical clinical problems all his life.

A second important factor was the times. The 1850s and 1860s were critical periods in the birth of Italy as a new unified nation, a period in history known as the *Risorgimento* (rebirth). The Napoleonic Wars, culminating in the Treaty of Vienna in 1815, had left the various city-states of Italy under Austrian hegemony. Unsuccessful uprisings against the Habsburg domination occurred in the European revolutions of 1830 and 1848. However, with France's help, Piedmont, under the great liberal leader Cavour, won its independence in 1859, and annexed Lombardy. Inspired by Garibaldi, the forces for unification swept forward, and the modern form of the Italian nation emerged after the Prussian defeat of France in 1870. Thus, Golgi grew up at a time when "the very air was full of the aspirations, enthusiasms and passions which marked the Italian Risorgimento" (Da Fano, 1926). He was a devoted patriot, and keenly felt Italy's provincial status compared with the centers of learning in Germany.

The third and most important factor in Golgi's life was Pavia. Pavia was a medieval town, whose university dated its earliest beginnings to the year 825. The university was refounded and enlarged in the fourteenth century, and had a distinguished history, even numbering Christopher Columbus among its students. Alessandro Volta was professor of physics there (1779–1819), publishing his discovery of the electric pile, the basis of the electrical battery, in 1800. Of more importance for our interest was a long series of distinguished scholars in biology and medicine. From the past, Spallanzani, a contemporary of Volta, had disproved the doctrine of spontaneous generation, and the anatomist Scarpa had left his name on Scarpa's triangle. Scarpa was an early advocate of the microscope (P. Corsi, unpublished manuscript), and passed this training on to Panizza, who was Golgi's teacher. An older pupil was Corti, who described the organ of hearing in the middle ear. Panizza died in 1867 at the age of 82, and the instrument-maker Amici, builder of microscopes at Pavia, in 1863, also at an advanced age, so Golgi was fortunate to benefit in his early training from their accumulated wisdom and close acquaintance with the developments in microscopy and histology in the centers to the north (P. Corsi, unpublished manuscript).

During his medical courses Golgi took a special interest in microscopy, and received advanced training in these methods from Eusebio Oehl, another of Panizza's pupils (P. Corsi, unpublished manuscript). An important influence in his training was the belief that biology could be reduced to physicochemical and molecular principles. This belief came to him through teachers who had been instilled with the ideals of achieving laws for physiology and histology that had arisen in the 1840s (see Chapter 3), and that we have seen were transmitted to generations of students everywhere (see Freud, Chapter 7). The professors of Pavia were well acquainted with these ideas from the mainstream of science in central Europe: Hoel, "the pioneer physiologist, . . . taught that only histology and experimental physiology could . . . throw a really full light on the normal and pathological conditions of life," and Tommasi, a prominent clinician, reaffirmed the teachings of Panizza and his students in insisting on "the necessity for placing the whole of medicine on sound anatomical foundations" (Da Fano, 1926).

These aspects of Golgi's training show that, despite remoteness from the main centers of research, Pavia nonetheless provided an excellent concentration of scholarly talent, well in touch with current trends and standards, ripe for a young scientist with the talent and zeal to make use of it. Such a favorable combination of factors is the more important the more remote the locality; the young student has to seize on the opportunities at hand, lacking the luxury of being able to visit a number of institutions, each rich in talent and facilities, as we have seen was (and still is) the pattern of training at centers of learning. The high quality of Golgi's training is also worth emphasizing in order to counter any presumptions that the later disfavor that befell his interpretations was due to deficiencies in his training, or to imprecise or even somewhat mystical beliefs. His views deserve a better hearing.

Golgi's Early Studies

For his graduation thesis, in 1865, Golgi "presented a work in which he discussed with great precision and criticism the possible causes of mental disorders and pointed out the necessity for classifying such disorders according to anatomical and aetiological factors" (Chorobski, 1936). This not only reflected the scientific climate of the day, as we have noted, but provided a general outline for his life's work. He began his career as a medical practitioner in the Hospital of San Mateo in Pavia, where he worked from 1865 to 1872. During this time he also started his scientific career. Legend has it (Ferraro, 1953) that he was stimulated to study the cellular composition of the nervous system by reading Virchow's *Cellular Pathology* (1858); by a mentor, Cesar Lumbroso, director of the psychiatric clinic, who believed that psychiatry could be reduced to a positive science (Chorobski, 1937b); and by his close friend Giulio Bizzozero, a younger classmate who in 1867 was appointed director of the Institute of General Pathology (at the age of 20!), and gave devoted support to Golgi's microscopical studies. Here again we see a happy combination of the right factors to support an eager young scholar.

Golgi's first paper, in 1868, was a postmortem microscopical study of pathological changes in the brain of a case of pellagra. There followed a microscopical study of brain tumors and, in 1870, a study "On the alterations in the vascular lymphatics of the cerebellum." These pathological studies were important for several reasons. They directed his attention to nutritional, connective tissue, and vascular factors in the brain. They brought him in direct conflict with established authorities in the field, from whom he did not flinch—he showed, for example, that the perivascular lymphatic spaces of Wilhelm His (see later) were artifacts due to tissue shrinkage. And they started him on the quest for better methods for visualizing brain cells under the microscope.

The work on the cerebellum led to a series of studies of normal brain histology, published in 1870–1872. His interest was focused particularly on the neuroglia. In the cerebellum and cerebrum he described how the glia give off a number of very fine processes: "Many of them are directed towards blood vessels on which they end by means of small expansions, either directly on their walls if they are capillaries, or in their lymph-sheath if they are of greater dimensions" (Da Fano, 1926; see also Chorobski, 1936). These remarks indicate that Golgi came to his studies of the brain with a keen interest in its nutritional requirements as well as its nervous organization.

At this point Golgi's career took a drastic turn for the worse. He had parted company with Lombroso (Da Fano, 1926), and in 1872 his friend and supporter Bizzozero left for Torino. Faced with an acute need to support himself, Golgi was forced to take a position as first resident physician in the Ospizio-Cronici (Home for Incurables) in Abbiategrasso, a small town some 25 kilometers to the northwest of Pavia and 15 kilometers southwest of Milan. It was a bitter disappointment not only to have to leave his beloved Pavia but also apparently to have to give up his scientific career as well. As Da Fano (1926) has remarked, "It would have crushed the aspirations of any man not endowed with his physical strength, force of character and extraordinary tenacity of purpose." He did not give up; according to legend, there in Abbiategrasso, "cut off from every form of scientific activity, his laboratory consisting of a microscope and of a few instruments collected in the kitchen of his home, working evenings by candlelight, he discovered his epoch-making chromate of silver method, *la reazione nera* [the 'black reaction']." (Chorobski, 1936; see also Da Fano, 1926; Ferraro, 1953).

The "Black Reaction"

In his early studies Golgi had started with the routine histological methods of that time, which as we have seen included dissociation of the tissue by fine dissection or maceration, and treatment with various agents for fixing (hardening) and staining the tissue. He soon found that the best staining of both nerve cells and neuroglia came from hardening the tissue in solutions of potassium bichromate [$K(CO_4)_2$] or osmic acid [H_2Os_4]. Osmic acid was scarce and expensive, and his straitened circumstances at Abbiategrasso forced Golgi to use the cheaper potassium bichromate or ammonia instead.

For staining, Golgi experimented with various agents, including silver. Silver reagents had come into prominence in the middle of the nineteenth century for their use in photographic development, following the invention of the daguerrotype around 1840. Histologists had tried these reagents for histological staining, but the results had not been significantly better than those obtained with other staining agents up to that time. We do not know how Golgi hit on the use of silver nitrate solutions for staining brain tissue blocks or slices previously subjected to prolonged immersion in solutions of potassium bichromate. All that is known is that Golgi announced the new method and its application in 1873 in a brief paper entitled "Sulla struttura della grigia del cervello" in the August 2 issue of the *Italian Medical Gazette* (in Santini, 1975):

ON THE STRUCTURE OF THE GRAY MATTER OF THE BRAIN

Researches carried out by Doctor Camillo Golgi, Head Physician of the Hospice for Incurables in Abbiategrasso

(Preliminary Communication)

Taking advantage of the method, found by me, of the black staining of the elements of the brain, staining obtained by the prolonged immersion of the pieces, previously hardened with potassium or ammonium bichromate, in a 0.50 or 1.0% solution of silver nitrate, I happened to discover some facts concerning the structure of the cerebral gray matter that I believe merit immediate communication.

I. [*Axis Cylinder*]

Starting with O. Deiters who, induced by the sole analogy with what he had observed in the spinal cord, was the first to teach that among the multiple prolongations of the nerve cells one, called by him nervous prolongation of the *cylinder axis*, had special characteristics and a particular significance as it was destined to continue directly into a nerve fiber, with increasing agreement it was always believed that a constant characteristic of the prolongation itself is to remain simple. Countering this firm agreement of the investigators I must now maintain that the above-mentioned prolongation, instead of remaining simple, gives rise to branches, and in good numbers, which likewise emit filaments, and these in turn give rise to others, thus resulting in a complicated system of threads widespread everywhere in the cerebral gray matter.

The prolongation in question, arisen either directly from the cell body, or from the root of one of the large protoplasmatic prolongations emanating from the cell surface, from its point of emergence up to the distance for which it can be followed by the usual preparation methods (20–30 μ), gradually thins until it becomes an extremely fine filament remaining, however, simple, usually rectilinear, regular, smooth. At the said distance the prolongation often exhibits a slight tortuosity; from there at times it remains simple for a certain distance without beginning to emit lateral filaments for a further 30 or 40 micromillimeters; more frequently the branchings begin immediately after the tortuosity and continue at quite regular tracts until the success of the black staining makes it possible to follow the prolongation. This maintains its regularity and smoothness but assumes a slightly meandering path (perhaps due to the shrinkage of the tissue) and besides, with an almost imperceptible gradation, often becomes thinner and thinner, finally becoming extremely fine. The maximum distance over which I could follow it was more than 600 μ (a distance more than six times longer than that at which Koschennikoff had allegedly seen the beginning of the medullary sheath) and up to this extreme limit, in well-stained preparations, I was able to see the detachment of the filaments.

As for the fact of the existence of the ramifications, far from resembling the other prolongations so notoriously branched in the most complicated way, it can, on the contrary, be distinguished from the latter even more decidedly because its way of issuing filaments is so peculiar as to constitute another of its given characteristics; in fact, its secondary filaments consistently arise sharply at a right angle and, in their aspect, their manner of running and branching do not differ at all from the former; in regard to direction, they run horizontally sometimes for a short tract and other times over a long tract, then generally tend to bend upward toward the periphery of the cortex and one can follow for a long distance. The behavior of the branches of the third and fourth order is entirely similar. No better comparison regarding the manner of branching and the general appearance of these filaments can be had than with the manner of distribution of the peripheral nerves, for example, the corneal nerves; this, it seems to me, can be of some value for the study of the physiological significance of these filaments.

At the moment I am not in a position to trace the complete history either of the properly named nervous prolongation or of filaments which arise from it; however, in relation to the former, I believe I can from now on refute the generally held opinion that it always goes on to constitute the *cylinder axis* of the medullary nerve fibers; that is, at least, not the general rule. The branching and the simultaneous progressive thinning are alone sufficient to invalidate that opinion; in a certain number of cases I was able to see that the prolongation in question, after running in a straight line for very long tracts (400–600 μ) and after having risen to a very great number of secondary branches, finally becomes of an incommensurable fineness, subdivided into three to four branches taking different direction, arising at a short distance from one another, tortuous, which branchlets I could follow only for a short distance. In spite of all this and particularly following the direct observations of Koschennikoff, Hadlich, Boll, etc., I do not intend to deny that sometimes the nervous prolongation continues directly with a medullary fiber without undergoing branching or other events; however, in my opinion, as regards the pyramidal cells, this would be an exception rather than the rule.

In regard to the final destination of the branches of the nervous prolongation I can only affirm that they certainly connect with granules of the gray matter (perhaps passing through the granules themselves) to which other filaments of identical aspect coming from other directions also project. Then I must mention as probable another fact which, once verified, could be of great importance for the study of the physiology of the nervous system; I mean *the anastomosis among the nervous filaments originating from the prolongation of the cylinder axis* [italics added], of several ganglion cells. In the cerebral cortex and in the gray matter in general there is certainly to be found a very widespread network of filaments anastomosing one with the other which for appearance and manner of running and branching, as well as for their connection with the granules, correspond completely to the filaments the derivation of which from Deiters' prolongation of the ganglion cells is easily verified.

II. Protoplasmic prolongations

Another series of interesting facts made me observe [*sic*] my new preparation method, and these concern the behavior of the so-called protoplasmatic or ramified prolongations.

Among the various opinions held by authors on this subject I will only mention those of Rindfleisch and Gerlach, between which there is some slight discord. The former holds that the protoplasmatic prolongations, after breaking up into a series of very fine fibrils, dissolve in an interstitial granular substance (diffuse nervous substance according to the old concept of Wagner, Henle, etc.) in which substance allegedly would also terminate, after breaking up likewise into bundles of fibrils of extreme fineness, the *cylinder axes* of many medullary fibers. Gerlach, with whom not long ago Butzke, Boll, and others associated themselves, is on the other hand of the opinion that the protoplasmatic prolongations, breaking up indefinitely into filaments, form a nervous reticulum *so fine as to be visible only under the strongest immersion systems*; from this reticulum by means of brushes of filaments the *cylinder axes* of the nerve fibers would arise, with the end result of a continuous nervous reticulum between these latter and the protoplasmatic prolongations.

On this point also I am essentially in disagreement with the observation of the above-cited authors.

The protoplasmatic prolongations, instead of breaking up indefinitely, either to dissolve in an amorphous fundamental substance (Rindfleisch) or to result in the formation of a reticulum (Gerlach), once they are reduced to the state of ramifications of the second, third or at the most of the fourth order, end instead at the cells of the interstitial tissue. What precise relationships, then, exist between the above prolongations and the cell bodies—if, that is, they retain their individuality, or closely connect themselves, almost blend with the cell bodies—I was unable to discover; probably both cases occur; in fact, at times it looks as if the prolongations cross the body of the interstitial cells to reach others further away, while at other times the prolongations definitely terminate in the cells; in the latter case it is probable that the cellular protoplasmatic substance fuses with that of the prolongations issuing to the same cell body.

The convergence of the protoplasmatic prolongations to the cells of the interstitial tissue can be recognized in a special way in the case of those of the apex of the pyramidal cells of the cortex. Already toward the middle of the cortical gray layer the apical prolongation of the large pyramidal cells, which generally are situated around the inner third of the same layer, often divides into two branches each of which is directed obliquely upward, giving off here and there very fine side branches, until, having arrived at the proximity of the surface, thinned, but still maintaining a marked thickness, it now ends up in the cells encountered here; now and more frequently it splits again in two, three or at the most four branches, each of which runs to be connected with a cell either of the surface or of the above-mentioned horizontal layer. The latter, then, are connected to each other by means of numerous filaments, so that at some places, near the surface of the cortex, there exists a very complicated network. In some regions it also appeared to me that a connection existed between the surface cells of the brain (which I described as flattened cells issuing prolongations horizontally, vertically, and obliquely toward the interior of the cortex) and those of the series described above situated at some depth within the cortex.

Regarding the secondary branches arising from the sides of the apical prolongations, these end at the small cells situated in the interstices.

The same fact occurs in the case of the basal protoplasmic prolongations, although it is very difficult to verify since these prolongations do not run to the nearest cell but go on for long distances, frequently running also in irregular paths; on one side, however, the elegant ganglion cells with prolongations of extraordinary length are seen; on the other side, particularly in the internal half of the cortex, large cellular bodies are seen from which emanate, or better, at which arrive an enormous number of filaments which for the most part are completely similar to the branches of the second, third and fourth order of the protoplasmatic prolongations, but only on very rare occasions can one see the connection between these cells with those.

I believe it is opportune also to mention the following fact which is probably very important for the physiology of the cerebral organ: to the cells to which the branches of the protoplasmatic prolongations run, other filaments also run from different directions which for their smooth uniform aspect and for a certain appearance of rigidity, as well as their pattern of running and branching, fully correspond to the above-described system of filaments which emanate from the nervous prolongation of the ganglion cells. Do they really belong to such a system? To me it seems probable, more so in view of the fact, observed by me, that the filaments emanating from the nervous prolongations connect with the granules; however, I do not believe I can give a pronouncement on this with absolute certainty.

[*Summary*]

When, with further research, I have better verified certain findings and discovered new details, perhaps I will be permitted to add to the reported facts appropriate and conclusive considerations; for the moment I limit myself to the following few comments:

Regarding the system of filaments emanating from the nervous prolongation of the ganglion cells, it seems to me that two hypotheses may be advanced, both supported by valid arguments and perhaps one at least in part as true as the other. The first is that they are the trophic nerves of the brain; the other is that they contribute in some way, which I do not believe I can specify, to the origin of the nerves. In support of the first we should have: their essentially nervous nature; their peculiar aspect and way of running and branching which recalls, as I already noted, the peripheral nerves; finally, their impinging upon the cells of the interstitial tissue. The second hypothesis could seem too arbitrary, and indeed, strictly regarding the brain I could advance in its favor no positive evidence of observation apart from the ramification of the nerve fibers which enter the gray substance from the medullary layers, ramification which is analogous to that of the nervous prolongation. However, it appears to me that in support of the new manner of origin or termination of the nerves to which I have just obscurely referred, the findings, more eloquent on such a peculiarity, which I obtained in the cerebellum and in the spinal cord may be of value.

In fact, in the former, besides the complicated ramifications of the prolongation of the *cylinder axis* of the Purkinje cells, I found: I. very complex ramification of the nerve fibers, which from the medullary rays crossing the granular layer run toward the external cortical layer, and, what is more important, a way of branching analogous to that of the nerve prolongations of ganglion cells both of the brain and the cerebellum, that is, at right angles and visible under the lowest magnification (80–100 diameters); II. insertion, at right angles, of some branches of the nerve fibers into a particular system of horizontal or curved fibers, which exist in great numbers in the deep half of the outer layer of the cerebellar cortex, to the constitution of which system of fibers take part some filaments emanating from the nervous prolongation of the Purkinje cells (my interesting observation on the cerebellum will be described in a subsequent publication). In the spinal cord I found likewise an elegant ramification of the fibers of the roots; but here also, far from the supposed brush-like ramification occurring, the secondary branches always arise isolated and at right angles.

In regard to the significance of the cells upon which converge the protoplasmatic prolongations, it appears to me that two suppositions can still be made: either they serve to establish the anatomical connection between the nerve cells, or else they are nutritional organs of the nerve cells themselves. Now it seems to me inopportune to list the arguments in favor of either hypothesis; I will only say why I believe I can propound in favor of the second, the more so since, I believe, it permits us also to explain the phenomena of functional connection which, not too long ago, one accepted only by admitting the direct connection or anastomosis between the cellular prolongations. And indeed if, as it is, the result of the excitation, even psychic, of the cerebral nerve cells is an alteration of nutrition—that is, an acceleration of the processes of reduction and an increase of absorption of the nutritional material—it seems obvious to me to suppose that, given the excitation of some groups of cells, the modifications which occur in these groups are participated in by other cellular groups whose roots (protoplasmatic prolongations) taken up nutrients from the same sources and are probably under the influence of the same nutritional nerve filaments.

In considering this paper one notes that the new observations on the structure of the nerve cell came wrapped in speculations about what still cannot quite be seen, and what could be the functional significance of the findings. This was to set the pattern for Golgi's subsequent studies of different brain regions, as well as for his attempt to derive overall principles of neuronal organization. It is important to distinguish carefully, therefore, between the experimental facts and the theoretical interpretations, in order to arrive at an accurate assessment of Golgi's contributions to the development of concepts of the neuron. A consideration of the entire corpus of Golgi's work goes beyond the scope of our inquiry. By discussing the main findings in the first paper cited above, we will see how many of Golgi's facts and concepts were present or implicit at this early stage; we will then discuss his collected works in the middle 1880s, which not only summarized his views but served as the primary means by which his method and his views became known to the outside world and stimulated the renaissance of anatomical studies of the nerve cell in the late 1880s.

Golgi's Discoveries

In section I of his paper, Golgi considers the axis cylinder, the part of the neuron we now call the axon. He confirms the observation of Deiters that the axis cylinder has special characteristics that differentiate it from all the other processes emanating from the cell body. He also confirms that the axis cylinder may continue to become a medullated fiber. However, the axis cylinder does not remain a simple prolongation, as Deiters maintained; instead, it gives off branches. Golgi characterizes the pattern of this branching: the way that the axis cylinder starts to become tortuous in its course; the branches tend to come off at right angles; the branching pattern resembles that of peripheral nerves; some of the branches bend back toward the region of origin, i.e., are recurrent.

In these observations, Golgi provided the first complete and accurate description of the path of the axis cylinder from its cell of origin to its entering the white matter. He also gave the first description of what we now call "axon collaterals" and their pattern of branching. As Golgi showed, these collaterals arise where the axon is still in its region of origin, and extend into and recur within that region. The discovery of the axon collaterals is one of Golgi's solid and enduring contributions to knowledge of the neuron.

Golgi's third finding regarding the axis cylinder was that, contrary to Deiters' belief, not all axis cylinders are connected to the white matter;

some give rise to many branches that all end within that local region of the brain. This was soon to become the basis of Golgi's distinction between two basic types of nerve cell: type I, those with long axis cylinders, and type II, those with short axis cylinders. The latter comprise what we now call "short-axon cells", and represent another important discovery by Golgi.

In section II of the paper Golgi considers the protoplasmic prolongations, as Deiters called them, or what we now call "dendrites." His new method allows one to see much more of the branching pattern of these prolongations. Thus, he is able to distinguish more clearly between the apical and basal prolongations (what we now call apical and basal dendrites) of cortical neurons. He is also able to see second, third, and higher orders of branching from a given dendritic trunk. Although he notes the "elegance of the ganglion cells with prolongations of extraordinary length," he does not further characterize the distinctiveness of the branching patterns for different cells. Thus, his actual observations on the dendrites were limited. As we shall see, this appears to be due, at least in part, to his notions about their functions.

Finally, we note two deficiencies in the paper that limit its impact. First, the description of the method is so brief as to be of little value to anyone wishing to take up the method and verify and extend the findings. This has been ascribed to the fact that the method was so capricious that Golgi himself could not depend on it and waited many years before publishing a full account of his procedures (cf. Clarke and O'Malley, 1968). Second, there is no illustration of nerve cells stained by the method. Given the dazzling effect of Golgi-stained nerve cells on later workers, it is odd that examples should be missing from this first paper. We have previously noted that anatomists of that era were often remiss in this regard, feeling that the written account was a better claim to priority than a drawing. Also, the earliest results may have been less complete, clear, and dramatic than the impression conveyed by later drawings, which, by Golgi as well as most other authors, tended to be composites or idealizations of the actual primary data.

Golgi's Speculations

If we turn now from facts to speculations, we find a characteristic of Golgi's contributions to neuroanatomy evident in this first report, and that is the way he saw his data within a framework of concepts about their possible functional significance. Now there is nothing inherently wrong in a scientist doing this; in fact, the best science combines acute observation of facts with a mind prepared to interpret those facts. Unfortunately, Golgi's imagination was most stimulated by those aspects he could see least well. The most critical of these were the fine terminal branches of axis cylinder branches (axon collaterals) and protoplasmic prolongations (dendrites).

With regard to the axis cylinder branches, he speculates that they certainly connect to the "granules" (i.e., cells) of the gray matter. He then states as "probable" that there are anastomoses between the "nervous filaments" (i.e., fine terminal branches) of the axis cylinder, so that "there is certainly to be found a very widespread network of filaments anastomosing one with the other" throughout the gray matter of the brain. In fact, the method was quite inadequate for establishing this; thinning of the terminal branches was mostly due to failure of complete staining, and the branches were too thin in any case for the purported anastomoses to be resolved clearly by the light microscope. This fateful misinterpretation was to become his reticular theory of nervous organization.

With regard to the protoplasmic prolongations, on the other hand, Golgi denied emphatically that any anastomoses take place between them, as had been postulated by Gerlach. Golgi's network thus was entirely composed of his newly discovered axis cylinder branches; he sharply differentiated it from Gerlach's network of protoplasmic prolongations (dendrites). Of course, the method was inadequate for assessing this question as well.

This left the question of the possible functions of the two types of processes. To Golgi the function of the network of axis cylinder branches was clear: the axis cylinders were the true "nervous" processes, and the network of their branches would subserve the physiological functions of the nervous system. The function of the protoplasmic prolongations was less clear. Golgi opted to deny them an important role in establishing anatomical connections between nerve cells, mainly on the argument that functional connections could only be mediated by anastomoses. This is an important point because it indicates that anatomists could not yet conceive of a functional connection (what we now call a "synapse"; Chapter 17) between two separate nerve processes.

Golgi favored instead the idea that the protoplasmic prolongations serve a nutritive role. This idea may be traced to his previous studies of glia. It may be recalled that he had described the way the fine glial processes terminate in relation to small blood vessels. In a somewhat analogous fashion, the protoplasmic processes seemed to terminate on cells of the interstitial tissue. We have seen that this idea of a nutritive role for the protoplasmic processes was an old and persistent one.

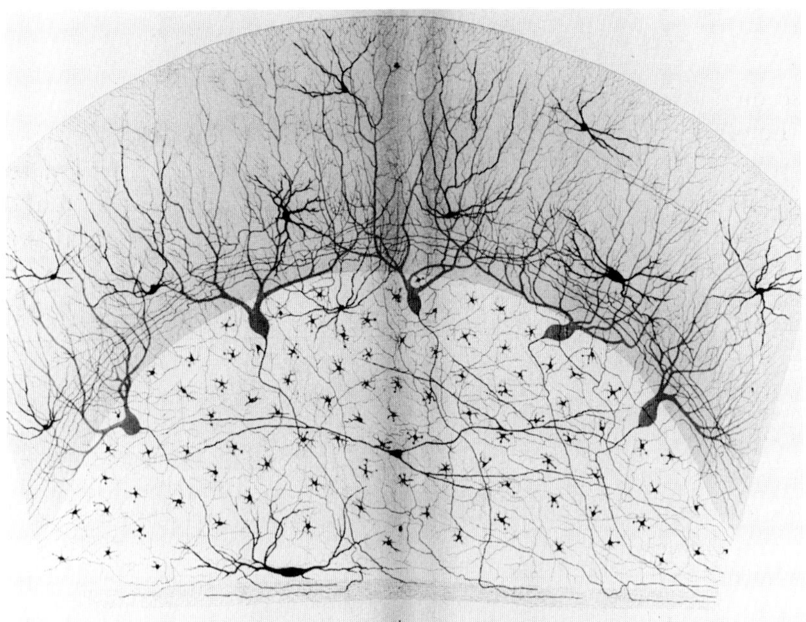

Fig. 12. A diagram by Golgi of the nervous elements of the cerebellum.

"*Fragment of vertical section of a human cerebellar convolution.*

The drawing shows especially the enormous complexity of relations existing between the nervous system fibers and the ganglion cells; it has to be considered as semi-schematic because it represents a synthesis of observations taken from several preparations; however, each element is drawn to correspond to reality with regard to localization, relations, shapes and ramifications of nerve fiber [axon] and cellular prolongations [dendrites], at least as they appear after black staining.

Even without descriptive labels [in the drawing], three cerebellar layers are easily distinguished: *molecular layer, granular layer, nerve fiber layer.*

Molecular layer. One can see very clearly, because of the intense staining, some of the small nerve cells characteristic of this layer. I want to draw special attention to many differences that, relative to the point of origin and successive path, are shown by the nervous prolongation (red thread) [axon], with which all these cells are provided. Regarding those that are situated in the inferior third of this layer, it should be noted that the same prolongation [i.e. axon] evidently joins with the layer of horizontal nerve fibers existing within, conforming exactly in its course and mode of ramification to individual fibers that constitute that plexus.

In the deep third is drawn, in red, a part of the complicated plexus, partly accentuated; into the fibers running in parallel at the margin of the layer in question are inserted many fibers that derive from the granule layer, by the same fiber emanating finally innumerable fibrils, which, with successive ramifications, extend toward the top. The plexus evidently is not as limited as it appears, but extends throughout all the thickness of this layer; the drawing corresponds to the most frequent mode of presentation in my preparations.

Along the deep border of the molecular layer are drawn with lighter color some

Golgi's Publications

Golgi studied several regions of the brain with his new method, and published the results in a series of papers over the following decade. The first region reported in detail was the cerebellum, in 1874, followed, in 1875, by the olfactory bulb, where he first gave a description of the method and showed illustrations of stained cells. In these early studies his idea of two main cell types, long-axon and short-axon, had already gelled. The example of the cerebellum is shown in Figure 12, where the long-axon type (later known as Golgi type I) is exemplified by the Purkinje cell, and the short-axon type (later Golgi type II) is represented by the large cell type that he discovered and that is now known as the cerebellar Golgi cell. For comparison, his view of the cellular composition of the hippocampus and dentate gyrus is shown in Figure 13.

Golgi was later accused of not illustrating diagramatically his concept of a reticulum or network, but the idea was quite manifest (certainly at least to him) in diagrams such as those of Figures 12 and 13. The network was

---

Purkinje cells. Their nervous prolongation [axon], after giving rise to a certain number of secondary fibrils [axon collaterals], finally reaches the layer of nerve fibers.

Layer of granules. Here are drawn: 1. The so-called granules, in much less quantity than actually exists, the nervous prolongation [axon], with which each of these elements is provided, is lightly accentuated. It may be noted that in man, the same elements are much smaller than in the rabbit, cat, and calf. 2. One nerve cell, identical to the small cells in the molecular layer located above, at the level of the body of the Purkinje cell. 3. Two quite large ganglion cells are shown, the one with a triangular shape, situated toward the middle of the layer, the other with fusiform shape, situated close to the border with the medullated [fiber] layer. The nervous prolongation [axon] of both these cells is lightly sketched. - This type of solitary cell having a variety of different shapes is quite different in the human cerebellum.

Layer of nerve fibers. This layer is portrayed only as a thin strip.

Among the horizontal fibers schematically rendered, it is possible to see some fibers reproduced in black. Following their path from below to above, some of them appear to find their way to the body of the Purkinje cells, these same prolongations maintaining their individuality although they give rise to some secondary branches; one can see others that instead cross the granular layer, subdividing in a very complicated manner, becoming lost in a plexus in which it is difficult, if not impossible, to see their ultimate behavior.

Many of the clearest ramifications of this secondary category of fiber certainly penetrate into the molecular layer, participating in the formation of the plexus which exists there; the same thing happens to some ramifications of the fibers emanating from the nervous prolongations [axons] of the Purkinje cells." (Golgi, 1886, Plate XI)

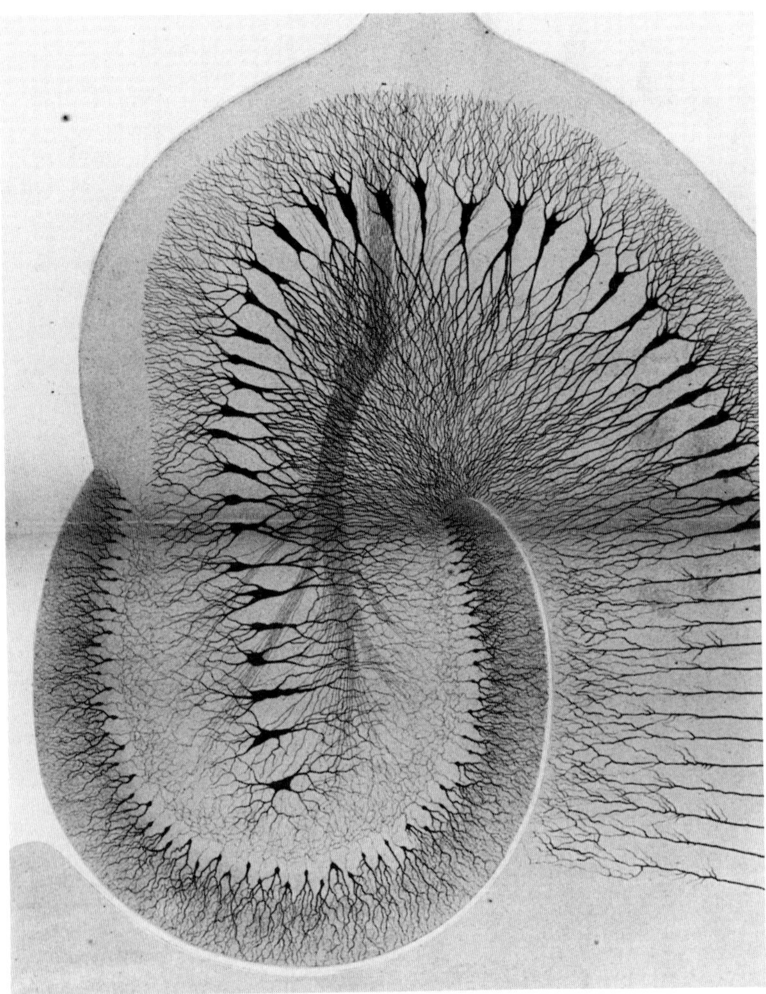

Fig. 13. A diagram by Golgi of the nervous elements of the hippocampus and fascia dentata.

"*Fragment of a vertical transverse section of the great foot of the Hippocampus of the rabbit.*

The diagram illustrates particularly the mode by which a fascicle of nerve fibers comes in relation to the small ganglion cells of the fascia dentata. - Between the [fascicle of] nervous fibers still maintaining themselves as individual elements and the nervous prolongations [axons] of the small cells, exists a complicated network, occupying a semicircular area, which, especially toward the deep part, has indeterminate borders.

It is on entering into this network, that, ramifying, a part of the nervous prolongations [axons] lose themselves, as well as all the fibers deriving from the fascicle. The latter, issuing from the semicircle formed by the fascia dentata, traverse the zone of the grey layer of the convolution, occupied by the bodies of the cells which belong to this layer, and go to join the fibers of the *Alveus* and the *Fimbria*." (Golgi, 1886, Plate XXII) formed by the collateral branches of the long axons and the terminal ramifications of the short axons. Incoming fibers made connection with this network, either directly through their terminal branches or indirectly through cells in the region, and the long axons carried the output from the network to other regions (see especially Fig. 13 and its legend).

In a period of just a few years the hippocampus, the motor and sensory areas of the cerebral cortex, the region of the corpus callosum, the olfactory lobe, the spinal cord, peripheral and central nerve fibers, and glia cells came under scrutiny. It was one of those wonderful periods of productivity that happen to a scientist who has a method and a mission. Nor did these studies of nerve cells define the limits of his energies and curiosity. Already in 1874, Golgi was opening a new era in histopathology by showing that in a case of chorea there were pathological changes in nerve cell structure in the brain. This was followed by studies of nerve cell degenerative changes and the histology of brain tumors. In 1878–1880, he discovered and reported the special organs in muscle tendons that now bear his name (Golgi tendon organs), describing their innervation pattern and correctly deducing that they must play an important role in muscular sensations. Also during this same period of intensive work on the nervous system came laboratory and clinical studies of blood transfusions (1879) and pathological changes in the kidney (1882 and 1884). And we shall see later that this was by no means the end of his labors.

This tremendous productivity rapidly brought him local notice. In 1875, he was called back to Pavia, becoming full professor of histology and general pathology in 1881. However, owing to the isolation of Italy, geographically, culturally, and linguistically from central Europe, Golgi was unknown to scientists elsewhere. To overcome this, he set about in the early 1880s to collect his main studies of nerve cells and have them translated into a widely used language. The first step was a translation into French, which appeared as several long reviews in the *Archives Italiennes de Biologie* of 1883 and 1884 (the slow emergence of Italy as a nation is reflected in the fact that this important biological journal was published in French). At about the same time, translations of parts of his work appeared in English (1883; 1885). Publication of the entire work *Sulla Fina Anatomia degli Organi Centrali del Sistema Nervoso* (*On the Fine Structure of the Central Organs of the Nervous System*) in monograph form in Italian took place in 1886. German translation had to await the publication of the *Opera Omnia* in 1903.

These works in the 1880s had the double merit of presenting a synthesis of Golgi's views on nervous structure and organization, and providing them in more accessible forms. Since these were the main means by which his work became known, it is useful to have some acquaintance with them. We here cite the passages in which he presents his conclusions regarding the structural and functional relations between nerve cells (Golgi, 1883):

> In conclusion, as regards the greatest part of the nervous centers, far from the described individual and isolate connections between cells and nervous fibers there is seen, on the contrary, an evidently direct disposition, by which is effected *the greatest possible complication in the relations between the two* [italics added]. And this law exists, not only as regards the several elements or groups of them, but also as regards entire provinces.
>
> Another observation occurs to me: The concept of the so-called *location of the cerebral functions,* should it be insisted on accepting it in a rigorous sense, would not be in perfect harmony with the anatomical data, or at the least, it should now be admitted only in a somewhat limited and conventional sense. It being demonstrated, for example, that a nervous fibre is in relation with extensive groups of gangliar cells, and that the gangliar elements of entire provinces, and also of various neighboring provinces, are conjoined by means of a diffuse network, to the formation of which all the various categories of cells and nervous fibres of these provinces contribute, *it is naturally difficult to understand a rigorous functional localization, as many would desire to have it* [italics added]. At the most, we might speak of *prevalent or elective* paths of transmission, and of provinces, not rigorously limited, which, as *prevalently or electively* excited, so prevalently do they react in a sense corresponding to the excitation effected.
>
> I would lastly allude to another question, already touched on in the descriptive statement precedently made, and which should have relation to one of the questions which we have proposed to solve; it is, whether in the nervous centers there exist elementary differences which may correspond to the different functional task devolved on them.
>
> As respects this question we can say that a difference truly exists, but it exclusively regards the different mode of deportment of the nervous prolongation. But from the point of view of the supposable relation existing between the anatomical differences of the elements, and their function, we cannot take into account either the form or the size of the cellular bodies. It is, however, true that there are prevalently large gangliar cells (of the first type) which, being provided with a nervous prolongation that puts itself into direct relation with the nervous fibres, should be designated as motor, or psycho-motor cells, whilst, conversely, there are prevalently small cells (gangliar cells of the second type), provided with a nervous prolongation which divides complexly to place itself in direct relation with the nervous fibres; these cells probably belong to the sensory, or psycho-sensory sphere; but these *relations have so many expectations that it is not possible to establish any general law* [italics added].
>
> That, in correspondence with the functional difference of the cells, there may at the same time also exist chemical or other differences, cannot be excluded in any manner; rather is it probable that they do exist; but from the anatomical point of view, I think I may assert that the difference described by me is, at the least, the most important.
>
> At the end of this study as to the mode of origin of the nervous fibres of

the centers, it appears to me useful to state, in a series of resumary conclusions, so much as directly or indirectly regards so important a question.

First. In studying the problem of the origin of the nerves, in the different provinces of the central nervous system, it becomes apparent that there exist some secondary differences, relative to the morphology, disposition and distribution of the elementary parts, as the relations between the cells and nervous fibres, there exist constant laws, and an absolute correspondence between the diverse provinces.

Second. In general, the nervous cells, by their form, the special aspect of the cellular body and of the nucleus, the mode in which the prolongations have origin from them, as also by the aspect, and the mode of ramifying of the prolongations, may, by an expert observer be differentiated from the other cellular elements; yet, no one of the characters assigned can be given as absolute so true is this that, holding as the basis of our judgement these data alone, it is not a rare case to find that we must remain uncertain whether some cellular elements should be considered as of connective or of nervous nature; and it is known that the elements are not few, relative to which the judgements of histologists are contradictory. There is, however, an absolute characteristic datum from which a cell may, with certainty, be designated as nervous, and this consists in *the presence of a prolongation (always unique) different from all the others* [italics added], and destined to be put into relation with the nervous fibres, or to be transformed into these.

Third. The so-called protoplasmic prolongations [dendrites] in no way, either directly or indirectly, give origin to nervous fibres, from these they always maintain themselves independent; they have, on the contrary, intimate relations with the connective cells, therefore *their functional purpose should be sought for from the point of view of the nutrition of the nervous texture* [italics added]; that is to say, they probably represent the paths through which the diffusion of the nutritive plasma is brought from the blood vessels to the gangliar cells.

Fourth. The gangliar cells of all the provinces of the nervous system, by a law which has no exception, are in relation with the nervous fibres by means of *one only of their prolongations* [italics added], that which, in homage to the author who first made it the subject of a particularized description, has been designated the prolongation of *Deiters*, or the cylinder-axis prolongation, but which we shall always call the nervous prolongation [axon]. Wherefore, from the point of view of their specific function, *all the central nerve cells may be considered as monopolar.*

Fifth. The fact, many times noted, that it is only by means of the nervous prolongation with which they are provided, that the gangliar cells are put into relation with the organs by which they extrinsicate their functional activities (nervous fibres of sense) is related to another fact of notable importance, which is that the difference between the nervous cells of sense and those of motion, principally, if not exclusively, relates to the mode in which, by means of this prolongation, their connection with the corresponding fibres of sense and motion is effected. *The relative differences as to the form, size and also, with some exceptions, as to the situation of the gangliar cells, falls into a very secondary rank* [italics added]. As an evident corollary of this law we ought to hold that, in performing the anatomical study of the nervous centers, *the function of the gangliar cells can, with secure foundation, be argued only from the deportment of the respective nervous prolongations* [italics added] and from the manner in which their connection with corresponding fasces of nervous fibres of known function is effected.

Sixth. All that has been asserted with regard to the nervous prolongation of the gangliar cells, first by *Deiters* and afterwards confirmed by the generality of anatomists who have occupied themselves with this subject, is erroneous, to-wit: that, maintaining constant simplicity, it passes directly to constitute the cylinder-axis or a nervous fibre. Instead of this, *the rule is, that this prolongation gives origin, at greater or less distances from its departure from the cell, to a more or less large number of filaments* [italics added], which are so many nervous fibrillae.

Seventh. The behavior of the nervous prolongation is not alike in all the gangliar cells; indeed in this respect notable differences may be shown; in many gangliar cells the nervous prolongation, subdividing complexly, takes part, in its totality, in the formation of a fine nervous network, which is found diffused in all the strata of the gray substance; in many gangliar cells, instead of this, the nervous prolongation, although it gives off some filaments, in like manner destined to take part in the formation of the above diffuse network, yet arrives in the medullary strata maintaining its proper individuality, and there, in fact, it forms the cylinder-axis of a medullary nervous fibre.

Eighth. In relation to the different mode of behavior of the nervous prolongation, in the gray substance of the nervous centers, two types of gangliar cells may be distinguished, viz:

(a.) Gangliar cells whose nervous prolongation, though it gives off some lateral threads, maintains its proper individuality, and passes on to place itself in direct relation with the nervous fibres [cells of long axon].

(b.) Gangliar cells whose nervous prolongation, subdividing complexly, loses its proper individuality and takes part *in toto* in the formation of a diffuse nervous network. These cells, therefore, would have only indirect relations with the nervous fibres [cells of short axon]

The arguments resulting from accurate studies of the two types of cells mentioned, give a sufficiently valid foundation to the decision, that the cells of the first type are of motor, or psycho-motor nature, and that those of the second type are, on the contrary, sensorial or psychosensorial.

Ninth. The two types of gangliar cells recognized by us, far from being found separately in this or that other region of the central organs, *are constantly found associated* [italics added] at the most in some zones, as regards their different function, there is noted a prevalence of one or of the other type, or it is observed that in the same zone, a series of cells belongs to the first type, whilst the others belong to the second.

Tenth. The nervous fibres, also, entering into the different strata of the gray substance, may, in relation to the behavior of the respective cylinder-axis, be divided into two categories, viz:

(a.) Nervous fibres whose cylinder axis, though it administers some secondary fibrillae (which subdividing are lost in the diffuse network), yet preserves its proper individuality, and passes on to place itself in direct relations with gangliar cells of the first type, and continues itself in the related nervous prolongation.

(b.) Nervous fibres whose cylinder-axis, dividing complexly loses its proper individuality, and in totality takes part in the formation of the diffuse network mentioned.

In the same manner as we judge, the two types of gangliar cells described, to belong, the one to the motor, psycho-motor sphere, and the other to the sensory, or psycho-sensory, so do we hold that the first category of nervous fibres belongs to the motor, and the second to the sensory sphere.

Eleventh. In all the strata of the gray substance of the central nervous organs, there exists *a fine and complicate diffuse nervous network* [italics added], in the formation of which these occur:

(a). The fibrillae emanating from the nervous prolongation of the cells of the first type (motor, or psycho-motor).

(b). The nervous prolongations of the cells of the second type, in totality, decomposing complexly (sensory, or psycho-sensory).

(c). The nervous fibrillae emanating from those nervous fibres which pass on to put themselves in direct relation with the gangliar cells of the first type (fibres of the first category).

(d). Many nervous fibres in totality, that is to say, those which, identically with the nervous prolongation of the cells of the second type, decomposing into very slender filaments, and thus losing their proper individuality, pass on to be gradually confounded in the network in question.

The network here described is evidently destined to establish a bond of anatomical and functual union between the cellular elements of extensive zones of the gray substance of the centers.

Twelfth. The several nervous fibres, far from being found in isolated, individual relations with a corresponding gangliar cell are, on the contrary, in the great majority of cases, found in connection with extensive groups of cells; but the opposite fact also is verified—that is to say—every (?) gangliar cell of the centers may be in relation with several nervous fibres, which have different destination and function.

Thirteenth. In the relations between cells and nervous fibres, rather than the described individual and isolate connections being verified, there is observed an evidently direct disposition, by which *the greatest possible complication of relations is effected* [italics added].

Fourteenth. As a necessary deduction from all that precedes, we should hold that, up to the present time, we have continued to speak too arbitrarily of isolated transmission between peripheral points and the supposed cellular individualities of centers. Taking account of the data above described, we may, without reserve, declare that, *from the so-called law of isolated transmission* [italics added], in so far as it is wished to apply it to the mode of functioning of the gangliar cells and the nervous fibres of the central organs, [*all*] *vestige of anatomical basis is now taken away* [italics added].

Fifteenth. Another corollary from what precedes is that the concept of *the so-called localization of the cerebral functions*, taken in a rigorous sense—(i.e., that certain determined functions may be referred to one or another zone, exactly limited)—*cannot be said to be in any manner supported by the results of minute anatomical researchers* [italics added].

Commentary

Here are summarized virtually the entire canon of Golgi's views on the cellular basis of nervous organization. The key point is the network formed by the axis cylinder branches (axon collaterals) of the gangliar cells (by "gangliar" cell he means all nerve cells with large cell body and thick axis cylinder). Golgi does not propose this network as an observation to be tested by further experiments; he proposes it as a law. The reason he placed so much emphasis on it appears to be that he saw it as the way to explain, at the cellular level, how nerve cells and their fibers could provide for the extensive interconnectedness that he felt was necessary for the nervous system to function *as a whole.* He believed that if the fibers (axons) and collaterals of the fibers provided this critical "nervous" function, the necessary nutritive function could be assigned to the "protoplasmic prolongations" (dendrites). The actual forms of the nerve cells were thus of secondary interest in relation to the mere fact of the interconnectedness of the fibers. The interconnectedness was so complex that no law about the relations between individual nerve cells could be established. We therefore have the paradox that Golgi provided the technological advance necessary to establish that the nerve cell belongs in the cell theory, and at the same time conceived a theoretical edifice that denied that possibility.

The very complexity of the network was, he declared, proof against two other "laws": the "law" that there could be isolated transmission between two nerve cells through any fiber connections, and the "law" that there was localization of functions (motor or sensory) in different regions of the brain. By the first he opposed most of the current (and subsequent) work aimed at analyzing spinal cord reflexes; by the second he opposed most of the work initiated by the discovery of Hitzig and Fritsch (1870) and carried forth by Ferrier (1876) of the localization of functions in the cerebral cortex; in both laws he ran counter to the whole effort of clinical neurology toward more accurate diagnosis and localization of individual tracts and centers underlying neurological disorders. As we shall see (Chapter 19), Golgi did not waver from these views for the rest of his life.

These views present a further paradox, that Golgi's focus was not on the function of the parts but the function of the whole. From this perspective, the actual structures of nerve cells were to a great extent irrelevant; the main thing that mattered was that they provided a network of connections sufficiently complex to mediate the extensive coordination that must be involved in cerebral functions. To the extent that this analysis is correct, it helps to explain why Golgi and his neuroanatomist adversaries spent so much time and energy at cross-purposes over what were the essential elements constituting the structural basis of brain function.

9

A Neuron Theory Begins to Take Form: His, Forel, Nansen

During the 1880s, the debates on the structure of the nerve cell continued in the universities of Europe. Then, in 1886, came definitive pronouncements by two well-known authorities, Wilhelm His of Leipzig and August Forel of Zürich, followed shortly by supporting evidence from an unsuspected quarter, a young anatomist in Norway named Fridtjof Nansen. Each of these moved the subject away from the preoccupation with unseen networks and set it squarely on the path toward the concept of the nerve cell as an independent cellular entity.

Wilhelm His

Few lives illustrate more persuasively than that of His the difference between the isolation and personal sacrifices of Golgi's early career and the advantages enjoyed by a young scientist growing up in the rich intellectual environment of central Europe in the latter part of the nineteenth century.

Academic Training: A Case Study

His was born in Basel in 1831. A grandfather, Peter Ochs, had been bürgermeister of Basel and a radical statesman during the Napoleonic Wars around 1800. The young His grew up in a family well-off and imbued with the ideals of public service (Mall, 1905). He began his medical studies in Basel, in 1849, and, after taking some courses in Bonn as well, decided to pursue his interest in microscopical anatomy. It was the custom of the time for a young scholar to decide on the authority in his field of interest and simply go and study under him, wherever he was. In His' case it was Johannes Müller, not an unpopular choice, as we have seen, so off he went to Berlin. There he studied under Müller and also by happy chance under Remak (see also Rasmussen, 1953). At that time Remak was not only carrying out the studies that led to his view that the axis cylinder arises from the nerve cell (Chapter 2), but was also helping to lay the foundations for the germ layer theory of the development of the embryo. His took Remak's course in embryology (Mall, 1905): "It made a profound and lasting impression upon the young student for it showed the relation between histology, embryology and comparative anatomy. . . . Remak's teaching helped him to formulate problems which occupied him during the following half century."

During his studies in Berlin, His became intrigued with the work of Rudolf Virchow, so off he went to Würzburg. There, as a fourth-year medical student at the age of 21, he did his first research project, a study of the microscopical structure of the connective tissue of the cornea. He also joined the circle around Kölliker, participating in a regular "journal-meeting," which sounds very much like a present-day "journal club," where the latest developments in anatomy and physiology were discussed (Mall, 1905). To finish his medical degree he did clinical rotations in Prague and Vienna. After passing his examinations in Basel, he settled down there to laboratory work. There were, however, sojourns in Paris, under the tutelage of Brown-Sequard, already known for his work on the sensory effects of hemisection of the spinal cord, and Claude Bernard, the founder of experimental neuropharmacology and successor, in 1855, to Magendie at the Collège de France, as well as a return trip to Berlin.

We have traced His' travels during his early years because they exemplify so well how the university system in Europe in the mid-nineteenth century provided opportunities for talented and enterprising students. Of course, the students also had to be sufficiently well-off to afford the travels; they had to speak German; and they had to have the necessary contacts through their professors at their home institutions. Golgi was outside this network, owing to family ties, limited means, and cultural, political, and linguistic barriers. Even travel was difficult; for example, direct rail communication across the Alps was not possible until the completion of the St. Gotthard pass in 1882.

If the Mediterranean lay in the penumbra of European academic activity, how much further away was America, and how much more keenly felt the distance. Consider the observations of Franklin Mall (1905), His' biographer and professor of anatomy at the Johns Hopkins University:

> How different is the study of medicine in Europe from that in America! There freedom reigns and students wander from place to place . . . able stu-

> dents select great men as teachers and thereby develop themselves. . . . [His] had received the best from his home, the school, the gymnasium and the university of his native city, had wandered for four years studying in the famous foreign universities receiving information and inspiration from the greatest masters—Muller, Virchow, Kölliker, and many others. . . . How much longer must we wait for similar privileges in America?

Johns Hopkins had been founded in 1876 to promote just these ideals for improving the environment for academic research in the United States, and Mall's feelings about the lot of students spilled over to faculties as well:

> In most of the continental universities any person approved by the faculty may teach and thus new blood is constantly being infused long before a fogy or a dog in the manger has been removed by a beneficent Providence. There is thus maintained a constant competition for better teaching. . . . In America, we frequently find recent graduates who tell us that they would follow an academic career if their future were assured as far as salary is concerned. Little do they realize that this attitude of mind alone should exclude such a career.

Mall himself was one of the early students in the United States who made the trip to Europe, to study under His; his remarks indicate how important were continental institutions as the seed bed for research training and as an ideal for academic enlightment. They served as the model for the development of academic research laboratories throughout the world well into the twentieth century; indeed, modern physics arose from just such a network of outstanding researchers and peripatetic students in central Europe during the 1920s. Only toward the end of the nineteenth century did the balance in the biological and medical sciences begin to shift to Great Britain and, following the devastation of the First World War, to the United States.

Describing Nerve Cell Development

In 1857, His, at the age of 26, won appointment to the chair of anatomy at Basel. Again, he was blessed with freedom to pursue his interests, and he knew how to use it, launching a comprehensive program of study that laid the foundations of the cellular basis of embryology. Central to this effort was the concept of the three germ layers as providing the origins for the different tissues and organs of the body. He devised a microtome for cutting serial sections of high quality through an entire embryo. He summarized his results in a definitive monograph on the chick embryo and a three-volume work, *Die Haute ünd Hohlen des Körpers* (*On the Membranes and Cavities of the Body*) (1865). In 1872, he was called to the chair of anatomy at

Leipzig, where he pursued his studies even more vigorously, aided by improved facilities and technical support. Soon he turned his attention to human development, and between 1880 and 1888 published another monumental three-volume work *Anatomie menschlicher Embryonen* (*Anatomy of the Human Embryo*).

During this period, at the peak of his investigative career, His focused his attention on the development of nerve cells in the spinal cord. He was well aware of the difficulties of visualizing nerve cell processes in the adult, and of the controversies surrounding the theories of Gerlach and the others who believed in anastomoses and continuity of the processes. He realized that analysis of the cells early in development, before they formed their processes and during the formation of the processes, would provide a way of testing the theory. The results were published in a paper entitled "Zur Geschichte des menschlichen Rückenmarkes und der Nervenwurzeln" ("On the structure of the human spinal cord and nerve roots") in 1886. In an early section of the paper, he describes the outgrowth of processes from the nerve cell:

> The nerve fibers extending from the cells start in the vicinity of a nuclear pole with a conically broadened base and show clear fibrillar stripes at their origin. Apart from an axis cylinder [axon] other extensions are barely noticeable. The cell body extends only a little over the nucleus and where it is possible to see it somewhat freely, it appears to be trimmed with several blunt points. Accordingly, the formation of the branched extensions [dendrites] occurs considerably later than that of the axis cylinder extension [axon].

Here is an unequivocal description of what is seen, not a speculation on what can be imagined. The early outgrowth of the axis cylinder (axon) followed by later outgrowth of "branched extensions" (dendrites) is a rule of nerve cell development that has generally been confirmed by modern studies. The text is accompanied by clear diagrams showing the motor cell with its axis cylinder growing into the anterior root of the spinal cord (Fig. 14), and the incipient "branched extensions" from the cell body (Fig. 15*A*). One feels in reading this paper that one is finally on the road to modern publication of experimental results and conclusions.

His next turned his attention to the posterior (dorsal) root of the spinal cord (Figs. 14; 15*B*). Here a controversy centered on whether the fibers of this root arise from cells within the spinal cord or from the cells within the dorsal root ganglia (see Freud, Chapter 7). His again came forward with observations and a conclusion:

> In an earlier communication, I presented the reasons which then favored growth of the sensible roots from the ganglia into the spinal cord. These

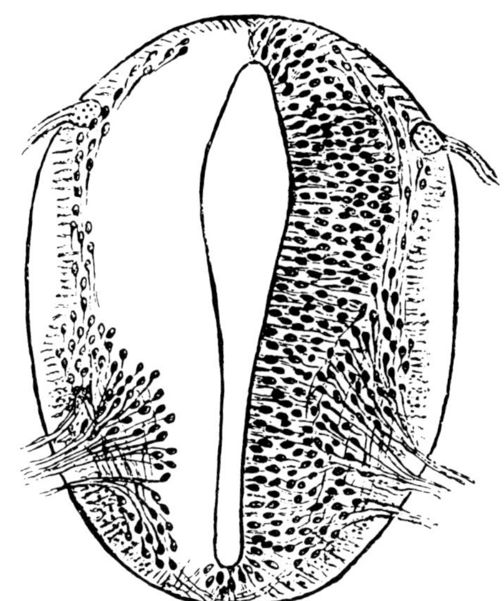

Fig. 14. "Section across the spinal cord of [a human] embryo. On the left is shown only the mantle layer." (His, 1886)

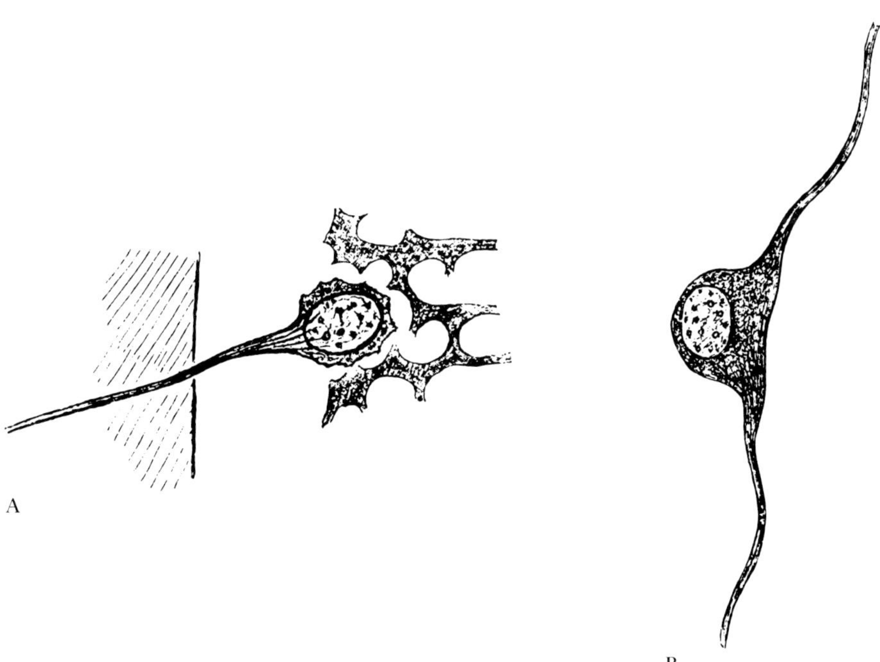

Fig. 15. A. "Motor cell from [human] embryo *R*; this can be seen to extend beyond the border of the spinal cord. The latter is indicated by a background lattice-work. Magnification c.1100. B. Single cell from a spinal ganglion of [human] embryo *N*. Magnification c. 1100." (His, 1886)

> were: 1) the trophic dependence of the root fibers on the ganglion as shown in experiments by Waller and von Bernard; 2) the early appearance of a fibrillation inside the ganglion not connected with the spinal cord; 3) the beginning shape of the upper root part becoming pointed towards the spinal cord; 4) the fact that the sensible fibers in the spinal cord have another fiber direction beyond these. I can now replace the above mentioned probable reasons with direct proof. The spinal ganglion cells of the embryo are bipolar formations, their dorsally directed extensions enter the spinal cord as root fibers, the ventral [ones] join with the motor roots and advance together to the periphery.

A further problem with the dorsal root ganglion cell was the fact that in the adult the cell appears unipolar, that is, the cell body gives rise to a single smooth process, which, after a short distance, divides into two branches, thus having a T-shaped form. As discussed in Chapter 7, this branching pattern was initially puzzling to anatomists, who, first of all, could not understand how it could be reconciled with the pattern of single axis cylinder (axon) and multiple protoplasmic extensions (dendrites) that seemed to be the rule elsewhere in nerve cells, and second, were hard put to give it a functional interpretation. Building on Freud's interpretation based on phylogenetic comparisons, His showed that, embryonically, the dorsal root ganglion cell started out as a bipolar cell, with the single axis cylinder growing into the dorsal root toward the dorsal horn of the spinal cord, and a single "protoplasmic prolongation" growing outward toward the periphery to become the sensory nerve fiber (Fig. 15*B*). The problem was discussed by His in an extensive footnote:

> As is known, Rudolf Wagner discovered bipolar ganglion cells in the spinal ganglia of plagiostomes already in 1846, and soon after Robin and Bidder independently confirmed this finding. Wagner certainly understood the importance in principle of this finding. . . . He fully understood the difficulty of proving the bipolar nature of the cells in the ganglia of higher vertebrates, [because of] the presence of the firm sheath. Even by dissociation of the ganglia, one could for the most part obtain only truncated forms of cells, apolar and unipolar. Among Wagner's illustrations there is a cell . . . which passes into an unquestionable T-shaped fiber. Later researchers were unable to find any bipolar cells in the higher vertebrates—only unipolar cells, as in particular Schwalbe also found in his careful research. But physiologically nothing could originate within such unipolar cells, and anatomically, too, they appeared contradictory, after it was shown through Holl's calculations that the number of ingoing fibers into a ganglion was the same as the outgoing fibers. Ranvier's discovery of the T-shaped nerve fibers inside the spinal ganglia must thus be regarded as the resolution of this question, although many ascribed only a secondary significance to these fibers. Through the above-mentioned results from the spinal ganglia of the embryo the bipolarity in fact now

appears as a general character of all these ganglia. . . . The shapes I have seen came closest to those which Freud describes for Petromyzon.

The primitive bipolar condition is retained in the lower vertebrates, which explains the observation of it by Freud in his work on Petromyzon, alluded to by His. In amphibians, reptiles, and mammals the adult cells are unipolar. The problem posed by the functional interpretation of the unipolar T-shaped branching pattern of the dorsal root ganglion cell was to play a significant role in the final stages of formulating the neuron doctrine, as we shall see (Chapter 15).

His finally dealt with the question of anastomoses between nerve cells. In the concluding section of his paper of 1886 he stated his position (cf. also Clarke and O'Malley, 1968):

> If now the nerve fibers originate without exception as extensions of ganglion cells, and gradually advance toward their central or peripheral regions, it follows as a necessary consequence that all other connections, if they are present, can only have originated secondarily. Previously, one was very inventive with such nerve connections in the center and the periphery. Schroeder van der Kolk has observed that connections of nerve cells among one another have long been recognized as illusions, but probably most of us believe silently that in some way the central nerve fibers serve for the mutual connections of cells; in the periphery, the termination of sensory nerves in so-called sensory cells has become the predominating dogma since the experiments of Max Schultze.
>
> The possibility that nerve fibers that penetrate epithelial layers also reach the insides of cells is *a priori* not to be disputed. The nerve endings discovered by von Hensen in the tails of tadpoles perhaps belong here. . . . On the other hand, we know that in an overwhelmingly large number of end structures, the nerve fibers as such run outward freely; these are the terminal fibrils of the corneal epithelium and the epidermis; the endings in Pacini corpuscles and in the end bulbs of Kraus; the plates in the tactile spheres of the beak of the duck; the terminals of the motor end plates, etc. A soft mass can accumulate around the ends of the fibers, as with the motor end plates, or, as in the case where the nerves end in connective tissue, it can form a more or less complicated system of capsules, which lends the end apparatus a more structured character. The example of the end apparatus provided with a connective tissue capsule (Pacini corpuscles, end bulbs, tactile corpuscles, touch bodies, etc.) offers a point of special interest, because it demonstrates that a type of stimulus is exerted at that site, and for this reason, an accumulation of special cell layers is induced. In the higher sense organs—in the retina, hearing organ, taste organ, and smell organ—according to the new observations of G. Retzius, Schwalbe, et al., we cannot follow further than the arrival of the nerve fibrils in the proximity of the so-called sensory cells, and *we shall ultimately have to accommodate to the idea that the transmission of a stimulus without direct continuity is possible in these organs* [italics added].

For centrifugally conducting nerves, *the motor end plates give the indisputable example of transmission of a stimulus without continuity of substance* [italics added]. It is even demonstrated here that between the stump-like ends of the axis cylinders and the contractile substance, an intermediate layer, the end-plate of Kuhne, is inserted.

I believe that one arrives at simplified notions with regard to the central nervous organs when one gives up the idea that a nerve fiber, in order to affect a part, must necessarily be in continuity with it [italics added]. For the course of one fiber, the law of isolated conductivity is indisputable; however, where a fiber ends in a stump, other conditions become valid for the transmission of stimuli from the stump. The multiplication of stumps, as the motor end-branches of Kuhne demonstrate, gains significance from this view. If the concept of the stimulus-transmitting significance of a nerve stump is justified, then for an explanation of the effect of one fiber on another, continuity of both pathways is not required, but rather, placement of the end stumps from both sides in the same area will suffice, with *interpolation of the stimulus-transmitting intermediate substance between* [italics added]. If we choose as an example the fibers of the pyramidal tract, their influence on the motor fibers [of the anterior spinal roots] will be understandable when it can be proven that they terminate in the proximity of the motor cells with single or divided stumps, and that they appear to move close to the ends of the branched extensions of the cell. Each of the bilateral pathways is enclosed up until its end, but between the two ends, the spinal cord interpolates itself as an open region, together with its interstitial substance, wherein the spread of, for example, chemical processes can take place in very different directions.

Gerlach . . . , whose concepts in many ways are like mine, believes in the existence of a nerve net as an intermediate link between fibers and cells within the grey matter. However, proof of such a net is to be drawn neither from his own observations nor those of others; rather, the positive observation, which Gerlach (1872) shows in his illustrations, is always just a multi-branched network of cell extensions, without true anastomoses of the intersecting branches. If now, in one way or another, a mass is inserted in between which connects on all sides the separately-ending nerve pathways, then this is the consequence: that within a given area, the stimulus travelling in one pathway can transmit itself to various neighboring pathways. According to this view, it can also be assumed that when there is inhibition of conduction in the nearest pathways, those that are further away can take over the conduction. Physiological knowledge of the circumstances of conduction in the spinal cord does not favor strict application of the principle of isolated conduction, and, at least within the grey matter, the realm of conduction possibilities is so large, that one maintains with difficulty the assumption of individual pathways.

These remarks, which agree in part with the tenets of Golgi (1883) . . . , based on histological experiments, are in no way intended to deal superficially with the whole problem of central and peripheral nerve endings, but I believe it is justified to bring up the problem again for discussion with new questions. *As a firm principle I thus put forward the proposition: that each nerve fiber originates as an extension from a single cell. This is its genetic, nutritive, and functional center; all other connections of the fibers are only indirect, or originate secondarily.*

In these passages we have taken a long stride out of the muddle of imagined images that has gone before. The evidence is assembled from a broad range of relevant experiments. His refers to Golgi, among the earliest signs of awareness of Golgi's work outside Italy. He notes the evidence of the free terminations of motor nerve fibers at the motor end-plate onto muscles, put forward by Kühne, as well as of sensory fibers in such structures as the Pacinian corpuscle. He argues that this evidence from the peripheral nervous system can be applied to understanding properties of nerve cells in the central nervous system, one of the first and clearest statements of a principle that was to serve many generations of anatomists and physiologists. His conception that nerve cells interact by *contiguity* rather than by *continuity* became an important focus of the ensuing debate on the nerve cell, and the remarks on the nature of interaction by contiguity anticipate Sherrington's formulation of the idea of the synapse (see Chapter 17). He states clearly for the first time that the nerve cell and all its extensions make up a single cell, supporting this proposition with the argument that in addition to constituting an anatomical entity, the nerve cell and all its extensions must be considered as a genetic (i.e., developmental), nutritive (i.e., metabolic) and functional (i.e., physiological) entity as well. Thus, he not only had a clear conception of the nerve cell as a cell, but he also had a clear understanding of the foundations upon which such a conception must be built.

August Forel

If Wilhelm His lived a resolutely focused life well within the cultural and professional confines of the main academic institutions of his time, those institutions were also able to accommodate researchers who were much more idiosyncratic in their careers and more varied in their contributions to diverse medical and social issues. Such an individual was August Forel. While His was absorbed in the neuroembryological studies leading him to see the nerve cell more clearly as an entity, Forel was pursuing a quite different series of studies that led to a similar conclusion.

Academic Training

Forel was born in 1848 near Morges, a village a few kilometers to the west of Lausanne on the shore of Lake Leman, in the predominantly French-speaking canton of Vaud in southwest Switzerland. He grew up a shy and introspective child, who early conceived an interest in natural science in general and a passion for insects in particular. As a youth in the late 1860s he read Darwin; in his memoirs he recalls (Forel, 1937):

> When I read *The Origin of the Species* it was as though scales fell from my eyes, while the light of a new and higher knowledge began to dawn upon them. . . . [I wrote in my diary]: "If Darwin is right, if man is a descendent of animal species, and if therefore his brain also is descended from the brain of the animal, and if, moreover, we think and feel with the brain, then what we call the soul in man is a descendant (an evolutionary product) of the animal soul, of the same fundamental structure as the latter, and, like it, entirely conditioned, in its simpler or higher development, by the simpler or higher development of the brain. Consequently, as Professor Le Felice once told us in an extremely interesting and stimulating lecture in Lausanne, psychology cannot in the last resort be other than a sort of physiology of the brain." The matter is not quite as simple as this account of it, but at that time it seemed to me perfectly clear and evident. Since then the notion has never left me. So far I have constantly found fresh confirmation of it, and have developed it further.

We may take this as representative of the effect of Darwin on many students of the time, and indeed on generations of students to the present.

Forel determined on medicine as a career. Lausanne and Geneva at that time had only academies, not full universities with medical schools, so he went to Zürich in 1866. Among his classmates there were the first two women students (Forel, 1937). During his medical studies he continued to collect insects, especially ants, observing their behavior in the field and studying their anatomy in the laboratory. These activities began to attract notice in academic circles, and resulted, at the age of 24, in the publication of his monumental book *Les Fourmis de la Suisse* (*The Ants of Switzerland*), which won prizes in Switzerland and Paris. Given his Darwinian outlook, Forel's thorough studies of the ants and their social organization must make him one of the pioneers in what we now call sociobiology (cf. Wilson, 1975); indeed, he was later to apply his idea of "the social instinct" among ants to human society (O.L. Forel, 1948).

Meanwhile, Forel, in 1871–1872, decided to complete his medical studies in Vienna and prepare a thesis under the tutelage of Theodor Meynert (see Kuhlenbeck, 1953). Meynert was then regarded as "the greatest living authority on the structure of the brain" (Forel, 1937); it was said that "Erst seit Meynert ist das Gehirn beseelt" ("Only since Meynert has the brain became animated") (Papez, 1953c). Meynert's comprehensive chapter on the anatomy of the cerebral cortex appeared in the same edition of Stricker's handbook that contained Gerlach's ideas on nerve nets (Chapter 6). It was to Meynert's clinic that Freud went when he left Brucke's laboratory (Chapter 7).

Although we have emphasized the advanced nature of science in central Europe during this the latter part of the nineteenth century, this was often achieved despite quite primitive facilities, poorly-run institutions, and eccentric personalities. When he arrived, Forel was shocked to find that Vienna in 1871 "was still a semi-oriental city . . . of . . . indescribable filth" (Forel, 1937); Viennese morals were "free and easy"; in the hospital ward "the greatest disorder prevailed, and the greatest uncleanliness"; Meynert's two children "were running about his study and playing." Meynert himself was a kind of genius, completely unpredictable in his leaps of imagination. "The longer I remained, the more I lost faith in his encephalogical schemata, and the fibrous connections which he perceived in the brain" (Forel, 1937).

Forel took further training in Paris, and then, after passing his medical examination, became an assistant to von Gudden in Munich. Because of Forel's interest in the anatomy of insects he wrote to Franz Leydig (see Chapter 6) to inquire about spending some time studying with him on the way to Munich. Leydig wrote back telling him not to come, but Forel went anyway (Forel, 1937):

> So, equipped with a microscope and a paraffin lamp, I arrived, at the beginning of November, in the ancient Swabian city of Tübingen, where Leydig was professor. Despite the advanced season, I succeeded in capturing some ants for dissection, though they had crept into the earth, and were already half-dormant. I took up my quarters in the Hotel zum Lamm. Facing my window were towering heaps of cabbages, and it was so dark that I could work only from eleven to one by daylight: the rest of the time I had to depend on my lamp for microscopic work. I entered my name for Leydig's course of lectures, and explained to him that I had brought my own preparations with me, and only wanted his advice. At this he became most amiable, excusing himself for his previous refusal to accept me, saying that others had often taken advantage of his researches. I now worked from early morning until far into the night, and in spite of defective lenses I succeeded in making some important discoveries regarding the antennae of the ants, which interested Leydig greatly.

Arriving in Munich in 1873, Forel found Gudden's laboratory to be in an "extremely primitive condition." Their first project was to construct a microtome large enough to accommodate the entire brain, and with it, "I succeeded in making the first thin microscopic section of the human brain" (Forel, 1937). Forel is anxious here to emphasize his role in constructing what came to be known as "Gudden's microtome" for cutting brain sections. Over the next few years he studied the anatomy of some of the deep regions of the brain. His description of the connections of the basal ganglia with the thalamus is commemorated in the "fields of Forel." He also produced "the first modern illustrations of the thalamus" (Meyer, 1971). Meyer (1971) also credits him with introducing such terms as medial, lateral, dorsal, ventral, etc., in a routine way in the description of brain anatomy.

The Method of Degeneration

The most important thing Forel learned from Gudden was the use of the degeneration method for studying connections in the brain. This approach had been pioneered by Augustus Waller (1816–1870), an Englishman. In 1850, Waller reported experiments in which he cut the nerves to the tongue, and observed decomposition of the nerve "tubers" around the taste buds in the tongue, beginning three to four days after the time of the cut and continuing to completion by approximately three weeks. He realized the great importance of this method for studying nerve connections: "By means of these alterations, we can most exactly determine the course and distribution of the whole nerve" (Waller, 1852).

He also realized that degeneration of the part of the nerve distal to (more peripheral to) the cut indicated that it had been deprived of its normal source of sustenance: "According to the interpretation of my researches, each of the fibres which is attached to one of the two poles of these cells (of the ganglion) finds in it the center of its nutritive life." This conclusion, of course, implied that the nerve fiber is an outgrowth of the cell body, and thus gave early support to that idea, which was just beginning to emerge in the work of Kölliker, Wagner, Remak, and others at that time (see Chapter 3). It also introduced the idea of the nerve cell body as the source of nutrition for the fibers.

Waller believed that, following a cut, the cell body and central stump of the nerve remained normal, but in the 1870s Gudden found that they also showed signs of atrophy. He launched a series of investigations in which he used this "secondary degeneration" to trace connections in the brain. Much of our basic knowledge of pathway connections between the main centers of the brain dates back to this period (see Meyer, 1971).

Forel worked with this method during his time with Gudden from 1873 to 1879. In 1879 he returned to Switzerland as the director of the Burgholzli Asylum and professor of psychiatry in Zurich. The asylum was not in much better condition than Meynert's ward had been, and the next years were absorbed in reorganizing it and setting up his laboratory where he continued the degeneration studies begun under Gudden. He also started to cultivate his many other interests, including hypnosis, which was attracting great attention at that time, and was to play such a large role in Freud's development of psychoanalysis, and even fascinated Cajal for awhile (Cajal,

1989). But Forel was turning over in his mind the implications of Gudden's degeneration method, and the fact that the degeneration was sharply limited to the cell whose fiber had been cut, rather than spreading diffusely to other cells. Exercising "his remarkable keenness of perception [which] allowed him to separate the facts from the hypotheses" (Clarke and O'Malley, 1968), he drew a far-reaching conclusion, which he has described in his memoir (Forel, 1937):

> During a holiday which was spent in Fisibach I also worked out quite a different idea, relating to the anatomy of the brain, which constituted a complete revolution of our views concerning the connection of the nerve-elements in the brain. At that time the problem was still quite obscure. We spoke of anastomoses between the ganglion-cells of the nervous system, without really knowing how such connections between the elements of cells which are originally quite independent of one another could be effected. But recently the Italian anatomist, Professor Golgi, had invented a new method of colouring, by which he was able to show that the so-called protoplasmic processes of the ganglion-cells are blind—that is, their terminations are not connected to anything. However, this author was so completely ensnared by the old notion of anastomoses that on showing that the so-called nerve-processes of the ganglion-cells undergo ramification, he now assumed a network of anastomoses for these ramifications, and even drew it. In my laboratory we succeeded in preparing specimens by Golgi's method, and we saw the blind terminations of the protoplasmic processes, but not the network of anastomoses connecting the nerve-processes.
>
> It was as though scales had fallen from my eyes. I asked myself the question: "But why do we always look for anastomoses? Could not the mere intimate contact of the protoplasmic processes of the nerve-cells effect the functional connection of nervous conduction just as well as absolute continuity?" I considered the findings of Gudden's atrophic method, and above all the fact that total atrophy is always confined to the processes of the same group of ganglion-cells, and does not extend to the remoter elements in merely functional connection with them. It is true that this assumption encounters a difficulty in the great length of individual nerve-fibres. But Ranvici has shown how these nerve-fibres, if resected, grow together again. The more I reflected, the clearer it seemed that we had hitherto been sunk fathoms deep in a preconceived opinion. The longer I considered it, the more untenable I found the theory of anastomoses. All the data supported the theory of simple contact, so at Fisibach, where I could be quiet, I decided to write a paper on the subject and risk advancing a new theory. I completed the paper, adding the evidence afforded by the experimental atrophies of the motor and sensory nerves (*Nervus facialis* and *trigeminus*—that is, the facial nerves of movement and sensation) and sent it to the *Archiv für Psychiatrie* in Berlin. However, this periodical was then appearing only at long intervals, so my paper did not appear until January 1887. I had made the further mistake of neglecting to give my new theory a name. People always like names!
>
> Without my knowledge Professor His of Leipzig had arrived at similar re-

sults, and had published them in a periodical which was issued more promptly, in October 1886, so that formally speaking the priority was his. He proceeded from the wholly dissimilar fact that in the embryo the nerve-fibres of the so-called spinal ganglia grew directly out of the cells. However, he had not realized all the connotations of the theory as fully as I had.

Forel's paper was entitled "Einige hirnanatomische Betrachtungen und Ergebnisse." The key passages are as follows (Forel, 1887; modified slightly from Clarke and O'Malley, 1968):

SOME CONSIDERATIONS AND RESULTS RELATING TO THE ANATOMY OF THE BRAIN

Now, where do we stand in relation to the *a priori* assumptions which still exist in the most recent textbooks and reports, that the ganglion cells represent, so to speak, nodal points (*Knotenpunkte*) between fibre systems? . . . one hears again and again discussion of the interruption of a fibre system by a gray nucleus; and most workers tacitly assume that apparently each ganglion cell is associated with at least two nerve fibres; that these, if not directly, yet indirectly are in direct *continuity* with nerve fibres by means of a fibre net, despite the fact that no certain evidence exists on this matter. One might point out, however, the so-called T-shaped division of the process of the spinal ganglion cells. But if it does exist, it must in any case be interpreted quite differently . . . and there can no longer be any doubt concerning the transition into a nerve fibre of the branch which is directed towards the spinal cord. However, this may be just as well explained by the fact that they simply pass through the ganglion rather than that they originate in its cells.

If however we pay more heed to comparative histology and embryology, we must arrive at quite different viewpoints. The nervous system which, as is well known, originates in epiplastic cells, is present in the lowest animals, first in the shape of isolated ganglia and neuroepithelial cells. The nerves are merely outgrowths of epithelial cells. To the best of my knowledge, *no one has yet seen, in the development of the nerve elements of vertebrates, any reliable anastomotic processes between the outgrowths of the ganglion cells, the fibres* [*axons*], *or the protoplasmic processes* [*dendrites*] *of one element, with those of others. Even the manner in which the nerve attaches itself to the muscle fibre, the so-called nerve ending in the transversely striated muscle, is a kind of cementing and does not represent a direct continuity* [italics added].

But now the fibre plexus. One ordinarily imagines it to be a true network, the most delicate branches of which are in direct continuity among themselves, but even Golgi's method cannot establish this point definitively, and Golgi expresses himself with extreme caution in this matter. The most delicate little branches of the nerve fibre are, after all, much too thin for it to be certain whether they can be seen lying on top of each other or anastomosing with one another, when the branches of some of the elements meet. However, when such enormous ramifications of the elements, which Golgi's method exhibits, meet, they must, of necessity, anastomose with each other in such manner that a dreadful feltlike maze must result, even if they do not form a genuine plexus of fibres. This felt could thus be a *phantom net.* And, indeed, how could we possibly imagine such a process in which these very delicate and innumerable cell processes, which originally were not connected with each other, should all meet exactly with their free endings in order to coalesce into a continuous network? Such an idea becomes even more improbable if we consider that this plexus of fibres must develop still further during the years of development, and this, after all, would not be easy to imagine in the case of a true anastomosis.

Gradually, I can see less and less reason why an actual, continuous union of the finest little branches of the nervous elements ought to be a physiological postulate. *If the branches of the trees of the various nerve elements interlock in the manner they actually do, this is quite sufficient for the transmission of stimuli. Electricity gives us such innumerable examples of similar transmissions* [*sic*] *without direct continuity that it could well be the same in the nervous system* [italics added].

I like to assume that all fibre systems and the so-called fibre net of the nervous system are nothing else than mere nerve processes, each of an individual ganglion cell. The nerve process proceeds from its base in the cell. It then branches in various ways and gives off fibrils at different points. Some are not far away [from the cell] (cells of the second [Golgi] category), some are both close to it and at a greater distance, but they remain temporarily united as medullary fibres. Ultimately [the branching] always takes the shape of extensively ramified, interlocked trees, but anastomosing [is found] nowhere.

Fridtjof Nansen

In the same year of 1886 when His and Forel were drawing their conclusions from years of investigations, a young Norwegian by the name of Fridtjof Nansen was peering into a microscope at Golgi-stained neurons for the first time in his studies of invertebrate nerve cells. These were published in his doctoral thesis in 1887; then, he was off to pursue his first love, polar exploration. In his thesis, Nansen provided a bridge between the network concept of Golgi and the view of the nerve cell as an individual entity; indeed, his name became linked by some to those of His and Forel as one of the early founders of the neuron doctrine. His views therefore merit our attention, the more so in that they come from one of history's most remarkable personalities.

Academic Training

Nansen was born in 1861 near Christiania (now Oslo). As a boy, Fridtjof and his brother led an active outdoors life, which instilled in him his two great passions: an intense interest in natural science, and a zeal for exploration and adventure. These steered his academic studies in the direction of biology. After a year at the university, he signed on board a commercial sealing vessel to make observations and train himself for "descriptive zoological research" (Brögger and Rolfsen, 1896). The voyage (spring, 1882) took them north to Spitzbergen and west to Greenland. Apart from his zoological observations of marine life, what really excited Nansen was the wild beauty of the glaciers and the drift ice, and the challenges of besting the elements and hunting the bear.

On his return, in 1882, he took a position as curator of the Zoological Museum in Bergen and began studies for a doctoral thesis. I am indebted to Professor Jan Jansen, Jr., for the following observations:

> The Museum in Bergen was really the leading Norwegian biological institution of the time. The director, Dr. Daniel Danielson, was also the head of the leprosy hospital in Bergen and for many years a member of parliament. In addition he published widely on topics from zoology to the treatment of leprosy. Better known internationally was his slightly younger colleague Armauer Hansen, who identified the leprosy bacillus in 1873. In 1877 Hansen visited Ranvier's laboratory in Paris, and later published a paper on "Nerve endings in leech voluntary muscles," concluding that there is no "ganglionic plexus." The prominence of scientific activity in Bergen at the time was underlined by a visit from Louis Pasteur in 1884 [see also Helle, 1987].

Bergen had been the largest city in Norway until well into the nineteenth century. The high level of biological research at its museum centered mostly on marine life in the coastal waters. The work there on leprosy was partly a consequence of economic conditions following the Napoleonic Wars. The ensuing prolonged trade depression had devastating effects on Norway, reducing the people who lived in remote habitations along the fjords to such poverty that leprosy "varied between one per hundred and one per thousand all along the west coast" (Derry, 1957).

For his thesis, Nansen chose as his subject the microscopic anatomy of a group of worms called the myzostomida, which are parasites of certain crinoid species. For this work he had an excellent microscope, a gift from his father, and one of the new microtomes that could cut serial tissue sections, that is, sequences of sections from which continuous reconstructions of the tissue could be made. His sterling qualities as an investigator soon attracted notice, so much so that in 1883, on the recommendation of an English zoologist (see Helle, 1987), he was offered a permanent position by Othniel March, professor of vertebrate paleontology at Yale College, who at that time was leading the earliest excavations of dinosaurs and other fossil vertebrates in the western United States. Nansen was tempted (Hoyer, 1957), but turned down the offer. This episode attests not only to Nansen's budding reputation, but also to the network of international contacts that aided in the identification of talented young scientists at that time.

Nansen's descriptions of the microscopic structure of the different organs of these worms were published in 1885. This work led him to focus his attention on the nervous system, and he launched into a comparative study of various invertebrates—worms, crustaceans, and molluscs—as well as some of the most primitive vertebrates—amphioxus and hagfish. He was impatient with his progress; Pasteur's visit in 1884 convinced him that he needed to visit other laboratories to bring himself up to date on new developments in microscopic anatomy. When he learned of Golgi's results—probably through the French or English translations noted before—he immediately recognized that he needed to learn this method. Obtaining leave from his curatorship, he set off on a study trip, financing his travels by having a gold medal he had won for his myzostomida work cast in copper instead (Helle, 1987). His stops along the way included Kiel, Berlin, Leipzig, and Heidelberg, visiting with zoologists, lithographers, and chemical suppliers (Helle, 1987).

Nansen spent a week in Pavia learning the Golgi technique; according to his daughter, he studied there "with Professor Golgi and Dr. Fusari" (Høyer, 1957). He then spent two months (April–June, 1886) at the Zoological Station in Naples. This station had been established in 1873 by a young German anatomist, Anton Dohrn, who had a vision of zoology as an experimental science and a conviction that crucial means toward this end were institutions where different animal species, many of them rare or hard to get, could be gathered systematically and studied by scientists from all nations. It was the first of its kind; scarcely 20 years later over 50 such stations had sprung up around the world (Brögger and Rolfsen, 1896), and have played an important role in the rise of modern biology (see Florey, 1985; Maienshein, 1985).

Nansen made full use of his time in Naples, applying the Golgi method to different species, scouring the literature for the relevant references and background for his thesis, and discussing the current controversies with fellow scientists from other countries. Not that it was all work; one of the visitors (presumably Apáthy; see Chapter 17) observed that, when it came time for social diversions, "He was the life and soul of all our little festivities" (Brögger and Rolfsen, 1896). On the other hand, "At other times he would be quiet and absorbed, and would sit by the hour without uttering a word." Out of those thoughts came visions of the future: the finest nerve processes of the crayfish brain; a zoological station for Norway; the ice-fields of the polar north.

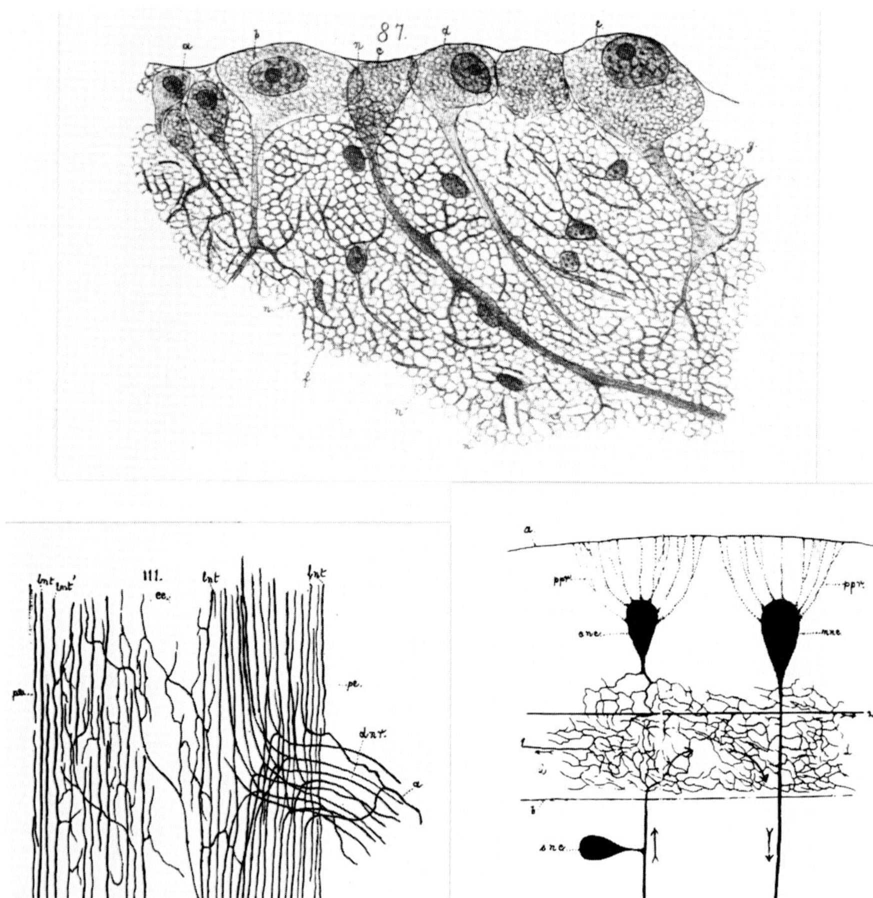

Fig. 16. Illustrations from Nansen's (1887) thesis.

"A. *Corella parallelogramma.* . . . Part of a longitudinal section through the brain. *a-g* Ganglion cells. *n* Neuroglia-nuclei. *n* Similar nucleus adhering to the sheath of a nervous process. (Fixed in osmic acid (1%), stained with *picro-carmine.*)"

B. Golgi stain, showing branching of dorsal root fibers within the spinal cord. "(Magnified 80 diameters.) Part of a chromo-silver stained horizontal section of the spinal cord of *Myxine*; exhibiting the dichotomous subdivisions of the nerve-tubes of the nerve-root. *dnr* Dorsal nerve-root. *a* Nerve-tube subdividing outside the spinal cord. *pe* Periphery of the spinal cord. *cc* Central canal. *lnt* Longitudinal nerve-tubes. *lnt* Longitudinal nerve-tubes giving off side-branches. *snt* Subdividing nerve-tube. *snt*' Subdividing nerve-tube crossing the central canal."

C. Nansen's concept of the neural basis of the reflex arc. "*Diagrame of the reflex-curve* The large arrows indicate the way the irritation of a sensitive nerve-tube has to pass to produce a reflex-movement. *SN* Centripetal (sensitive) nerve-tube. *dd*

Nansen's Thesis

Back in Bergen, Nansen worked diligently with the new Golgi method. In scarcely a year he drew together all his findings into a thesis, "The Structure and Combination of the Histological Elements of the Central Nervous System" which was published in 1887.

The thesis is a remarkable document. It is written in English; Nansen obviously intended that it should be widely read outside Norway. At its publication, Nansen was barely 26 years old; among the main contributors to the theory of the neuron, he was one of the youngest. The thesis runs to 215 pages, with 11 plates containing a total of 113 figures. The illustrations of nerve cells are beautifully executed; in a number of cases Nansen notes that they are "drawn under the camera lucida, from the microscope directly upon the stone" (i.e., the stone used in the engraving process; see Fig. 16*A*).

Of the 190 pages of text, over 70 were devoted to an exhaustive survey of the literature dealing with the microscopic structure of the nervous system, with separate sections for the structure of the "nerve tubes," the "ganglion cells," "Leydig's dotted substance," and "the combination of the ganglion cells with each other." Some of this material was covered earlier in the review of the work on Leydig's "dotted substance" (Chapter 6). Nansen then describes his own research on these four questions. His method is characteristic: after an exhaustive description of the details of microscopic structures in many different species, he assesses the results against the background of the literature and then draws his conclusions. Sometimes he sides with the "authorities," sometimes bluntly opposes them, always giving the impression of living up to the ideal of the fearlessly objective scientist.

Dotted substance or interlacing of nervous fibrillæ in the central nervous-system. *MN* Centrifugal (motoric) nerve-tube.

"The small arrows indicate the way small parts of the irritation of the centripetal (sensitive) nerve-tube pass to arrive in other parts of the central nerve-system. 1. Nerve-tube passing to the brain. 2. Longitudinal nerve-tube running along the spinal cord, whilst giving off side-branches. *snc* The nutritive centre of the centripetal nerve-tube (i.e. spinal ganglion cell). *cnc* The nutritive centre of a part of the fibrillæ forming the dotted substance or interlacing of nervous fibrillæ (i.e. ganglion cell of the central nerve-system). *mnc* The nutritive centre of the centrifugal nerve-tube (i.e. ganglion cell of the central nerve-system). *ppr* Nutritive (i.e. protoplasmic) processes sometimes issuing from the nutritive centres, and penetrating towards the periphery of the central nerve-system or towards blood-vessels to absorb nutrition. *a & b* Periphery of the central nerve-system." (Nansen, 1887)

The positive contributions of the thesis may be summarized as follows (see especially Jansen, 1982/1987 for a full discussion). According to Retzius (1896), "Nansen was the first to employ the Golgi process in the study of the nervous system of invertebrates." He was also one of the first outside Pavia to publish results using the method. In the invertebrates, he illustrated and interpreted the function of the unipolar cells more clearly than before. He extended Golgi's finding of nerve tube branches (axon collaterals) to invertebrates, as well as his distinction between cells with long nerve tubes with side branches (long axons with axon collaterals) and cells with only short nerve tubes ending in branches (short axons and axon terminal branches). In the primitive fish he described for the first time the way that a sensory fiber of the dorsal root divides, sending one branch rostrally (toward the head) and the other caudally (toward the tail) (Fig. 16*B*). He correctly deduced that these and other findings must apply to higher vertebrates as well. He surmised that the ganglion cell body is the nutritive center not only for the cell and the protoplasmic processes but also for the long nerve tubes (axons) as well.

The most important contribution to the concept of the nerve cell concerned the question of the relations between nerve cell processes where they interweave within the central cell-free regions (the "dotted substance" of Leydig) of the invertebrate nerve ganglia. Here Nansen's stand was unequivocal; first, between the protoplasmic processes (dendrites): "A *direct combination between the ganglion cells, by direct anastomosis of the protoplasmic processes does not exist.*"

Second, between the side-branches of the nerve tubes (axon collaterals): "*The branches of the nervous processes do not anastomose*—They contribute to form a reticulation, or rather interlacing of nervous fibrillae."

Finally, he extends these observations to neuroglial cells: "*The processes of the neuroglial cells do not anastomose.*"

These blunt conclusions, based in part on evidence from the Golgi stain, have put Nansen firmly among the contributors to the neuron doctrine. In addition, his characterization of the relations between the intervening processes as involving "combination" rather than "continuity" anticipates later concepts and terminology (see Chapters 16, 17).

Not content solely with structure, Nansen concluded his thesis with speculations on the implications of his findings for nervous functions. His concept of the neural basis of the reflex is illustrated by the drawing in Figure 16*C*.

> The *reflex-curve is*, consequently, *composed of the following constituents*: 1) *centripetal* (sensitive) *nerve-tube*; 2) *the central web or interlacing of nervous fibrillae or tubes* [Fig. 16*C*]; 3) *the centrifugal* (motoric) *nerve-tube.*

> This theory will necessarily give a new view of the functions of the central element; but it will, I think, explain a great many relations which have been rather difficult to understand. The dotted substance (the interlacing of nervous fibrillae) must be a principal seat of the nervous activity, through this substance or interlacing is the reflex-actions etc. communicated to the consciousness, which even possibly has its seat in this substance itself (especially that of the brain). According to this view there can of course, to some extent, be a *localisation* in the central nerve-system but *no isolation*. This view will also I think possibly be able to explain the fact that other parts of the brain can take up the function of lost parts. This is not, however, the place to enter into such physiological details, we have especially taken up the histological side of the question and in this respect we can state, as a fact, that a plaiting or interlacing (not reticulation) of nervous fibrillae extends through the whole central nervous system of all animals (which possess a central nervous system) and that probably all peripheral nerve-tubes, entering into or issuing from the central nervous system, are connected with this central fibrillar interlacing by branches. We will then ask the physiologists if it is not probable that it is this interlacing of nervous fibrillae (or tubes) which especially produces the feeling of unity in the nervous system, in other words that it is the principal seat of self-consciousness?

This argument, from the details of microscopic structure to the level of consciousness, gives evidence of a mind with a tremendous capacity for both analysis and synthesis. Unfortunately, along with the correct conclusions from the experimental evidence went some flawed interpretations that limited the impact of his work and ideas. Most serious was the notion that the ganglion cell body and the protoplasmic processes (dendrites) served primarily nutritive functions (see Jansen, 1982/1987). Nervous conduction passed only through the nerve tubes (axons) and their side-branches (axon collaterals) and terminal branches, as is illustrated in Figure 16*C*. This part of his theory seems to be derived from Golgi. (Nansen's stand against anastomoses between these processes, and in favor of combination rather than continuity, would appear to demonstrate his independence from his mentor, though it may also reflect Golgi's own equivocation on the nature of the reticulum formed by these interlacing processes.)

Despite these limitations, his speculations on the nervous basis of mental abilities makes fascinating reading (Nansen, 1887):

> Whether the ganglion cells of the central nerve-system have any function besides being nutritive centres is, of course, extremely difficult to decide.
>
> It is not impossible that they may be the seat of *memory*. A small part of each irritation producing a reflex action, may on its way through the dotted substance be absorbed by some branches of the nervous processes of the ganglion cells, and can possibly in one way or another be stored up in the latter.

> Howsoever that may be, and whatever the function of the ganglion cells is, this new theory of the combination between the centripetal and the centrifugal nerve-tubes gives, if approved, a quite new view of the importance of the dotted substance (or the interlacing of nervous fibrillae of the vertebrates) and will, in my opinion, explain many facts as to its occurrence. If the theory is correct, then, the dotted substance must be a principal seat of the nervous activity, and—the higher an animal is mentally developed—the more complicated and extensive must we expect to find its dotted substance; this is in the fullest harmony with the facts already known. We need only refer the reader to the ant, or the bee, to compare the extremely complicated and highly developed dotted substance of these small inteligent [*sic*] animals, with the dotted substances of less developed insects, or to compare the dotted substance of the insects or crustacea with that of annelides, etc. etc. I am sure that my readers will very soon arrive at the conclusion, that the more complicated the structure of dotted substance is—the more highly is the animal mentally developed; in other words, we may conclude that *the more the inteligence of an animal is developed—the more intricate becomes the web or plaiting of nerve-tubes and fibrillae in its dotted substance*; the protoplasmic processes etc. of the ganglion cells are of no great importance in this respect. In this manner we can explain how it is, that unipolar cells occur in the nervous system of animals (e.g. insects and crustacea) which are mentally even highly developed; these animals have an extremely intricate web of nerve-tubes in their dotted substance, and this web is probably the principal seat of inteligence.

Nansen: A Summing Up

In considering the thesis, the reader cannot help but wish that on his travels Nansen had taken more time to include stops in places like Wurzburg; a few minutes with Kölliker would surely have given him a more balanced view of the issues and the evidence bearing on them. The careful reader in addition finds certain aspects of the text puzzling; at many places the author states that his studies are incomplete, and that he will publish further results in the future. Even more puzzling, although the English is fluent, the thesis is full of minor grammatical and typographical errors, indicating that it had not been carefully proofread.

The answer is to be found in the Arctic. At that time, the Arctic and the Antarctic were the two last great parts of the Earth remaining to be discovered. They exerted the same fascination as space travel does in our time, with the difference that, whereas space travel requires huge government-supported enterprises, Arctic exploration was open to any individual with the zeal to put together a team and go for the prize. Ever since his sealing expedition in 1882, Nansen had been "brooding over a plan I believe it must be possible to carry out. It is to cross the interior of Greenland on skis" (Høyer, 1957). In 1883, a Swede, Nordenskiöld, had made a foray into the west coast of Greenland, and in 1886 Peary and Maigaard penetrated the eastern coast. Nansen, then in Italy, realized he must finish his thesis quickly or lose the race. In November 1887, he travelled to Stockholm to get Nordenskiöld's blessing and support. The die was cast. The following passage is crucial for understanding the pressures on the young scientist during the time he was finishing his thesis (Brögger and Rolfsen, 1896):

> The first six months of 1888 passed in one incessant rush. At the beginning of December 1887 he is back in Bergen. At the end of January, he goes on snow-shoes from Eidfiord in Hardanger, by way of Numedal, to Kongsberg, and thence to Christiania. In March he is in Bergen again, lecturing on nature and life in Greenland. One day—or rather night—we find him camping on top of Blaamanden, near Bergen, to test his sleeping bag, and a week later he is on the rostrum in Christiania giving his first trial lecture for his doctor's degree, on the structure of the sexual organs in the myxine. [The subject of the second lecture was: "What do we understand by alternation of generation, and in what forms does it occur?"] On April 28, he defends his doctorial thesis: *The nerve elements: their structure and connection in the central nervous system*—and on May 2 he sets off for Copenhagen, on his way to Greenland. 'I would rather take a bad degree than have a bad outfit,' he used to say to Dr. Grieg in those days. He succeeded in getting both good, but only by straining every nerve. On the one hand he had his scientific reputation to look to, on the other, his own life and the lives of five brave men; for he was fully convinced that, of all the dangers which were pointed out to him, the most serious by far was the danger of a defective outfit. On the outfit, more than on anything else, depended victory or defeat, life or death.

And so Nansen was off, to lead the first expedition to cross the interior of Greenland. This was followed by a sensational three-and-a-half-year polar voyage in his ship the *Fram,* through the ice floes north of Russia, almost to the North Pole, the furthest north that had been reached to that time. A portrait of the young Nansen and his wife conveys some of the strength and intensity that carried him, and her, through these exploits (Fig. 17). On his return, in 1894, he was an international celebrity. He played a significant role in helping Norway gain her independence in 1905; he served as Ambassador to England, then High Commissioner for war refugees following the First World War, for which he received the Nobel Peace prize in 1922. He was widely recognized as one of the greatest humanitarians of modern history, and one of the first world statesmen to dedicate himself to liberating mankind from war.

Nansen never gave up his interest in science; following his Arctic explorations he was appointed professor at the University of Oslo and made important contributions toward founding the new science of oceanography. However, his muted scientific legacy has to be understood in the lime-

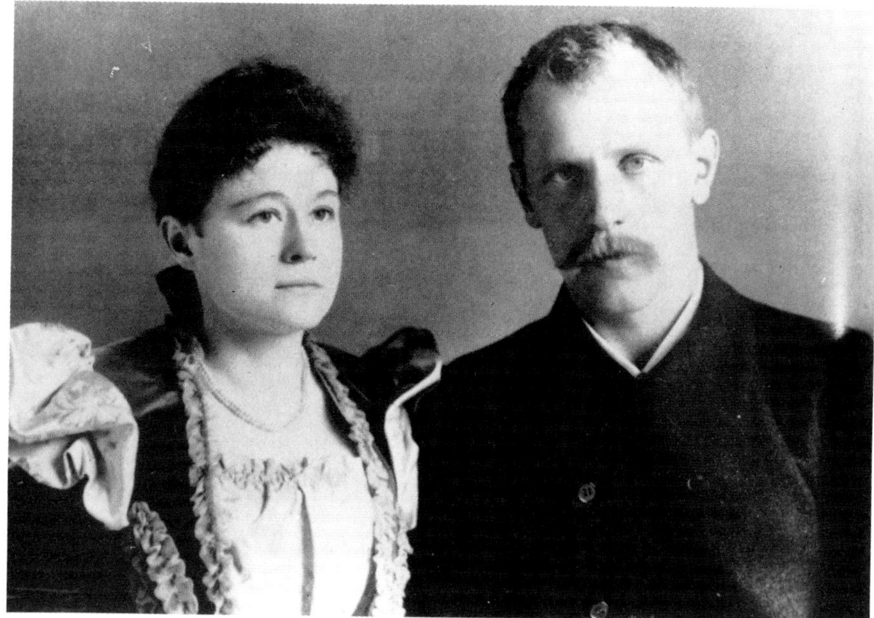

Fig. 17. Portrait of Fridtjof Nansen and his wife, Eva, in 1885, following his return from the first land expedition across Greenland. (Høyer, 1957)

light of his amazing and varied career on the international scene. In response to Nansen's instant international acclaim upon his return from the voyage on the *Fram,* a two-volume biography appeared (Brögger and Rolfsen, 1896). Gustav Retzius, the recognized authority on invertebrate nerve cells, was asked to write the chapter on Nansen's scientific work. In the early 1890s the two had corresponded about the work on nerve cells, and Nansen had expressed the hope of returning to his studies, but his role on the world's stage was overtaking him (Brögger and Rolfsen, 1896; Jansen, 1982/1987). Retzius' characterization of the significance of Nansen's work on nerve cells was appreciative but restrained; no mention was made of his contribution to the neuron theory. Perhaps Retzius knew better than most that the thesis was an unfinished work. Nonetheless, when the neuron doctrine was finally promulgated, Waldeyer listed six major authorities: Cajal, Kölliker, His, Nansen, Lenhossék, and Retzius (see Chapter 14). It thus seems undeniable that he earned his place among the great scientists of his time.

10
Ramón y Cajal: The Shock of Recognition

Up to this point we have seen that the problem of the microscopic structure of the nerve cell had engaged many of the leading scientists of the nineteenth century; among them, Purkinje, Schwann, Kölliker, Helmholtz, Virchow, and His were particularly well known. These are among the greatest scientists of their respective countries, and among the founders of modern biology. We turn now to consider the central figure in our epic, the person universally regarded, already during his lifetime, as the chief architect of the neuron theory. This achievement has made him one of the founders of modern neuroscience, some would claim *the* founder. Moreover, in this achievement he attained recognition, again, within his lifetime, not only as the greatest of all Spanish scientists, but also as one of the greatest scientists of all time, ranked among the modern pantheon of Copernicus, Vesalius, Galileo, Newton, and Darwin.

These claims are stated here as facts, because few would dispute them; few biological scientists have had the immediate and electrifying impact that Don Santiago Ramón y Cajal had on the science of his times. I am partisan to these claims. However, a full appreciation of Cajal's contributions has been limited by the unavailability of most of his primary writings in English, and an unfamiliarity with his relations with his field, particularly in the critical early years. Thus, there is lacking an objective assessment of the social and intellectual context of his endeavor; the trials and errors in developing his techniques and ideas; the places where he built on the work of others, and where his own precise additions to facts and theories of nervous structure were made. Translations of several major works are available (*Degeneration and Regeneration of the Nervous System,* 1928/1959; *Studies on the Cerebral Cortex,* 1955; *Neuron Theory or Reticular Theory?*, 1933;

Nobel Lectures for 1906, 1967; *Cajal on the Cerebral Cortex,* DeFelipe and Jones, 1989). His monumental *Histologie du Système Nerveux* (*Histology of the Nervous System*) (1909, 1911) is available only in the French translation, but nonetheless is an indispensable starting point for cellular studies of the nervous system. All of these works are extremely valuable for providing access to Cajal's mature views synthesized from his own and others' work. However, they do not give direct insight into the origins and evolution of his work and concepts.

The task of assessment needs to begin with translations of the early works. Most of Cajal's early papers were published in Spanish in essentially private journals that are virtually inaccessible today. Two of the most important early papers (Cajal, 1888b; 1889c) were reprinted in the original Spanish many years ago but have not been generally available. A big step forward has been the recent translation of all of Cajal's writings on the cortex (DeFelipe and Jones, 1989). Here I shall provide translations of the two early papers, as well as of other writings that complement the work covered in DeFelipe and Jones. I shall then begin the next stage of a critical reassessment of this work, building on DeFelipe and Jones, and Piccollino (1988), with particular reference to the neuron doctrine. I shall attempt to show that a detailed analysis of Cajal's earliest contributions to knowledge of the structure and organization of nerve cells, including consideration of his errors as well as successes, leads not only to an increase in our appreciation of the magnitude of his achievement but also to a deeper understanding of the neuron doctrine itself.

Most of what we know about his formative years comes from his *Recuerdos de Mi Vida,* published originally in Spanish in 1901 and 1917, translated into English under the title of *Recollections of My Life* in 1937, and recently reprinted (1989). It is one of the most thorough and forthright works of self-evaluation by a scientist, and provides valuable clues to the origin of his scientific career. It has been the basis of several engaging accounts of Cajal's life (see Cannon, 1949). Most previous readers have considered the early account of his childhood "captivating," but the later account of his career "tedious," overburdened with scientific minutiae. In fact, we will see that the early part provides useful information about the qualities responsible for his later achievements, and in the later part he directly and thoroughly addresses many of the issues that are at stake in understanding how the neuron doctrine emerged.

Early Years of Mischief and Rebellion

Santiago Ramón y Cajal was born in 1852 in northeast Spain in the village of Petilla, in the region of Aragon, near the French border. Cajal's childhood was dominated by the tension between his unruly nature and his stern and demanding father. His father, at the time of Cajal's birth, was a struggling village surgeon, but was possessed of a great ambition to better himself. Through dint of stern will, hard work, continuous study, and severe sacrifice (by himself and his family) he obtained the title of Physician and Surgeon, followed by Doctor of Medicine, establishing a good reputation throughout the region. During this period, the family moved several times, affording plenty of scope for the young Santiago to get into one mischievous scrape or rebellious incident after another, so much so that the elder Cajal began to despair of his son achieving the goal of the medical career he had determined for him, and apprenticed him for awhile to a shoemaker and to a barber. In his memoir Cajal remonstrates against the severity of his father and the brutality of his schoolmasters. At the same time, he recognizes that, for someone as headstrong as he was, their discipline served as the anvil to the hammer of his will.

An interesting impression gained from this account is the many talents struggling for expression in the boy. Among his playmates he excelled at "games of strength and agility." He loved the out-of-doors, exploring new woods and streams (we have seen that Nansen shared this love). A curiosity about nature was early evident. He was especially fascinated by birds, and built up a large collection of nests and eggs. Another trait was shyness, an "antipathy for social intercourse," coupled with a need for solitude, to be alone with his own thoughts. As a student he fared erratically, partly because of the resentment aroused by his rebellion in his masters, partly because of his loathing for rote exercises; but his memory was extraordinary for things he cared about. As a youth he showed a talent for sketching and painting; seized by "graphic mania," he decided to be an artist, but this idea was quashed by his father. Nonetheless, his artistic talent was to become part of the intuition he had for the shapes and relations of nerve cells, and the extraordinary clarity and vividness with which he portrayed them.

Despairing of his son ever finishing school, the elder Cajal finally took matters into his own hands and gave his son an intensive home tutorial on the human skeleton. This took place in a barn behind the house, often with osteological material gathered locally in the moonlight, but it schooled the young student in the minutest details of each bone, observed, remembered, and sketched from every angle. It kindled his imagination, mobilized his memory, focused his energies, reconciled him to the rigors of formal education.

He proceeded to take the bachelor's degree in Ayerbe, and enrolled in the medical school at Zaragoza, the largest town of the region just to the south. The family soon followed, around 1870. There the father finally achieved his lifelong goal of an academic appointment as a professor of dissection. Cajal in his memoirs recalls his father's "determination to make his son a skilled dissector" (Cajal, 1989): "And with such a master who could shirk? Three years passed over us in that humble dissecting room . . . as we took apart piece by piece the intricate mechanism of muscles, nerves and blood vessels. . . . Henceforth, I saw in the cadaver, not death, . . . but the marvellous workmanship of life." Cajal's watercolors of these dissections excited in his father a plan to publish them as an atlas of anatomy, but there were no means in Zaragoza for reproducing them, so the plan came to nought. However, Cajal's skill gained him his first appointment, as an assistant in dissection, giving him a little income and setting his foot on the path toward a career in anatomy.

With this new purpose Cajal moved more steadily through his studies, though not without distraction. His incredible energy and restlessness would never allow that, and took him through several "manias," which he details in his memoirs. One was "graphomania," during which he was obsessed with writing verse and prose of a romantic hue. This culminated in a "biological novel," patterned after Jules Verne, in which the hero voyages through the body, engaging in many epic struggles along the way. Such juvenilia, of course, pass into oblivion, but the discipline of the writing presages the future author of articles, monographs, and textbooks.

His second mania was gymnastics. Suddenly obsessed with being the strongest among his peers, he enrolled in a muscle-building class, and trained himself in gymnastics. He developed "monstrous pectoral muscles," the "strut of a side-show Hercules"; his handshake "unconsciously crushed" the hands of friends. Fortunately, as he was about to become "an incurable victim of athletic brutalization," the aberration passed, but his strong physique would carry him through several severe illnesses.

Finally was a mania for philosophy. As if to transfer his energies from muscles to brain cells, he threw himself into the study of philosophy, devouring the works of the great thinkers like Berkeley, Hume and Kant ("By good luck, those of Hegel . . . were not in the University library"). Interestingly, he favored idealism, of the Berkeleian variety. This mania passed, too, though he notes that it played its role in preparing him mentally for a career of scientific investigation.

Cajal graduated in medicine in 1873, at the age of 21. He spent a year locally in army service, then was sent with an expeditionary unit to Cuba, at that time under Spanish rule. This turned out to be a disaster. He fell ill with malaria; forced to continue working, his health deteriorated, and he barely made it back to Spain alive.

Slow Beginnings

Starting in Zaragoza

Cajal's prospects on his return to Zaragoza in late 1875, at the age of 23, were quite modest. He obtained an assistantship in anatomy and took up his studies again in order to apply for a professorship. This required him to pass the examination for a doctorate. According to Penfield (1926), it was on a sojourn at this time in Madrid to study for the examination that "for the first time he saw a microscope." From Cajal's memoir (1989) it is at least clear that it was the first time he had actually studied microscopic anatomy, and, with no training or experience, but with typical determination, he decided at once that he would set up a microscopical laboratory for himself in Zaragoza. Using every peseta saved from his service in Cuba, he purchased a French Verick microscope, a popular make of the time, which included a water-immersion lens and the ability to magnify ×800, and other necessities. He also bought anatomical and microscopical manuals, and began to subscribe to several journals. Since he did not read German, he had to rely mostly on French translations, although he eventually purchased Stricker's *Handbuch* of 1872 and Waldeyer's *Archiv* (Cajal, 1989).

It is hard to comprehend fully how isolated Cajal was in his interest in microscopy at that time in Spain. He quotes an anecdote told by Kölliker, that on a visit to Spain in 1849, Kölliker was astonished to discover that the director of the Museum of Natural Sciences had put on display a fine microscope, but hadn't the faintest idea how to use it. Cajal (1989) observes that much the same applied in the 1870s to his professors, most of whom regarded the instrument as an obstacle to progress in biology, just as Bichat had thought in 1801 (see Chapter 2)!

The next several years were a mixture of slow advancement and bitter disappointment. His social ineptitude hampered his ability to compete for the available professorships. The best he could do was a position as temporary auxiliary professor in 1877. In 1878, he suffered a pulmonary hemorrhage, due to tuberculosis in the aftermath of his malaria. It seemed that his career, if not his life, was at an end, and he fell into a deep depression. But competent medical management by his father, and a few months at the baths, restored his health. His spirits, too, bounded back; he took up a new hobby, photography. Soon after, he married a young woman who, though lacking education, was to be a mainstay of his life; he cites with pride an acquaintance who observed, "Half of Cajal is his wife." In 1879 he was appointed director of Anatomical Museums in Zaragoza.

Cajal was now ready to embark on his career as a microscopist. Working as he did in his home-built laboratory, he acknowledges that his first efforts were "pretty weak": a study of the origin of pus cells in inflamed mesentery (1880), and a study of nerve endings in voluntary muscle (1881). These had the merit of giving him experience in the use of different stains (including silver nitrate and gold toning); his impecuniousness also required him to engrave the illustrations with his own hands directly on the stone (as did Nansen; see Chapter 9), a skill that was later to stand him in good stead.

Advancement to Valencia

In his unsuccessful attempts at advancement Cajal had nonetheless acquired admirers, and in 1883, at the age of 31, he was appointed to the chair of anatomy at Valencia. This seaport in the Mediterranean was known as the Athens of Spain, and Cajal luxuriated for the first time in a cosmopolitan environment. No sooner had he settled into his new duties than the cholera of 1885 broke out. Like many microscopists all over Europe, Cajal was captivated by the new study of microbiology and inspired by its pioneers—Pasteur, Koch, and others—to discover the causes of dreaded diseases in the search for microbes under the microscope. Responding to the crisis, Cajal carried out a study of the disease for the Provincial Government in Zaragoza, in the summer of 1885, including experiments involving inoculations of animals. This work had two positive effects on Cajal: it stimulated an interest in pathological microscopic anatomy, and it resulted in a gift from the Zaragoza government of a "magnificent" Zeiss microscope (beside which, he writes, his Verick seemed "a rickety door bolt").

Back in Valencia, he took up his microscopical studies with renewed determination. The next study, in 1885, was on "anastomotic cells of stratified epithelium," his first publication in a foreign (German) journal. Then followed (1887 and early 1888) several papers on the microscopic structure of muscle fibers, in insects and in mammals. He also prepared a handbook with 203 woodcuts, all executed by himself, on histology and microscopic technique, the first such in Spanish, a project to which he devoted himself with patriotic fervor.

If, as they say, "the past is prologue," these years in Valencia present a murky view of the future. All in all, Cajal's career at that time, measured against his high aspirations, would seem to be best characterized as something of a muddle. On the positive side, he had finally the security that came with the chair; his laboratory was upgraded by the new microscope; he had started publishing his articles in foreign journals and seeking out criticism from foreign scientists; he was extending his mastery of microscopic techniques; his handbook on histology had established him as one of the leading Spanish microscopists.

There were, however, significant entries on the debit side of the ledger. His life was still essentially bounded by the walls of a provincial town in an underdeveloped country. This on the face of it would seem to have made Cajal's situation in Valencia similar to Golgi's in Italy, but there were differences: Spain was more remote from central Europe, and it lacked virtually any tradition in science and learning—a lack that Cajal felt keenly. It not only put him at a disadvantage in keeping up with the latest techniques, but it also meant that his fecund imagination produced a hodgepodge of untested ideas. One example he cites is his belief in spontaneous generation—this despite his research in microbiology, and knowledge of Pasteur!

Another example is found in his work on muscle. Cajal (1989) himself draws attention to it as a cautionary tale, and it has also been cited for that purpose in another context more recently by Huxley (1977) regarding a controversy over the reticular theory of muscle. Since this was one of Cajal's first sallies into the international arena of ideas, and since it involved several protagonists who were soon to play large roles with Cajal in establishing the neuron doctrine, it will be worth our close consideration. I am much indebted to Sir Andrew Huxley for drawing my attention to this episode in nineteenth century biology.

The Reticular Theory of Muscle and the Principle of the Uniformity of Nature

The microscopical study of the structure of skeletal muscle began with a paper in 1840 by William Bowman, who first described the muscle fiber and its characteristic alternating striations. In the 1870s a series of studies from different laboratories described the patterns of striation and the ways they changed during contraction, and suggested what the underlying mechanism might be. For many of the studies, insect muscles were favored because of the very prominent birefringent striation patterns. One of the early workers was Wilhelm Krause, the same Krause who later befriended Cajal in publishing his first papers, on muscle, in the journal that Krause edited (see later).

Around 1885, two new developments occurred. One was the introduction of staining with gold chloride, which revealed a diffuse network of thin fibrils within each fiber. The other was the finding of similarly appearing networks within many other types of cells, including cells that were actively motile, such as amoebae or white blood corpuscles. From this discovery arose the seemingly logical idea (Klein, 1878; Carnoy, 1884) that the striated skeletal muscle fiber was merely a specialized example of a universal contractile mechanism expressed in a more general and accessible manner in simpler types of cells. This idea, which Huxley (1977) characterizes as an example of the application of "Principle of the Uniformity of Nature," quickly established itself, with strong adherents. One of the first, B. Melland (1885), a student in England, wrote a paper entitled "A simplified view of the histology of the striped muscle," in which he presented the basic argument that if one finds that the protoplasm of motile cells consists of a fibrillary network, then that network must be responsible for the contractile property; the same must apply to the similar network in skeletal muscle; therefore, the additional striations of skeletal muscle must be artifacts. He wrote: "Everyone who has considered the subject must admit the essential identity from a physiological point of all those tissues which possess in a special degree contractility. The contraction of a white blood-corpuscle or amoeba is essentially the same phenomenon as the contraction of an involuntary fibre-cell or a striped muscle-fibre" (Melland, 1885; in Huxley, 1977).

This idea attracted Arthur van Gehuchten, a young Belgian microscopist. In two long papers, in 1886 and 1888, in the journal *La Cellule,* his very first publications, he reported his studies of both invertebrate and vertebrate striated muscle, and arrived at a similar conclusion: "The muscle cell is an ordinary cell in which the reticulum [of fibrils] is organized in a regular manner and the chyle [protoplasmic matrix] is invested with myosin." (in Huxley, 1977).

Cajal (1989) describes his own participation in this subject as follows (see also Huxley, 1977):

> There was current in histology at that time one of those diagrammatic conceptions which temporarily fascinate the mind and influence young workers decisively in their inquiries and opinions. I refer to the reticular theory of Heitzmann and Carnoy, which was applied very ingeniously to the striated substance of muscles by Carnoy himself, the author of the famous *Cellular Biology,* and afterwards by the Englishman, Melland, and the Belgian, van Gehuchten. Impressed by the ability of these scientists and by the prestige of the theory, I had the weakness to regard the contractile substance, as they did, as a tiny lattice of delicate fibres (the *preexistent filaments* seen in preparations with acids and with gold chloride) united transversely by the net postulated at the level of the line of Krause. As for the primitive fibrils, they were supposed to be the result of post mortem coagulation. Later on I changed this opinion, which was vigorously criticised by Rollet, Kölliker, and others, who declared rightly that the so-called artifacts could be observed even in the living muscles of certain insects.
>
> I insist upon these details because I wish to warn young [men] against the invincible attraction of theories which simplify and unify seductively. Ruled by the theory, we who were active in histology then saw networks everywhere. What captivated us specially was that this speculation identified the complex

> structural substratum of the striated fibre with the simple reticulum or fibrillar framework of all protoplasm. Whatever the cell might be, amoeba or contractile corpuscle, the physiological basis or rather the active factor, was always represented by the network or elementary skeleton.
>
> From these illusions no histologist is free, least of all the beginner. We fall into the trap all the more readily when the simple schemes stimulate and appeal to tendencies deeply rooted in our minds, the congenital inclination to economy of mental effort and the almost irresistible propensity to regard as true what satisfies our aesthetic sensibility by appearing in agreeable and harmonious architectural forms. As always, reason is silent before beauty. The case of Phryne (Greek hetaira who, when placed on trial, won an acquittal by displaying her extraordinary beauty to the judges) repeats itself continually. Nevertheless, no error is useless so long as we are attended by a sincere purpose of emendation; and being convinced that enduring fame accompanies only the truth, I wished to be correct at that price. Hence, later on, I reacted vigorously against those theoretical conceptions, under which reality is lost or distorted.

Even an authority like Willy Kühne was deceived on this issue. Kühne's (1862) classical studies of the neuromuscular end-plate, showing that the nerve terminals remained discontinuous with the underlying muscle, had provided one of the few redoubts where advocates of discontinuous connections between cells could hold out against the network view (see Chapter 17). However, as early as 1864, he had noted "chemical similarities between muscle and the protoplasm of ameboid cells" (Huxley, 1977), and in his Croonian Lecture of 1888 he supported the reticular view of the contractile mechanism.

The idea did not last long. Gustav Retzius, who introduced gold chloride for the staining of muscle fibers in 1881, was never fooled by it. Nor, as one would expect, was Kölliker. In his 1888 paper "On knowledge of striated muscle fibers" he subjected the concept to a devastating attack, upholding the view that the striations of the myofibrils contain the essential contractile mechanism of skeletal muscle.

The idea, and the principle behind it, may be regarded as an example of what Peter Medawar has called "nothing-butism"—that a particular property is "nothing but" an unnecessarily complicated instance of some other simple property. That Cajal and the others should fall prey to it is perhaps understandable; after all, as Huxley (1977) points out, the "Principle of the Uniformity of Nature" seemed manifest in the cell theory itself. The experience was obviously sobering for Cajal, and must have been a precautionary warning to himself when he soon thereafter formulated his concepts of the nerve cell. The same may be said of the others; Retzius, van Gehuchten, and Kölliker, together with Cajal—key players in the emergence of the neuron doctrine—had this experience in common, and it must have placed extra burdens of skepticism on them all when they turned to assessing each other's work on the nerve cell.

The Breakthrough

Cajal's life might well have gone on like this, becoming a footnote to the history of histology, but for the Golgi stain. As we have seen, mention of the method had begun to appear in the literature by the mid-1880s, but the fact that the stain was capricious in its selectivity, as well as being erratic in the structures actually visualized, mitigated against its adoption. Nonetheless, a number of microscopists here and there tinkered with it. One of these was Don Luis Simarro, a Valencian psychiatrist and neurologist working in Madrid, who learned the technique on a trip to Paris. Upon his return, he included it among the techniques he was using to investigate changes in neurons associated with different nervous diseases.

Cajal, by chance, made a trip to Madrid in early 1887 and, as was his custom, went around to different laboratories to learn what was new. This led him to pay a visit to Simarro. As so often in those days, his laboratory was in his home: "It was there, in the house of Dr. Simarro . . . that for the first time I had an opportunity to admire . . . those famous sections of the brain impregnated by the silver method of the Savant of Pavia." (Cajal, 1989).

At the time, Cajal was beginning to study nervous tissue, starting with the use of carmine as a stain, but seeing little more than had anyone else of the nerve processes with that approach. Drawing on his talent for dissection, he had started to dissociate mechanically individual nerve cells and their processes, after the manner of Deiters, using fine needles combined with dispersion of the cells by maceration in weak fixative solution. It seems he had got about as far as Deiters had. Thus, we must suppose that he had at least a relatively clear image of a Deiters-like cell with its axis cylinder and protoplasmic extensions in his mind, when he first encountered a Golgi-stained cell. There must have been an instant resonance of images; a shock of recognition.

The effect on Cajal was deep and immediate; as he describes it himself (translated by Sherrington, 1935a):

> Against a clear background stood black threadlets, some slender and smooth, some thick and thorny, in a pattern punctuated by small dense spots, stellate or fusiform. All was sharp as a sketch with Chinese ink on transparent Japan-

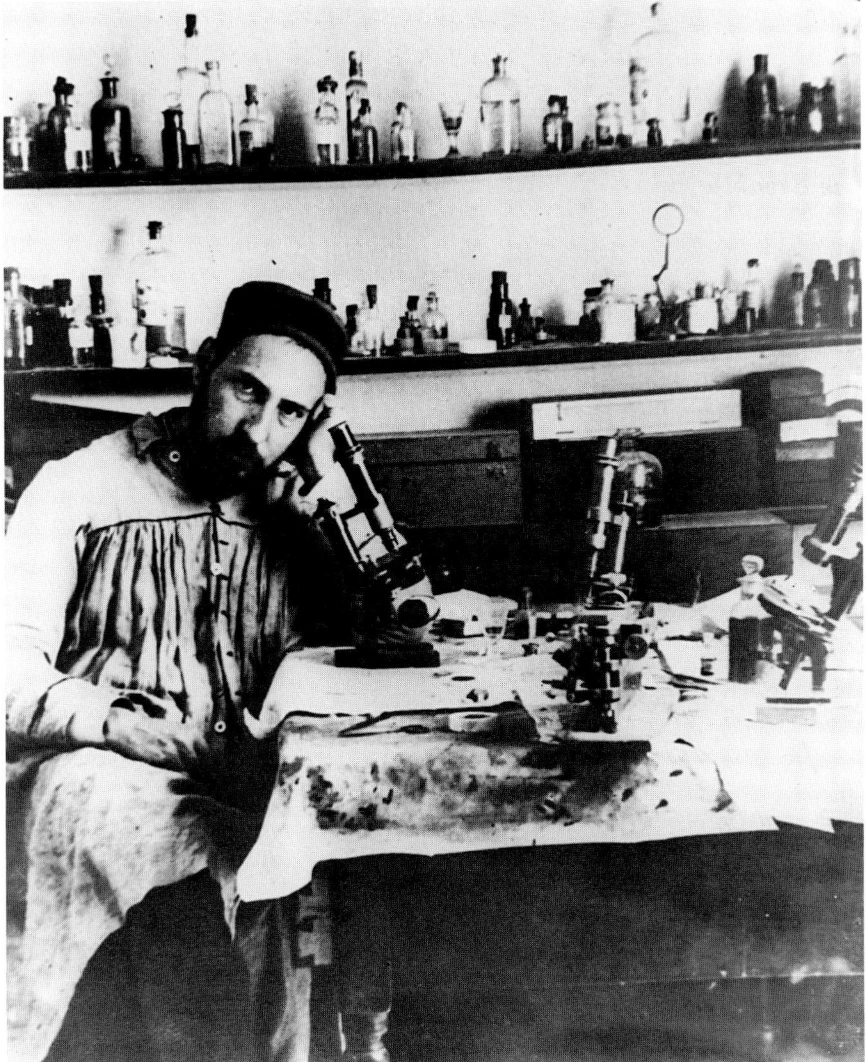

Fig. 18. Portrait of Cajal in his laboratory, around 1890. Courtesy of P. Rakic, originally from P. Yakovlev.

paper. And to think that that was the same tissue which when stained with carmine or logwood left the eye in a tangled thicket where sight may stare and grope for ever fruitlessly, baffled in its effort to unravel confusion and lost for ever in a twilit doubt. Here, on the contrary, all was clear and plain as a diagram. A look was enough. Dumbfounded, I could not take my eye from the microscope.

Cajal returned to Valencia and immediately tested the method on different parts of the brain in a variety of animal species. The results convinced him that "the new method of analysis had before it a brilliant future, especially if there could be found some way of overcoming its highly capricious and uncertain character" (Cajal, 1989).

Before he could address this problem, he had to make a career choice, between accepting the chairs of anatomy in Barcelona or in Zaragoza. Despite the attraction of his native region, he feared the personal frictions within too small a faculty; but more important, he knew that, "For a man dedicated to one idea and resolved to devote his whole activity to it, great cities are preferable to small ones" (Cajal, 1989). Then, as now, Barcelona was "a city of architecture, ideas, cuisine and manners" (Vecsey, 1990). It offered laboratory facilities and publishing means not available in Zaragoza, and a peaceful atmosphere for exploiting them. It was a felicitous move; by the autumn of 1887 he was installed in Barcelona in excellent new quarters and surrounded by congenial and highly regarded colleagues. His first self-imposed task was to finish his *Manual of General Pathological Anatomy*. By early 1888, he was ready to pursue his destiny. The intensity he brought to that task is evident in the portrait of Figure 18.

11

The Early Discoveries of Cajal

Cajal's Strategy

> The year 1888 arrived, my greatest year, my year of fortune. For during this year, which rises in my memory with the rosy hues of dawn, there emerged at last those interesting discoveries so eagerly hoped and longed for. Had it not been for them, I should have vegetated sadly in a provincial university without passing in the scientific order beyond the category of more or less estimable delvers after details. As a result of them I attained the enjoyment of the sour flattery of celebrity; my humble surname, pronounced in the German manner (Cayal), crossed the frontiers; and my ideas, made known among scientific men, were discussed hotly. From that time on, the trench of science had one more recognized digger.
>
> How did it happen? . . . (Cajal, 1989)

Cajal's very first results with the Golgi stain had largely confirmed the findings of Golgi, as far as they went. Cajal realized that if he was to make any significant progress beyond this he would have to solve the problem of the "capricious and highly uncertain character" of the method. This he did through two strategies. One was to use very intense staining reactions. Although this introduces increased amounts of metallic deposit that can obscure the image, it has the double advantage of revealing better the finest processes, and of permitting the use of thicker sections, thereby enabling one "to follow a nervous conductor from its origin to its termination" (Cajal, 1989). One can gain some appreciation for this approach by comparing Golgi's renditions of processes in the cerebellum, where the processes are thin and faint (see Figs. 12, 13), with Cajal's drawings, where the processes are much more clearly demarcated (see below).

The second strategem dealt with the problem that the Golgi technique does not stain myelinated fibers well, because the myelin sheath prevents the entry of the silver into the fiber. Cajal reasoned that he could get around this obstacle by working on embryonic and young animals, before myelination takes place. This has the further advantage that a series of young animals studied at different ages can reveal the mechanism by which the nerve cells grow their processes and establish their final positions and relations with each other. This was the ontogenetic (developmental) method. It was, of course, the method of Wilhelm His, but he had lacked this new staining tool for revealing the growth of the processes into the later stages of development. The very fact that, as we have seen, the methods up till then had favored the study of adult humans and other large mammals, where the nerve cells are large, had tended to leave the ontogenetic approach underappreciated. Against that background, Cajal's use of it was the more innovative.

Part of Cajal's genius was in realizing the importance of developing the Golgi stain into a method on which one could have some reliance. Many of those who tinkered with it gave it up and became suspicious of its results, Simarro himself among them; Cajal (1989) quotes a letter from him in 1889:

> "I received your last publication on the structure of the spinal cord, which seems to me an important work but not *convincing*, because of the method of Golgi, which, even in your hands, who have perfected it so much, is a method which *suggests* rather than *demonstrates*."

The First Publication (May, 1889)

Once Cajal had got the Golgi stain working to his satisfaction, and had begun to apply it to animals of different ages and also to many different species, the results came quickly. Cajal saw immediately that if he was to obtain the recognition he sought for his discoveries, he needed to have an avenue for rapid publication of a considerable volume of material. In characteristic fashion, he determined to set up his own journal for this purpose, calling it *Revista Trimestral de Histologia normal y patologica* (*Trimestral Review of Normal and Pathological Histology*). He tells us that the costs of publication "entirely swallowed up my income," and that the 60 copies of each issue were sent almost entirely to "foreign scientists" (presumably free of charge) (Cajal, 1989). "Naturally," he writes, with his usual directness, in the first year (1888) "all the articles, six [actually seven, according to the enclosed bibliography] in number, sprang from my own pen," as well as the lithographic plates.

The first article in the *Revista* was Cajal's journal article on the nervous system using the Golgi stain. It is of special interest to us. As so often happens, the early work on a subject in science carries the seeds of much of the later thought. Cajal's article is entitled "Estructura de los centros nerviosos de las aves." Apart from a section on details of the methods, we cite it here in virtually its entirety (Cajal, 1888b):

STRUCTURE OF THE NERVOUS SYSTEM OF BIRDS

The investigations of Golgi into the texture of the nervous centers have opened a new era of study which appears to be unlimited, since the analytical method described by this author permits the resolution of some problems of structure, and has served in addition to raise new and difficult questions. Such, for example, are the connections of the cells, impossible to discern in the best preparations of the centers, and such are moreover the disposition and termination of the lateral branches of the nervous prolongation, whether sensory or motor, to which all the corpuscles give rise.

We do not have the pretension of resolving these problems: we intend for now only to expound the results of our new investigations into the nervous system of birds, particularly the cerebellum, which will be the object of this first communication.

The analytical method we have utilized is the one that Golgi (1885) [ed: 1886] recommends in his memorable work and the one followed in the notable investigations of Fusari (1887), Tartuferi (1887) and Petrone (1888). . . .

Of the three methods of fixation that Golgi recommends in order for the pieces of tissue to receive the action of the silver nitrate, the third has given us the best results (immersion of the fresh pieces in Muller's solution for two or more days; immediate submersion for 24 or more hours in a mixture of osmic acid and Muller's solution). This method is very suitable for impregnation of the small cells of the molecular layer [of the cerebellum], as well as their nervous prolongations. We have sometimes used the second method of fixation (immersion of the fresh pieces for two days in a mixture of solutions of bichromate and osmic acid), which is the only one which reveals in an acceptable manner the expansions of the dwarf corpuscles of the granular layer. Finally, the first method of Golgi, used occasionally, reveals very well the Purkinje cells and their nervous prolongations. . . .

The bird cerebellum

The bird cerebellum consists of a thin grey cortex and a white nucleus that supplies transverse laminae radiating forward, above, and backwards. The form and disposition of these laminae remind us of those of the medial lobe or vermiform eminences of mammals, which can be considered homologous to those of the bird cerebellum.

The most instructive parts of the cerebellum are the perpendicular anteriorposteriors of the laminae, the ones which appear in the surface of the section constituting a veritable tree of life. Furthermore, the disposition of the grey and white layers of each lamina, and the form and connections of their elements, perfectly remind us of the mammalian cerebellum and the descriptions of its cells which Golgi (1885) and Fusari . . . have made. However, in the birds (hen, duck, pigeon, etc.), certain elements appear more clearly, and some dispositions that would be very difficult to appraise in the human are exaggerated and modified in a prominent manner.

In each lamina of the cerebellum we encounter: First, a superficial or molecular layer; second, an underlying granular zone, and third, an axis or layer of white substance.

a) The Superficial or Molecular Layer—Is the thickest of the three and looks finely granular under low magnification. Its thickness in the pigeon is .45 to .50 mm. Golgi's procedure in the pigeon reveals three classes of corpuscles: the large Purkinje cells, the small stellate cells and the bifurcated neuroglial corpuscles.

1. *Purkinje cells.*—Are located at the junction of the molecular layer with the granular layer. In the pigeon their size varies between 18 and 20 micrometers in width and 32 to 36 micrometers in length. They are pear-shaped with the greatest mass seen below, and present two prolongations: an axis cylinder and expansion below, and the protoplasmic trunk and expansion above. The *cylinder* or nervous prolongation [Fig. 19B] arises in a lightly stained core, crosses the granular zone in an oblique way and continues without diminishing in thickness, before broadening itself into a fiber of the white matter. At a variable distance from its origin, it emits two or more expansions of frequently retrograde course, which, after becoming tortuous and varicose and branching off various times, terminate freely (apparently at least) under the *descending fringes* (see below). The superficial prolongation is thick, always single (as opposed to the mammal where it is usually multiple) and, at a variable distance from its origin, divides in two or more branches, in its turn decomposing into thinner ones, that after an ascendant and flexuous trajectory terminate, be it slightly thicker or not, in the same cerebellar surface. Many fibers arriving at the surface are doubled, terminating much lower and describing small terminal arcs. We distinguish these fibers from those exhibited by the Purkinje cells of mammals, which are thicker and less numerous and lacking in transverse or secondary ramifications. Moreover, the surface of the latter appear bristling with thorns [puntas] or short spines [espinas] that in their ends are represented by light roughnesses. (Essentially, we believe that these eminences are the result of a tumultuous precipitation of the silver; but the constancy of its existence and its presence, even in preparations in which the reaction appears with a great delicacy in the remaining elements, inclines us to judge that this is a normal condition.)

2. *Stellate cells.* [These stellate cells near the Purkinje cell layer are now called basket cells.] These are small, globular, and irregular, situated at different levels within the thickness of the molecular layer, and supplied with numerous protoplasmic prolongations [dendrites]. However, the special character of these cells is the unique arrangement of their nervous filament [axon]. This arises from the cell body, and also quite often from a thick, protoplasmic expansion [dendrite], and directing itself horizontally, describes a long trajectory, runs for a considerable distance through the molecular layer, giving off numerous branches, some ascending and others descending. The ascending ones are thin, and after various ramifications they terminate in the

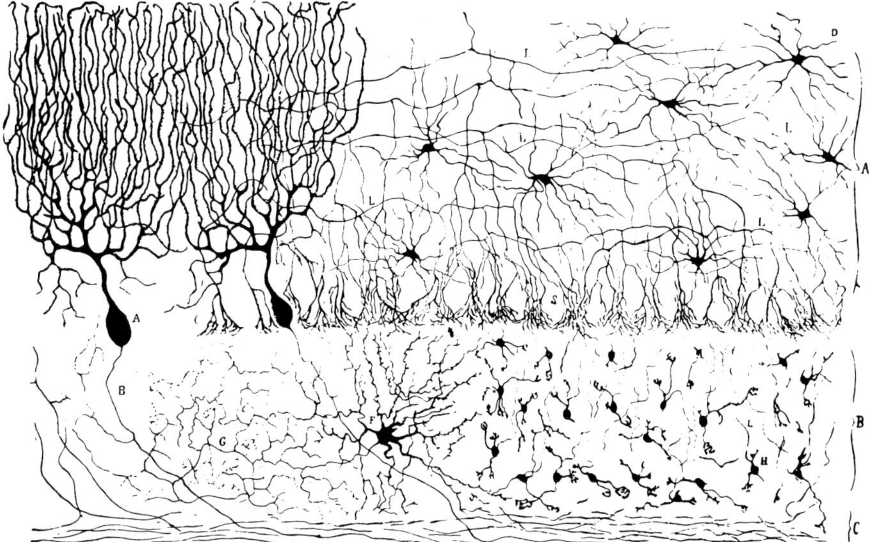

Fig. 19. Cajal's first illustration of his results using the Golgi stain:

"Vertical section of a cerebellar convolution of a hen. -Impregnation by the Golgi method. A represents the molecular zone, B designates the granular layer and C the white matter.

"A, the body of a Purkinje cell. -B, prolongation of Deiters [axon] of this cell. -D, small stellate cell. -L, nervous prolongation of these elements. - C, descending fringe [basket] in which the branches emanate from the axis cylinders.- S, space left by the descending fringes in which reside the body of the Purkinje cells. -H, dwarf corpuscles of the granular layer with an axis cylinder [axon] L directed upward. -F, large stellate cell of the granular layer. -G, its highly ramified nervous prolongation [axon]." (Cajal, 1888a)

molecular layer in a manner still unknown, perhaps by free endings, since we have never found anastomoses between these fibrils and the branches of the *cylinder* [axon] of more superficial cells. The descending branches always arise at a certain vertical angle from the trajectory of the nervous prolongations [Fig. 19B]; descending, they grow visibly thicker, ramify at acute angles, and terminate in fringes [tufts] of short and varicose fibers [baskets] which envelope completely the bodies of the Purkinje cells. Due to their abundance and thickness, these fringes form a virtual layer in the transitional zone between the molecular and granular layers. The fibers that form them do not anastomose among themselves and, apparently, end freely, oriented downwards, after becoming considerably thickened and repeatedly varicose [Fig. 19C].

Never, in numerous preparations, have we been able to observe the prolongation of one of these varicose fibers of the fringes extending into the subjacent granular layer. With regard to the termination of the *cylinder* [axon], it appears to take place through a descending fringe [basket] somewhat more robust than the others, but without any new features. This singular manner

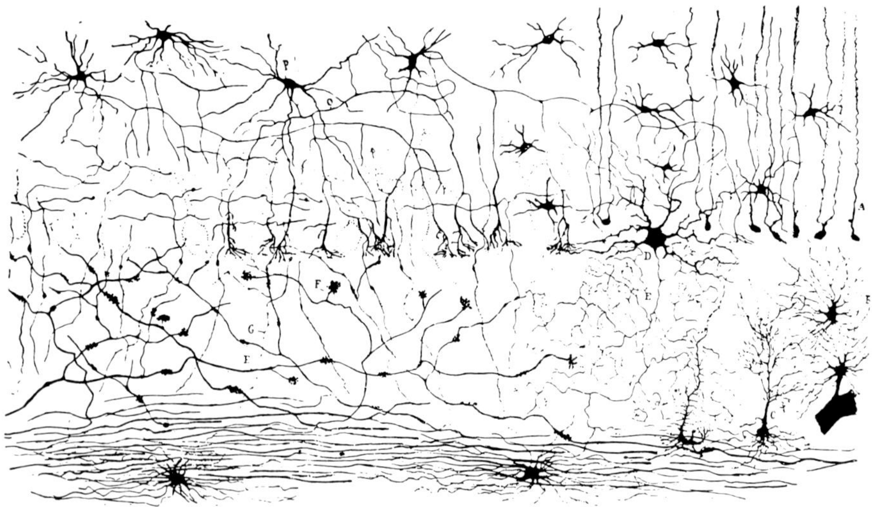

Fig. 20. Another view of Golgi stained nerve cells by Cajal:

"Section of a convolution of the cerebellum of the pigeon. -Silver impregnation by the Golgi method. -(For more clarity some Purkinje cells and some stellate cells, as well as some axis cylinders [axons] have been deleted.) -The same layers are represented as in the former figure.

"A, neuroglial cells of the molecular layer. -B, neuroglial corpuscles of the granular zone. -C, arboriform neuroglial cell. -D, large stellate cell with its axis cylinder [axon] E, abundantly ramified. One can see that many of its branches terminate in varicose arborizations. -E, nodular [mossy] fibers with an arborizing branchlet F. -G.Vertical varicose fibers. -P, stellate elements of the molecular layer. -O, an axis cylinder [axon] belonging to cell P." (Cajal, 1888a)

of termination of the *cylinder* and these same dispositions of the descending fringes or tufts are apparent in the human, except that there the fringes [baskets] contain few fibers (two or three somewhat larger and unequal), and the arcs formed by the *cylinder* in its horizontal trajectory are much smoother or incomplete. We do not wonder that Golgi has not mentioned these arrangements, since we ourselves learned to see them in mammals only after having discovered them in birds. We may add for the sake of completeness a very frequent arrangement of the *cylinder* [axon]. Immediately after its origin, it describes a complete horizontal circle around the cell; sometimes it is a semicircle, so that the fiber courses in the opposite direction; finally, on some occasions these circles, or more or less extended arcs of the cylinder, occur near its termination [Fig. 20].

3. *Neuroglial cells.*—Are small and emit one or two filaments which, from the limit of the molecular zone where they reside, extend in a flexuous trajectory to the cerebellar surface. As can be seen, these elements are almost identical to the figures by Golgi in the mammalian cerebellum [Fig. 20A].

b) Granular Layer.—Contains three classes of cells: *small globular cells, large stellate cells, and neuroglial cells.*

1. The *granules or dwarf cells* of this layer are very numerous and so small that they are no larger than 6 to 8 microns in the hen. They are difficult to stain with the ordinary Golgi procedure (first method), but they color frequently enough using the second method of this author (first immersion in osmium bichromate mixture and then silver impregnation). The body of these cells is spherical or oval, rarely triangular, and from it divide three or four thin protoplasmic expansions [dendrites] which terminate after a short distance as a very tiny and varicose arborization that perfectly reminds one of the ramification of the *cylinder* [axon] in a motor plate [neuromuscular junction] impregnated by gold. Golgi has seen without a doubt this arborization in the human, but he has taken it for a cluster of granulose material, which is not strange, since in mammals this arborization is very delicate and frequently looks continuous. As well as these singular expansions, one sees a very thin fiber that presents the aspect of an axis cylinder [axon]. This fiber originates frequently from a protoplasmic stem, and after a flexuous and ascendant course, terminates, sometimes dichotomizing, under the Purkinje cells. We have never seen such fibers penetrate into the molecular zone nor bend underneath as if in search of white matter, for which reason we are inclined to think that, in judging the connections of these prolongations [axons] with some element, they must be with the Purkinje cell, perhaps by intermediation of the small lateral branches of the nervous prolongations. But this cannot be more than a mere conjecture.

2. *The large stellate cells* lie only partly in the same row as the Purkinje cells, and consequently one could as well consider some of them to be elements of the molecular layer, whereas others lie at distinct levels in the thickness of the granular layer; these must be related to the white matter. As Golgi has noted, these cells are characterized by the elegance of arborization of the nervous prolongation [axon]. Figures 19 and 20 show two of these cells and their axis cylinders [axons]. Each one of these is seen to ramify at almost a right angle and give rise to an almost infinite number of tenuous filaments that substantially fill the granular zone and whose course undulates to supply undoubtedly the surfaces of the small dwarf corpuscles. In this arborization, the individuality of the cylinder is lost, leaving two or three rather voluminous branches, that, arriving at the white matter, disseminate between its fibers, probably continuing with the finest conducting tubes. The small lateral branches terminate apparently freely in a fiber drawn out and pointed, and, more frequently, in a varicose horseshoe-shaped arborization. In summary, it is impossible to confirm definitely that these granular arborizations are the terminations of the aforementioned branches; it could also be that they continue further, and that the analytical method employed here is powerless to reveal them in their new course.

3. *The neuroglial cells* are divided into two types: stellate and arboriform. The *stellate* cells lie within the granular layer, nearly always connected by a thick pedicle to the surface of the capillaries, where it forms a discontinuous investiture. Its prolongations are granular, very flexuous and ramified, accommodating themselves to the curved surfaces of the dwarf corpuscles [Fig. 20B]. The *arboriform* cells [Fig. 20C] are situated partly in the white matter and partly in the gray matter, where they are further separated into two

zones. These give rise to a thick part of irregular form whose expansions penetrate between the conducting fibers, and a narrow part prolonged into a branched stalk which crosses to supply short and delicate branchlets, nearly perpendicularly within the granular layer.

c) Layer of white matter.—The conducting fibers are compressed into bundles of varying thickness which at certain points separately penetrate the granular zone up to the molecular zone. The fibers that leave the white matter and course through the granular zone are of four types: 1, nervous prolongations [axons] of the Purkinje cells; 2, nodular ramified fibrils [axons]; 3, perpendicular varicose filaments [axons], and 4, axial filaments continuous with the cylinder [axon] of the large stellate cells.

1. *Fibers of the Purkinje cells.* This is thick, with a slightly flexuous course and usually oblique in relation to the plane of the white matter, with smooth contours; one sees that it enters the superior part of the granular zone and is continuous with the Deiters filament [axon] of the Purkinje cells [Fig. 19B].

2. *Nodular [mossy] fibers.* These are the most robust of all the fibers that pass through the granular layer, and are characterized by presenting, at intervals, varicose nodules, which consist of an irregular accumulation of silver precipitate. Examination of random nodules [Fig. 20], in sections very lightly impregnated, enables one to see that these are true arborizations, short and varicose, which embellish certain sites in the manner of an investment of moss or thicket. At many sites, this granular arborization is supported by a short fine stalk which gives it the appearance of a flower [Fig. 20F]. These nodular fibers ramify repeatedly at very acute angles, giving the arborization a large extension throughout the granular zone. Frequently, from the principal stalk emerge secondary branchlets which run nearly parallel in the granular layer for a considerable distance. The daughter branches (which may number as many as 15–20) are much more delicate than the trunk, give rise as well in their trajectory to mossy arborizations, and after several divisions, advance up to the zone of the descending fringes or tufts, where they either truly terminate or the impregnation ceases in a constant manner, but they never reach as far as the molecular layer. We consider as very probable the union of these fibers with the extremities of the tufts, or that there does not exist narrow contiguity between the one and the other; it is therefore certain that the nodular fibers are the most abundant of the granular zone and unique by virtue of the fact that an extraordinary number of them maintain some relation with the notable quantity of descending fibers emanating from the cylinder [axon] of the stellate cells of the molecular zone.

3. *Vertical varicose fibers.* These fine varicose fibers are directed from the white matter up to the molecular layer, where they terminate at various levels. Within the granular zone its trajectory is rectilinear and without ramifications, but arriving at the molecular zone ultimately at the piriform [Purkinje] cells, it seems to enlarge and divide into two or more branches that course horizontally, terminating in a manner that is not easy to describe [Fig. 20G]. Nearly all of these fibers exhibit in their passage through the granular zone and at a point proximal to the Purkinje cells an ellipsoidal enlargement which appears to be rather thick and varicose.

4. *The fibrils of the stellate cells* are very fine and disappear among the fibers of the white matter so that it is not possible to follow them even for a short distance.

5. *Neuroglial cells.* These elements naturally contained in the white matter are stout, with prolonged thin fibers, and completely resemble those of the white matter of the cerebellum of mammals [Fig. 20].

Finally, in the white matter at the point of general emergence of the lamellae there exist thick cells (30–40 micrometers) provided with thick protoplasmic expansions that in cell body form are stellate or triangular. These elements possess a nervous prolongation which appears to maintain its individuality and course to a junction with the peduncular fibers.

Connections of the Cerebellar Elements. Here one has an arduous question whose solution cannot be achieved solely with data so limited and incomplete beyond measure. The Golgi procedure, so excellent for impregnating the protoplasmatic expansions [dendrites] of the nerve cells, is highly inconsistent with relation to the staining of the nervous prolongations [axons], which almost always appear stained only over short lengths. Judging the course and connections of a fiber can only be done by comparative study of a great number of good preparations.

The first result that we have gathered in preparations of the cerebellum of birds, is that in these creatures, as in mammals, the nerve cells do not anastomose directly, in other words by their protoplasmic expansions [dendrites]. This phenomenon, that so contradicts our physiological and anatomical hypotheses about the connections of the nervous centers, has not escaped Golgi, who in some manner tries to explain it, postulating in the core of the center's grey substance a network of axial [axonal] expansions (the branches of the prolongations of Deiters) that is termed the *diffuse reticulum,* and through which the cells could be interlaced in an indirect manner. We have carried out meticulous investigations on the course and connections of the nerve fibers, of the cerebral and cerebellar convolutions of the human, monkey, dog, etc. *We have never been able to see an anastomosis between ramifications of distinct nervous prolongations* [*axons*], *nor of the filaments emanating from the same expansion of Deiters* [*axons*]; *the fibers are interlaced in a very complicated manner, engendering a intricate and dense plexus, but never a network* [italics added]. The above observations on the structure of the bird cerebellum corroborate as well this result of seeing no relations between the dwarf corpuscles and the border stellates, and never an anastomosis between the Purkinje cells and the small stellate cells; it could be said that *each element is an absolutely autonomous physiological canton* [italics added]. This does not negate the indirect anastomoses (by branches of the filaments of Deiters) [the thin secondary filaments Deiters imagined to arise from the dendrites; see Chapter 4], but simply asserts that, because none can be seen, our judgment must be suspended on this point, or inclined to the belief that there are none, abandoning our anatomical prejudices.

A no less difficult problem, intimately connected with the above question, is the investigation of the connections made by the prolongations of Deiters [axons] that lose their individuality, with the fibers of the white matter. It is known that cells of the motor category (those of Purkinje) exist in the cerebellum, whose cylinder maintains its individuality until the white matter, and cells where this is not maintained (small stellate cells, large stellate cells, and dwarf corpuscles), which, accepting the hypothesis of Golgi, can be considered to be sensitive. But, where are the descending fringes continuous with the fibers of the white matter? And which of the infinite fibers into which the cylinder [axon] of the large stellate cells divides is continuous with a nervous fiber? This is what we have not been able to determine. It is doubtless that many of the fibers of the descending fringes, varicose and branching, are terminal arborizations, since they are constantly presented in the same way and with that aspect of discontinuous spheres characteristic of the nervous terminations; and, it is also certain, that almost all of the varicose and arciform expansions presented by the lateral filaments of the nervous prolongation of the large stellate cells show a terminal arborization (analogous to that exhibited by the trunk of the bipolar cells of the retina) in view of the fact that the procedure of Golgi never reveals a subsequent contination. Here must apply one of two hypotheses: either the procedure of Golgi is insufficient to show the bridges of union between these fibers with those of the white matter; or the connection between these and the axis cylinders can be mediated and can carry out the transmission of the nervous action in a manner like the electrical currents in an inductor coil.

Comments on the Paper

The first thing to note about this paper is that it is written in a modern format. It begins with an introduction that sets out clearly and succinctly the problem to be addressed. The methods are described in sufficient detail for a reader to repeat the experiments. The results then follow, organized in a logical framework according to different layers. The description is tied to plates that illustrate the major findings. There is a final discussion in which the author assesses how far the results have gone in resolving the questions posed in the introduction. We have left behind the personal and anecdotal styles of most of the earlier papers we have considered, as well as the wallowing in endless detail; here all efforts are focused objectively on an immediate problem. It is remarkable that Cajal, situated outside the mainstream of the science of his times, had this modern sense of how to write a scientific paper. He certainly would appear to deserve credit for helping to establish the modern format for scientific papers in neuroanatomy.

The next point of interest is that this paper, concerned with connections between cells and the mode of termination of the lateral branches of axis cylinders, is not on the spinal cord. Cajal follows Golgi in addressing these questions in the brain itself. To shift the battleground was a master stroke of strategy. The layers of nervous elements and the differentiation of cell types are much more sharply delimited in the cerebellum and other regions such as the retina, olfactory bulb, and tectum; the next paper in the *Revista* in fact is Cajal's first paper on the retina.

A third point about this study is that it was carried out in birds. We have noted that in the previous tradition it was natural for medically trained researchers to study directly the human brain. However, the rise of embryology under von Baer was based largely on the chick embryo, where the different stages of development could be readily analyzed, and the work of His in the 1880s had continued the use of the chick for analyzing the development of the nervous system, as we have seen. Cajal was well aware of this, of course, and he may also have turned his boyhood fascination with birds to practical use as well. In any case, it became part of his professed strategy to take a comparative approach to the study of a given region; certain elements could be seen to better advantage in different species, and, as he stated (see above), this was crucial in identifying certain elements in the bird so that this knowledge could be used to unravel more complicated relations in humans and other species.

The two illustrations in this paper give the clearest renderings in the literature up to that time of nerve cells and the full extension of their processes. These sharply etched images with their definite origins and endings may be compared with Golgi's delicately rendered fibrils disappearing into the background (Figs. 12, 13, Chapter 8). As in the case of Golgi's diagrams, each illustration is a composite of drawings of individual cells from many different histological sections. As Cajal states in his section on methods, different variations on the histological procedures were best for visualizing different types of cells. In the illustrations, these different elements are arranged *as Cajal conceived that they should be.* The drawings thus are based, on the one hand, on accurate but isolated experimental observations, and, on the other, on the author's intuition and imagination in synthesizing the arrangement of the separate elements. It is apparent that Cajal's images appear much more "drawn from life" than the stylized elements arranged with almost crystalline regularity by Golgi. All of Cajal's skills as a draughtsman, all his graphomania and his thwarted artistic ambitions, expressed themselves in these representations of the fantastic forms of nerve cells and the ways by which they were related. These first illustrations are early versions of what was to become the beautifully realized forms and pathways that have provided later generations of neuroscientists with their basic visual images of the neuronal organization of the nervous system. In these drawings Cajal the scientist and Cajal the artist unite; contemplate the overall impression of the diagram of Figure 19 and ask yourself if his view of the cerebellum is any less vivid than his countryman's view of Toledo.

New Findings and Interpretations

The new observations by Cajal may be summarized as follows:

1. *Purkinje cells.* Cajal confirms Golgi's basic description of the many-branched protoplasmic prolongations (dendrites). However, there is no emphasis on how elaborate this tree is, or the fact that it is flattened into a single plane. A new observation is that the branches are covered with small structures that he calls thorns or spines. This was the first report of *dendritic spines,* the smallest branches given off by a nerve cell. Cajal realizes that these might be artifacts, spurious deposits of silver, but believes that they represent normal structures. In fact, this issue was only resolved, like so many other questions, by the electronmicroscope in the 1950s. Cajal also confirms Golgi's discovery of the lateral branches (axon collaterals) of the prolongation of Deiters (axon) of the Purkinje cells, and the fact that the prolongation of Deiters is continuous with the nerve fibers of the white matter. There is not a clear realization, however, that this is the main pathway out of the cerebellar cortex.

2. *Stellate cells.* Star-shaped cells scattered throughout the superficial (molecular) layer had been seen and repeatedly illustrated by Golgi. He had noted their protoplasmic prolongations (dendrites); he had also seen their axis cylinder coursing laterally, but had not been able to visualize their terminations. Cajal focuses on the cells nearest the Purkinje cell body layer and discovers that their axis cylinders give rise to two types of branches: some end freely within the molecular layer, but some descend and end as a special tuft of branchlets that surround the Purkinje cell body. Cajal called these *descending fringes*; they soon came to be called *basket endings,* and the cells giving rise to them a variety of stellate cell called *basket cell.* Why Golgi had not seen them is not clear; perhaps it required heavier impregnation with silver than he was willing to use. It happens that this is one of the most specialized type of terminal in the entire nervous system; furthermore, it is made by an entirely local nerve cell, a type not even conceived of by the classical anatomists, absorbed as they were in the large motor cells of the spinal cord. Golgi had assumed that these axis cylinders ramify and unite with the lateral branches of the axis cylinder of the Purkinje cells, contributing thereby to the nervous reticulum. But Cajal brilliantly exploited his discovery of the fringe. Never mind that it arose from a practically unknown kind of cell; it was a clearly defined local terminal arborization, and it clearly made contact with the Purkinje cell without there being any anastomoses between the arborizations or between them and the Purkinje cell bodies. If there was one structure that persuaded Cajal of "contiguity without continuity," this was it.

3. *Granule (dwarf) cells.* Golgi had described these cells—their small cell bodies and tiny protoplasmic prolongations with thickened terminations—but had not been able to visualize more than the stump of an axis cylinder. Interestingly, Cajal cannot do much better. He likens the thickened terminations to the motor nerve endings at a neuromuscular junction, a quite misleading comparison between dendritic branches on the one hand and axonal branches on the other. As for the axis cylinder, he sees it ascend as far as the layer of Purkinje cell bodies but then loses it: he concludes, incorrectly, that these fibers never penetrate the molecular layer; discovery of the ascending axon that divides into the parallel fibers of the molecular layer is still to come. He is forced to conjecture that these fibers must connect to the Purkinje cells, perhaps with the lateral prolongations of their axis cylinders. This is as close as Cajal ever comes to admitting any possibility of fiber-to-fiber connection, and would not have been necessary if he had heeded his own advice and not let his imagination exceed the evidence.

4. *Large stellate cells.* This cell type was discovered by Golgi. Cajal confirms the branching pattern of the protoplasmic prolongations (dendrites), as well as the profuse ramifications of the axis cylinder (axon). The latter defeat him: some "lose their individuality," thus leaving the possibility of entering a diffuse network; others seem to enter the white matter, which is not the case. Wisely, though, Cajal emphasizes that the methods were not yet adequate to the task.

5. *Mossy (nodular) fibers.* A new finding by Cajal was the fiber that enters from the white matter and branches and terminates in an enlargement called a nodule, thicket or mossy excrescence. It came to be called "mossy fiber." Far from realizing that this is one of the two main types of fiber carrying information to the cerebellar cortex, and that its main connections are made with the terminal tufts of the granule cells, Cajal is misled by the fact that he can visualize these fibers up to the layer of Purkinje cell bodies, and therefore indulges in the same flawed speculation, as before, about the possibility of a connection to the descending tufts of the stellate cells.

The Question of Anastomosis

In response to the first question at which this study is aimed, Cajal supports Golgi's conclusion that the protoplasmic prolongations (dendrites) end freely and do not anastomose, but now goes further and draws the crucial conclusion that this also applies to the axis cylinders (axons) and their branches as well, in contradiction to Golgi. The fibers interlace, but never form a continuous network. The general concept Cajal offers is that "each element is an absolutely autonomous canton." Whether he had a Swiss canton in mind, we do not know; it was a somewhat opaque simile, taken from political life. One can only speculate that if he had used instead a word like "unit," the new doctrine, of the nerve cell as an independent unit, might have been born instantly. That is certainly what he intended. Interestingly, after this leap into the future, he has to remind himself that he cannot rule out indirect anastomoses through the enigmatic secondary filaments of Deiters.

The Connections of the Nerve Fibers

Even though terminal arborizations could be seen for some fibers, it still left many fibers inadequately visualized and with undetermined fates. Lending confusion to this problem was the traditional idea that the axis cylinder (axon) of a nerve cell was expected to enter the white matter. If, for example, the descending fringes end at the Purkinje cell bodies, how could their axis cylinders connect to the white matter? Cajal is not ready fully to believe that this connection does not have to exist.

12
The Laws of Cajal

Extending the Evidence

In the same May issue of the *Revista* appeared Cajal's first paper on the retina, "Estructura de la retina de las aves" ("Morphology and connections of the elements of the retina in birds"). This study supported his conclusion that there is no anastomosis between the nerve cells. It may be noted that the ganglion cells, whose long axons carry the output of the retina, do not have axon collaterals; thus, Golgi's hypothesis actually cannot be tested in these cells. Cajal later wrote that the retina was "the oldest and most persistent of [his] laboratory loves" (Cajal, 1989; quoted in Piccolino, 1988). The retina served him well in formulating his general laws (see later), but it also contained sources of misconceptions that have only been cleared up by modern work (Piccolino, 1988; see also below). The two other papers in that first issue of *Revista* reported observations on "Nervous terminations in the muscle spindles of the frog" and "Texture of the muscle fiber of the turtle," the latter a continuation of his earlier interest in muscle.

The August issue of *Revista* contained three more papers, on the cerebellum and retina, and on the brain of the electric eel (Torpedo). The paper on the cerebellum was particularly concerned with the organization of the elements in the molecular layer. Here were reported, first, the discovery of the axis cylinder (i.e., axon) of the granule cell, arising as a very thin fiber to enter the molecular layer and divide at a right angle to give rise to the *parallel fibers,* which course horizontally in the molecular layer perpendicular to the dendritic trees of the Purkinje cells. The second discovery was the *climbing fiber,* which enters from the white matter and climbs over the Purkinje cell body to branch and terminate over the Purkinje cell dendritic tree. Cajal (1989) later wrote: "This fortunate discovery, one of the most beautiful which fate vouchsaved to me in that fertile epoch, formed the final proof of the transmission of *nerve impulses by contact.*"

In August 1888, there also appeared a review entitled "Estructura del cerebelo" ("Structure of the cerebellum") in the *Catalan Medical Gazette,* his last publication that year. He summarized here his findings and interpretations in the cerebellum, and was able to take the problem of the connection between the fringes and the Purkinje cells a step further (Cajal, 1888e; modified from Clarke and O'Malley, 1968):

> The contacts between [Purkyne cells] and the [descending fringes (i.e, basket endings)] are . . . so numerous that it is possible to say that each of the Purkyne cells lies on a cushion of ramifications of the cylinder [axons]. Now then, could not these very extensive and intimate connections be the means which nature provides to allow the nerve current to pass from one cell to the other; for example, from the stellate [basket] cells that have hitherto been considered sensory, to those of Purkyne which have been supposed to be motor? Would it not be possible likewise to determine, as with the procedure of indirect contiguity, that those innumerable arcuate endings of the branches of the cylinder of the plump or starlike little bodies of the granular layer, . . . that are never without them, stimulate the surface of the granular or dwarf cells?
>
> Although anatomy does not prove the existence of direct connections, this hypothesis of the transmission by contact appears as likely as any other, and has the advantage of harmonizing better with the discoveries that have been made in the structure of the central nervous system through the use of Golgi's black stain.

Here we are aware that Cajal was beginning to see the relation between nerve cells and their fibers in a new light. The fringe (basket ending) was conceived of as passing activity (nerve current) to the Purkinje cell body. Two generalizations immediately extended from this. One was that the axis cylinder (axon) terminals *send* activity, and the cell body (and the neighboring surfaces of its protoplasmic expansions, i.e., dendrites) *receives* activity. This may be regarded as the first step toward the law of dynamic polarization of the neuron (see Chapter 15). The other generalization was that other cells, despite different shapes and sizes, could be similarly organized; his examples, using modern terminology, were the connection of the axon terminals of the large stellate (Golgi) cells onto the granule cells, as well as the climbing fibers and the Purkinje cell dendrites mentioned earlier. Cajal was thus freeing himself from Golgi's terminology of motor and sensory cells within each region, and moving toward a more general theory of nervous organization.

Writing with the benefit of hindsight, Cajal (1989) characterizes his frame of mind at this point in the following manner:

> The conclusions of my investigations concerning the cerebellum contradicted completely the ideas current at that time regarding the minute anatomy of the gray matter. Obviously my views were too revolutionary to be readily accepted. By this time, however, I nourished the certainty that I was not mistaken; for actually, the laws which I enunciated were the simple expression of the facts, without any mixture of the subjective. It was not now a case of one hypothesis more, but of a legitimate induction with all the guarantees of certainty which could be desired, as distinguished histologists and neurologists later recognized. I had been too well punished by the error which I had committed in my temerarious interpretation of the structure of muscle tissue to proceed lightly or to allow myself to be led astray by a mere theoretical conception, whether my own or that of someone else.

Attacking the Reticulum

The seminal publications in 1888 were supported by preliminary observations on a number of other regions in a variety of species. The main regions studied in the early years of 1888–1889 were, in addition to the cerebellum and retina, the spinal cord, optic lobe (tectum), cerebral cortex and olfactory bulb. The results poured forth faster than he could write them up, so that publications for each region were spread out during the period of 1889–1891.

Buoyed by his interpretations of the cerebellum and retina, and chastened by the lessons of his experience with muscle, Cajal felt ready to mount a more direct attack on the reticular theory. He compared Gerlach's concept of an anastomatic network of protoplasmic prolongations, to which are connected the terminals of incoming axis cylinders (see Fig. 8) with Golgi's concept of an anastomatic network restricted to the terminals of the incoming fibers and the axon collaterals (see Fig. 13). He analyzed the claims with mordant accuracy, much as a general pours over the map of the enemy's forces to plan his attack—indeed, Cajal's language and metaphors constantly evoke images of the battlefield. Cajal, the artist, understands the attractions of these diagrams (Cajal, 1989):

> I have already pointed out that the suggestive power of certain formulae which are extremely diagrammatic depends on their convenience. The hypothesis of the network once being accepted, nothing is easier than the objective study of a group of neurons or of the behaviour of the terminations of a bundle of fibres; the whole matter is reduced to taking for granted that the final axonic branchlets, after several dichotomies, are lost or disappear in

> the aforesaid interstitial network; in that sort of unfathomable physiological sea, into which, on the one hand, were supposed to pour the streams arriving from the sense organs, and from which, on the other hand, the motor or centrifugal conductors were supposed to spring like rivers originating in mountain lakes. This was admirably convenient, since it did away with all need for the analytical effort involved in determining in each case the course through the gray matter followed by the nervous impulse. It has rightly been said that *the reticular hypothesis, by dint of pretending to explain everything easily and simply, explains absolutely nothing; and, what is more serious, it hinders and almost makes superfluous future inquiries regarding the intimate organization of the centres* [italics added]. Only by dint of evasions, irrelevances, and subterfuges could this conception (which, moreover, was upheld almost exclusively by Golgi and his immediate disciples) be adapted to the exigencies of physiology, where the doctrines of reflexes, instinctive actions, functional localization in the cerebrum, etc., described paths or channels of conduction through the cerebrospinal axis.

It was apparent that if the reticular theory, as embodied in either Gerlach's or Golgi's ideas, were to be definitively disproved, it would ultimately have to be on its own ground, the spinal cord, which as we have seen had served as the main region for studying nervous organization for half a century of histological investigation. Cajal devoted much of his energies in 1889–1891 to applying the Golgi method to the spinal cord. The results were published in a total of 13 papers during those three years, almost as many as on all other subjects combined. This reflected the complexity of the subject and the large number of pathways and connections involved. For these studies the use of embryonic tissue was particularly important.

The essential outcome was that incoming fibers, from the dorsal roots or from the white matter of the spinal tracts, terminate with free endings in the grey matter of the spinal cord. The cells of the cord could be divided into distinct categories on the basis of where they send their axons: motor cells, into the anterior (ventral) root; tract cells, into the spinal tracts; and commissural cells, to the opposite side. No anastomoses were seen, involving either the axis cylinder terminals or the protoplasmic prolongations; all ended freely. These findings will be considered in more detail in Chapter 18.

Toward a New Concept of the Nerve Cell

Near the end of 1889, Cajal brought together his new ideas on the nerve cell and its organization in a review article. It was published in a Spanish review journal *La Medicina Practica* (*Practical Medicine*) under the title "Conexión general de los elementos nerviosos." This article is of special interest with regard to Cajal's contributions to the neuron doctrine for two reasons. First, it represents his first attempt to review all his findings with the Golgi method and synthesize new concepts. Second, it was Cajal's last publication before undertaking his famous journey to Berlin; it therefore gives us a snapshot of his mind, and a summary of his own unique contribution, on the eve of his setting out on the journey that was to merge his life with those of his colleagues in the mainstream of science in the rest of Europe. We cite this article (Cajal, 1889c) in nearly its entirety.

GENERAL CONNECTIONS OF THE NERVOUS ELEMENTS

One of the most interesting problems of Anatomy is the determination of how the cells of the [nervous] centers are related with each other and with the nervous fibers of the white matter. Is this connection made by contiguity, that is to say by simple contacts between cellular expansions, or rather by means of anastomosis? Do the sensory nervous fibers end in the centers by free arborizations, as do the motor [fibers] in the periphery, or are they substantially linked with the cells?

The doctrine of intercellular anastomoses due to Gerlach and supported by Deisters [*sic*], Meinert [*sic*], etc., is still today the most generally accepted; it being very notable however, that, so far, no one has been able to provide direct and absolute evidence [supporting such] a doctrine, [and] it can be said that if it is still maintained in science, it is not because of its own support, but *because of the prejudices and impositions of Physiology that require a substantial continuity between cells in order to explain more easily nervous transmission through the grey matter* [italics added]. Thus, it is not surprising that in the last few years some authors, such as Forel, Golgi, Ranvier, Obersteiner, have begun to doubt the exactness of this hypothesis, and have [begun] to consider other possible mechanisms of cellular connection. In this line, Forel affirms that the nerve cells are linked by means of their processes by simple entertwining, like the branches of trees in a dense forest; and Obersteiner considers also as possible that the nerve cells transmit their reciprocal reactions by contact or engagement of their processes.

The so-called Golgi methods of impregnation have overthrown completely the hypothesis of direct anastomoses or by protoplasmic processes [dendrites]. Based on his observations in the cerebrum, cerebellum and spinal cord, Golgi has proved that the nerve cell always maintains its individuality; but, still influenced by the doctrine that he combats, he accepts, as if by compensation, the existence of an interstitial nervous reticulum, which, according to him, would be made up of the collateral ramifications of axis cylinders [axons] of cells, and of the final ramifications of the nerve tubes that end in the grey matter. In short: a fibrillar lattice that surrounds the nervous elements, but in which participated only one kind of cellular process: the prolongation of Deiters, or axis cylinder [axon].

Golgi himself implies clearly, in both his drawings and writings, that the cited reticulum is a simple anatomical hypothesis suggested by him to explain the linkage of nerve fibers with central cells, and the functional solidarity of these cells among themselves. But for ourselves, who have never been able to see such a reticulum, neither in the cerebrum nor in the spinal cord, cerebellum, retina or olfactory bulb, etc., we believe that it is time to separate from histology all physiological obligations, and simply to adopt the only opinion that is in harmony with the facts, namely: *that the nerve cells are independent elements which never are anastomosed, either by means of their protoplasmic expansions [dendrites] or by the branches of their prolongations of Deiters [axons], and that the propagation of nervous action is made by contacts at the level of certain apparatuses or dispositions of engagement* [i.e., synapses], whose objective is to make fast the connection, multiplying considerably the surfaces of influence. The proofs of this point of view will be found in nearly all our previous works. Here we cannot give a detailed [account], since we would go beyond the limits imposed by ourselves; rather, we are going to expound, in general terms, the nature of these connections and the main varieties that they present.

At the outset, we must affirm that, for effecting these connections, we consider the protoplasmic expansions [dendrites] and the axis cylinders [axons] to be of equal significance; that is to say, in our view, both play the same role of relating contiguitively the nerve elements; the only difference lies in that the axis cylinders [axons] are destined to carry the nervous action to remote territories, being therefore, long conductors; while the protoplasmic expansions [dendrites] transmit it to nearby elements, [which are] almost always of the same type, being, as a consequence, short conductors. When the long conductors . . . transmit an [action] current outside of the grey territory in which it commences, they are protected by an insulating sheath of myelin; but they lack this protection when they course and end within the grey cortex where they have their origin.

The distinction between protoplasmic [dendritic] and nervous [axonal] expansions is not, therefore, fundamental, nor is it based on different physiological properties; nor is the presence or lack of myelin around the cellular processes, since on the one hand we see that the protoplasmic processes of the central nerve cells lack this sheath, on the other hand, we observe that the peripheral protoplasmic process [dendrite] of the dorsal root ganglion cells possesses [a myelin sheath] like the central process. And, finally, let us add that there are cells (the sympathetic cells) whose protoplasmic expansions have the function of axis cylinders, lacking always a medulated sheath.

The shape, dimension and degree of differentiation of the expansions vary a great deal in the nervous regions, so that it is possible to distinguish several kinds of cells. Proceeding from the simplest to the most differentiated, anatomically and dynamically, we shall expound the characteristics of the connections of the: 1), *sympathetic cells*; 2), *bipolar cells*; 3), *multipolar cells with short cylinder* [*axon*]; and 4), *multipolar cells with long cylinder* [*axon*].

I. *Sympathetic cells.* As is well known, most authors consider the sympathetic cells of mammals to be multipolar, and are inclined to think that each expansion represents an axis cylinder or fiber of Remak. We have had occasion to study these cells, with the method of Golgi, in an extremely favorable region, the intestinal villi, and are inclined to think that all the cellular expansions have a protoplasmatic character. Like the latter, they are thick and have an uneven outline; they ramify at acute angles, losing their original orientation, and never appear to be enveloped by a myelin sheath. A portion of such prolongations anastomose with each other (perhaps reuniting or crossing their component protoplasmic filaments, but without a meeting of the same); and part of them, after repeated ramifications, terminate in fibrous cells or in the contiguous mucosal surface.

In short: the sympathetic cells represent cells in which there exist no anatomical differences between protoplasmic [dendritic] and axis-cylinder [axon] expansions, both having the two roles of establishing *internervous* and *extranervous* connections. . . .

II. *Bipolar cells.* All of these are sensitive elements, be they of general sensitivity (dorsal root ganglion cells), or of special sensibility (peripheral ganglion cells, represented by the retina, nasal mucosa, etc.).

The dorsal root ganglion cells are bipolar cells in the fish, by contrast with mammals, birds, amphibians, etc., in which they are unipolar; in these, at a short distance [from their origin] the single expansion is divided into two branches, one central and the other peripheral, running in the same manner as the two expansions of the dorsal root corpuscles of the fish, etc., so that this modification lacks significance.

In any bipolar or ganglionic cell the thicker appendage or fiber is directed towards the periphery, therefore it could be considered as a protoplasmic [dendritic] branch, and this disposition is evident in the bipolar cells of the retina and olfactory mucosa; and the thinner and longer is directed towards the nervous centers where they end by free arborizations on the surface or on the expansions of central nervous cells.

The final arborization of the cylinder [axon] is connected always with the first level or with the most immediate cellular formation of the centers; in this way, the bipolars of the retina send their axis cylinder [axons] to seek connections in the ganglionic layer which is its most proximate center; the olfactory bipolars are directed to the glomeruli of the olfactory bulb, which likewise represent the nearest protoplasmic outpost of the cells of this organ; and the medullary bipolars send theirs to the posterior bundle, where, after bifurcating into ascending and descending branches, it sends to the first cellular plane of the spinal cord (posterior horn) numerous free arborizations. . . .

III. *Multipolar cells of short ramified axis cylinder* [short-axon cells]. An example of this interesting type of cell is found in the grey molecular layer of the cerebellar convolutions. There exists here a stellate cell, of small size, provided with numerous and divergent protoplasmic arborizations [dendrites], whose contours are rough, tooth-like, and with a thick, arciform axis cylinder, oriented transversally with relation to the length of the cerebellar convolutions.

This axis cylinder [axon] does not go to the white matter, nor is it surrounded by myelin, but it exhausts itself by numerous descending small branches, which show the very singular particularity of forming, around the bodies of the Purkinje cells, nests of terminal varicose ramifications which, sometimes following for a certain interval the origin of the cylinder [axon] of these cells, end by a paintbrush. It is impossible, given this interesting connection, not to suppose that, by means of the terminal brushes, the stellate cells of the molecular layer transmit their action to the Purkinje cells.

The protoplasmic branches [dendrites] probably establish connection between each other by numerous contacts and perhaps also by means of their rough bristles [spines] with the infinite longitudinal fibrils that make up the molecular layer, fibrils that we have demonstrated to originate in the axis cylinder of the granules.

To this same type of cell of short axis cylinder, which does not extend beyond the limit of the grey region where it arises, are related also the granules of the granular zone of the cerebellum and many of the small cells of the posterior horns of the spinal cord The granules are dwarf corpuscles, spheroidal, which emit: various short protoplasmic expansions [dendrites], terminating in small and varicose arborizations, and an axis cylinder [axon], which is directed upward to the superficial or molecular layer, where, at different levels, it divides into two terminal branches of opposite direction (longitudinal fibrils). Since the granules are extremely numerous, the fibrils thus arising (that are perfectly parallel and oriented in the same direction as the cerebellar convolutions) are of such a large quantity that they literally fill all of the molecular layer of the cerebellum.

By means of these longitudinal [parallel] fibers the granule cells are connected with the infinite ascending protoplasmic branches [dendrites] of the Purkinje cells that receive and hold them up by means of their bifurcations and protuberances, somewhat as a telegraph pole supports the conducting wire. The granule cells are probably connected between themselves by their protoplasmic branches, since we have often seen granule cell bodies tightly embraced by rings of terminal arborizations of neighboring congener elements.

The large stellate cells of the granular zone are related also with these, by means of arborizations of their cylinder [axon], whose role seems to be to establish solidarity between a considerable number of elements, since the shortness of the protoplasmic [dendritic] arborization of the granule cells only allows them to be connected with the nearest cells.

Other cells seem to behave in the same manner as the above; but we have not succeeded in carrying out studies sufficiently complete to permit establishing their paths of connection. These include the small corpuscles of the posterior horn (substance of Rolando, Clark's column, etc.), the small cells of the cerebral cortex, the diminuitive elements of the olfactory bulb, those of Ammon's horn, etc.

IV. *Multipolar cells of very long and medullated axis cylinder* [*long-axon cells*]. This is one of the most abundant varieties. To this belong almost all elements of the grey cortex of the cerebrum (pyramidal cells), the Purkinje cells of the cerebellum, the large pyramidal cells of Ammon's horn and the olfactory bulb, those of the anterior horn of the spinal cord, the spongioblasts and ganglionic cells of the retina, etc.

The protoplasmic [dendritic] arborizations of these cells are extremely extensive, often extending through almost the whole grey cortex where the cells, such as for example Purkinje's cells and large pyramids of the cerebrum, are located. For us there is no doubt that all of these protoplasmic branches have as their object, not conveying nutrient fluids to the cell body, as Golgi has said, but rather establishing contacts of transmission, either with protoplasmic [dendritic] arborizations of similar cells, or with nerve fibers of different origins. This function of *taking currents* from nerve fibers seems to us undubitable in two examples: 1, in the olfactory glomeruli (rounded granular masses which are arranged in rows around the bulb), the fibers of the olfactory nerve end by arborizations, and precisely in these parts, where, after overcoming great distances and obstacles, the thick protoplasmic [dendritic] shafts of the large pyramidal cells [mitral cells] and of the smaller elements located in the molecular layer [tufted cells] come to form their terminal arborization. Here the contact is exclusive, and it is made in a narrow area and, in order that the influence be more direct, Nature has enormously multiplied the ramifications or surfaces of engagement; 2, the other example we find in the Purkinje cells, whose protoplasmic [dendritic] arbor, transversally flattened, goes up to the cerebellar surface, placing each branchlet in intimate and almost exclusive contact with an infinite number of longitudinal fibers (axis cylinders [parallel fibers] of the granule cells).

With less evidence although with some certainty, this connective function also appears in the ganglion cells of the retina and pyramidal cells of the cerebrum. In effect, in the retina and at the level of the internal reticular [inner plexiform] layer are arranged in contact: 1, the ascending protoplasmic arborizations [dendrites] of the ganglion cells; 2, the descending axis cylinders [axons] of the bipolar elements ramifying and terminating in tufts. In the cerebrum, notwithstanding that it has not been possible to establish connections very securely, because of our ignorance with respect to the major part of the fine fibers which plough through the grey cortex, one can conjecture it is the crown in which terminate the thick ascending protoplasmic expansion [apical dendrite], relating itself with the nerve fibers of the superficial layer; while the protoplasmic branches [dendrites], both lateral and descending, serve to make direct contacts with neighboring corpuscles.

With regard to the axis cylinder [axon] of this type of cell, it is directed to the white matter, covered with myelin, and either leaves the nervous centers in order to arborize in muscles (motor fibers), or terminates in distant provinces of the same centers, in an unknown manner. Our studies show that in the white matter of the cerebellum, retina, spinal cord, one sees fibers emanating from the white matter and terminating in free arborizations among the nerve cells; but it has not been possible to determine if such arborizations proceed from the ganglion cells (the so-called sensitive-sensorial), or from the thick multipolar elements with very long *cylinder* [axon] which we have studied.

From the point of view of the ramification of the nervous prolongation [axon], these cells present several variations. Certain cells exhibit a cylinder [axon] which only ramifies at the site of termination (anterior root cells of the spinal cord [i.e., motor neurons], elements of the ganglionic layer of the retina, cells of the electric lobe of the cerebrum of the torpedo, etc.). There exist others whose *cylinder* bifurcates immediately, or emits a certain number of fibers of almost the same thickness, each one of which becomes enveloped in myelin and penetrates into the white matter. This variety [of axonal ramification] that we had verified in some cells of the grey cortex of the cerebrum of the bat (in the human, the great distances make it difficult to follow the fibers), has been found recently in the embryonic spinal cord, as it pertains to nearly all the cells which form the white matter of the [posterior] columns. Finally, three is a much more numerous category of cell whose *cylinder,* without dichotomizing or losing its individuality, furnishes, near its origin, several collateral branches, of whose manner of termination we are ignorant, but which in general seem to be lost between the nerve cells, perhaps in search of making connections by contiguity. The large Purkinje cells and nearly all the pyramids of the cerebrum and Ammon's horn behave in this fashion.

Such arrangements of the *cylinder* [axon] must involve some differentiating physiological properties; but this is in fact not easy to determine. Golgi has supposed that the cells whose axis cylinders conserve their individuality, despite their ramifications, have a motor character, and that those whose cylinder exhausts itself in ramifications possess a sensitive character. But, concerning the character of the exhaustion, it is not more than a question of the length of the *cylinder* (all cylinders ramify and lose their personalitiy [*sic*], but some do it near and others far from their origin); cells exist of evidently sensitive character, whose *cylinder* conserves its individuality up to its termination; such are, for example, those of the bipolar cells of the olfactory mucosa, the ganglionic cells of the retina and the large pyramidal cells [mitral cells] of the olfactory bulb, etc. As we see, the question of the physiological distinction of cells based on the histological data is more difficult than it seems, so that we ourselves will not venture some divisions of physiological character; and thus we consider that the length and manner of arborization of the cylinder [axon] have no relation to the direction and nature of the current that they must transmit, but *with the distance at which are located the elements that must receive the nervous excitation and with the number and shape of these elements.*

Such is the summary of the investigations that we have been carrying out over the past three years in nearly every region of the nervous system. Certainly some of these opinions are anatomical hypotheses which will have to be further rectified or transformed; but even so, they are the only ones that are in harmony with the recently discovered facts, and we believe that, better than any others, they could serve Physiology in investigating the dynamic relationships of the nervous elements.

13
Joining the Mainstream

Despite the burst of discovery, the publications so painfully paid for and strategically posted to leading authorities in nervous system anatomy, there was little response. Of all this, the outside world knew almost nothing. Combing the periodicals of 1889, Cajal was alarmed to find his work either ignored or dismissed "contemptuously." He lived, he recollects, in "a state of restlessness and suspicion," fearful of being regarded as "deluded" or a "pretender" (Cajal, 1989). He realized that the authorities to whom he had sent his papers did not read Spanish, and that he would have to have key works translated into French (since he himself did not know German), and published in well-known German periodicals. This he began through Wilhelm Krause, whom he knew through correspondence from his work on muscle, editor of the *Internationale Monatsschrift für Anatomie und Physiologie* (*International Monthly of Anatomy and Physiology*).

The Berlin Congress of 1889

Even more than translations, Cajal knew that he must meet the authorities in person and persuade them by actual demonstrations of his stained cells and fibers. He therefore applied for membership in the German Anatomical Society (Cajal, 1989),

> to which belonged anatomists, histologists, and embryologists of many nations, especially of the German confederation and of Austria-Hungary. This association met each year in a different university city. During the sessions, the members discussed current anatomical problems; demonstrated, in support of their views, the gross and microscopic preparations which they had

> procured; explained the details of the methods used; in fine, pointed out to the lovers of investigation the fertile directions and the veins recently opened up for scientific exploitation. Finally, concurrently with the work of the congress, the manufacturers showed the recent developments in instruments for observation and experiment.

As this passage indicates, international meetings had become a routine part of academic and scientific life by the latter part of the nineteenth century.

The next meeting of the German Anatomical Society was to be at the University of Berlin in early October of 1889. Cajal, who had never travelled outside Spain except for the ill-fated voyage to Cuba, prepared carefully, saving the funds for the trip, arranging numerous visits with leading authorities along the way, assembling his best material, and taking along his own Zeiss microscope to present them.

At the Congress, Cajal paid little attention to the talks, but devoted his efforts to setting up several microscopes provided for demonstrators, as well as his trusted Zeiss, to show his slides of the cerebellum, retina, and spinal cord, which, as we have seen, were the main focus of his work up till then. When the demonstration time began, Cajal, speaking in his broken French, attracted only a few skeptics. But once they began to examine the material, they realized that they were seeing nerve cells and fibers stained with a sharpness and clarity not seen before, what one would call a technical breakthrough. What started as a possible fiasco ended, in those brief hours of demonstration time, in everything Cajal had hoped for: the chance to present the evidence to the leading authorities—he mentions His, Schwalbe, Retzius, Waldeyer, van Gehuchten, "and especially Kölliker" (Cajal, 1989)—and gain their acceptance of his results. Since these authorities had all tried the Golgi method and had been frustrated by inconsistent results, a crucial element in Cajal's success was the opportunity for him, at the Congress, to discuss the details of the method, and reveal to them "all the little secrets" by which he had achieved his clear and reproducible results. Thus, far from keeping to himself the secrets of his success, Cajal was eager to share them. This was not only in the best and truest tradition of science, it also reflected both Cajal's unselfish nature and his determination to have the credit that was due him. It is interesting to speculate what might have happened if Golgi had followed the same course 15 years earlier, and had not only shared his secrets at such a Congress but had also had the benefit of their discussion of his interpretations.

Cajal not only rejoiced in the acceptance of his results but was much gratified by the kindness shown to him personally by these imposing authorities who had until then seemed distant and forbidding. He recalls, for example, that at the end of the demonstration session, Kölliker took him in a "splendid carriage" to his "luxurious hotel," entertained him at dinner, and apparently introduced him to every histologist and embryologist he could lay hands on (Cajal, 1989). Through these meetings, Cajal obtained instant personal acquaintance with the main figures who were to share with him the final fashioning of the doctrines of the nerve cell.

Making Connections in Europe

Cajal's horizons were widened not only by the Congress but also by the visits he paid on the trip. On the way to Berlin he visited in Lyon, Geneva, and Frankfurt-am-Main. He met Carl Weigert, renowned for his stain of myelinated nerve fibers; Edinger, whom Cajal regarded as "the greatest authority in comparative neurology" (Cajal, 1989), and Paul Ehrlich, who had introduced a technique for staining living nerve cells (see below).

The return trip was similarly carefully arranged. Cajal first spent several days in Göttingen with Krause. Cajal was always grateful to Krause for befriending him in his early period. The two got on very well personally. From Krause, Cajal learned of German academic life, and his reaction (recalled in Cajal, 1989) makes an interesting parallel to that of the American, Franklin Mall, cited earlier (Chapter 9).

> In our conversations at table we exchanged observations about the organization of our respective universities. It filled me with astonishment to learn that professors were chosen almost freely, without competitive examinations. The absence of a uniform plan of teaching also shocked me, as did what resembled the systematic abandonment of that spirit of unity and centralization, so highly regarded in Spain as a result of the servile imitation of the French university organization. Each science had its own quarters which received the name of institute, and included the lecture room, the laboratory for the professor and his students, the library. etc. There were no examinations except at the end of the course. Finally, the professors, classified into the categories of *Privatdozent, professor extraordinary* (*ausserordentlicher Professor*), and *regular professor* (*ordentlicher Professor*), instead of being engaged according to a uniform scale of salaries, were paid by the state and the city on the basis of their merits, besides receiving in addition honoraria from their pupils.
>
> Suppression of examinations, university autonomy, remuneration from the students, appointment without competitive examination and often by a sort of contract! Here was a series of reforms which, if applied to Spain, the classical country of routine and favouritism, would have reduced us before ten years had passed to a state of savagery. It is with reason that Paulsen has said that every country has the university system that it requires, that is, the best possible in view of the condition of social ethics.

From Göttingen, Cajal made his way south to Italy, where

> I did not have the pleasure of finding the illustrious Professor Camilo [*sic*] Golgi in Pavia. He was in Rome, whither he was taken at certain times of the year by his responsibilities as a senator. We may note in passing that in Italy it is customary for the most renowned men of learning to receive, among other rewards, investiture as members of the Upper Chamber. The absence of the master disappointed me very greatly. I am perfectly certain that, if I could have shown him my preparations and expressed to him at the same time my admiration for him, future polemics and vexations [*sic*] misunderstandings would have been avoided.

Ironically, in Turin he did meet Bizzozero, Golgi's early close friend; we do not learn whether they discussed the disparities between Cajal's and Golgi's positions. One can only regret that the two did not meet on this one possible occasion. Cajal was still willing to be the student paying homage to the master, as he did to the authorities in Berlin. But they were far more disinterested in the issues than Golgi. The moment passed; henceforth, Cajal was a master, too, and there would be no more pilgrimages to Pavia.

Testing the New Results

Although Cajal had "won over" the skeptics by his demonstrations at the Congress, it really meant no more than that they accepted his material as persuasive evidence bearing on the form and connections of nerve cells. To accept the evidence as valid, free of artifacts, and a basis for drawing interpretations regarding the significance of Golgi-impregnated nerve cells and fibers for nervous function required taking what they had learned from Cajal and returning to their laboratories to verify the results themselves. We will focus only on several of the people whose judgment was most critical in assimilating Cajal's findings into the tradition of central European histology.

Kölliker

When last we discussed Kölliker (Chapter 5), he had finished the fifth edition of his textbook, in 1867, in which he was forced to admit that the available evidence made possible, even likely, the presence of anastomoses between nerve cells. It seemed to confirm his counsel of despair, in 1853, that nerve fibers might never be traced within the spinal cord (see Chapter 3). He therefore put the burden on any method to prove that anastomoses did *not* take place.

Kölliker reached the age of 70 in 1887. He was still very active, the senior statesman of histology, and kept a hawk-like eye on the vast range of publications in the field he had played such a large role in founding.

When Golgi's work was translated into French in 1883–1884, followed by *Organi Centrale del Sistema Nervoso* (*Central Organs of the Nervous System*) in 1886, Kölliker was one of the first to read and assimilate the new findings; in fact, with characteristic forthrightness, he made a trip to Pavia to see for himself, not a vacation jaunt for a man in his seventies. Kölliker was not above making pilgrimages to hunt down the truth! The visit was the occasion for the famous photograph of himself, Golgi, and Bizzozero (Fig. 21). He tested these findings in his own laboratory, and published his observations and judgment on the new method in a paper in 1887, one of the first on the Golgi method to appear in German (Kölliker, 1887).

GOLGI'S STUDIES OF THE FINER STRUCTURE OF THE CENTRAL NERVOUS SYSTEM

On May 21 I gave a lecture to the Würzburg Physiological-Medical Society on Golgi's studies which will be published in more detail in the Society proceed-

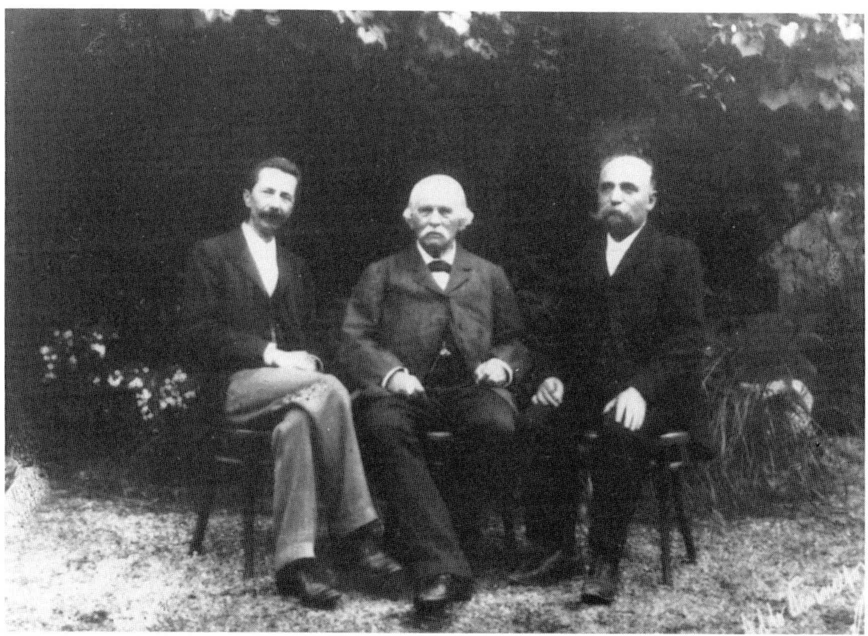

Fig. 21. Portrait of Guilio Bizzozero, Albrecht Kölliker, and Camillo Golgi, at Golgi's home in Pavia, during Kölliker's visit to Golgi in 1887 to learn about the Golgi technique first-hand. Bizzozero was a schoolmate and long-time friend and colleague of Golgi. (Kindly supplied by Professor P. P. C. Graziadei)

ings; therefore I shall only briefly draw attention here to the main points which arise from this difficult problem.

Golgi was kind enough to send me one of his preparations this spring, and I, too, likewise succeeded in obtaining nearly the same results according to his silver method. I have had preparations from the human cerebrum and cerebellum and from the medulla of a young cat (from Golgi), and of my own from the human cerebellum and from the cerebrum of the horse. Based on the facts, I must admit that Golgi's method remains unsurpassed in displaying nerve cells with their processes, and after all I have observed, I do not doubt that Golgi's pictures on the whole are true to nature, especially those of the protoplasmic prolongations [dendrites] of nerve cells which I have carefully studied.

The Golgi method stains neuroglia cells very beautifully; there are many places where the two kinds of elements [nerve cells and glial cells] are easily distinguished, whereas in other cases it is uncertain, as with the elements of the granular layer of the cerebellum. Stained by the Golgi method, the glial cells in the brain appear as stellate, richly branched formations, without anastomoses of the extensions; I cannot at this point prove, however, that such anastomoses are lacking everywhere, including in the medulla.

Of Golgi's assumptions I reject mostly one, which is that the protoplasmic prolongations [dendrites] of the nerve cells are not of a nervous nature. Golgi's main support for this striking assertion is that these prolongations partly lie in areas and go to places where no medullated nerve fibers [axons] are found, and he cites as such: 1) the surface layers of the grey matter of the brain, and 2) especially the fascia dentata of the Cornu ammonis [hippocampus]. Concerning 1) I already showed in 1850, and in all editions of my histology book, that in the most superficial parts of the cerebral cortex a large number of dark-bordered fibers [axons] occur; and 2) concerning the fascia dentata no one has (despite all efforts) as far as I can see shown nerve fibers in its grey cortex, and yet these exist here in great numbers, as shown even by an experiment performed with my old method (hardening in chromic acid, making the section transparent in dilute caustic alkalis). As I write this today (May 29) I have also, courtesy of Weigert, received two preparations of Ammon's horn, according to his method, which show the same.

These arguments of Golgi's, and a third one, that the protoplasmic prolongations of the nerve cells also extend to areas where only nerve fibers occur (here Golgi cites the spinal cord and the white matter of the brain) do not seem convincing to me, for in such places the extensions might go directly into dark-bordered, fine fibers [fine axons].

I agree with Golgi, on the other hand, that there is no anastomosis of these branched prolongations [dendrites]. In the Purkinje cells of the cerebellum, which, following Golgi's method, show a wonderful richness of ramifications, I have not seen a single certain case of a connection between the prolongations, despite all effort, and all these sooner or later, partly right on the surface, bend back towards the rust-colored layer. Saying this certainly does not provide proof against anastomoses; still, there are so many that such connections can only be accepted when supported by precise evidence.

What Golgi reports about the axis cylinder extensions [axons] of the nerve cells is very peculiar. These are said to occur in two ways. Concerning the centrifugally oriented motor cells, the extension should completely and with constant thickness become the axis cylinder of dark-bordered fibers, from which a certain number of finer branched extensions deviate to a nervous network which, according to Golgi, connects nerve fibers and nerve cells. Into this nervous network go, besides the just-mentioned fine extensions, also 1) fine, branched extensions from the motor nerve fibers which come from the axis cylinder extensions of the motor cells, 2) extensions of the centripetally excitable (sensible) nerve cells, characterized by Golgi as nervous, but which dissolve in a fine network, 3) and finally, branched fine extensions of the centripetally acting (sensible) dark-bordered fibers.

Despite full acknowledgement of the important achievements of Golgi, it seems to me that the existence of such a complicated nerve net is not sufficiently well substantiated. I can certainly concede that the axis cylinder extensions of the Purkinje cells give off small sidebranches, as I myself see these in Golgi's and my own preparations, and am also inclined to assume that the extremely rich ramifications which Golgi indicates in what he calls the nervous extensions [axons] of certain cells of the cerebellum and of the fascia dentata do occur; however, I do miss in Golgi's studies any evidence to support the assumption that the motor nerve fibers give off such small branches, and that the sensible fibers completely dissolve in fine ramifications. In objects made transparent with dilute caustic alkalies, and in preparations of the grey matter of the brain made with Weigert's method, we see neither dark-bordered nerve fibers [axons] nor a dissolution of these into fine branches, even though these can often be followed far, which makes a very weak basis for assuming the existence of such ramifications. It is, however, possible that the finest of the small dark-bordered fibers become unstained unmedullated elements and make ramifications, but at this point we do not have any evidence to support such an assumption.

For my part, I would like to [support] a hypothesis which until now has remained in the background [but] deserves more attention, which is that the connecting links between distant nerve centers are by means of dark-bordered nerve fibers [axons], which come directly from the final extensions of the ramified nerve cell extensions, perhaps because each of these extensions goes to a particular nerve fiber or because several of these become the axis cylinder of a single medullated nerve fiber. Such an assumption, supported also by certain observations, would closely follow the requirements of physiology, and also render unnecessary the hypothesis, which until now has not been supported by facts, that the ramified nerve cell extensions anastomose as such. These observations just mentioned are the old findings by myself and Corti, that the ramifications of the nerve cells of the retina give rise to several varicose optic fibers and that, according to Corti, in the elephant even several nerve cells of the retina are connected directly through optic fibers.

In closing, I would like to say that Weigert's method of revealing dark-bordered nerve fibers [Weigert's myelin stain], and Golgi's procedure for showing the ramifications of nerve cells, are the most important achievements which the finer anatomy of the nervous system can point to in our time.

In summary, Kölliker recognized that Golgi's stain was a big step toward a clearer picture of the nerve cell, but it still left the key questions unanswered. Furthermore, Golgi's interpretations confused the picture. Kölliker rejected Golgi's assertion that the protoplasmic prolongations (dendrites) do not have a nervous function, citing his own work going back to 1850. He accepted the evidence against anastomoses between the protoplasmic prolongations, but found the whole issue of Golgi's network of branches from the axis cylinders (axons) unresolvable, favoring instead a hypothesis of interconnections that did not require anastomoses. One assumes that more definitive results were precluded by the inconsistency of the Golgi method; Kölliker obviously did not devote himself as exhaustively to the development of the method as did Cajal, nor did he exploit the use of embryonic animals, which was so crucial to Cajal's success.

Against this background we may surmise that, when Kölliker first met Cajal, he was interested in seeing new results and clearer results with the Golgi method, but he would have been most skeptical about their reliability. We can now better appreciate that Kölliker already knew of the Spaniard because of the controversy about the reticular theory of muscle, into which Cajal had plunged in his first histological papers in 1887 and early 1888. In 1888, Kölliker published a 21-page review entitled "On knowledge of striated muscle fibers" in which he reviewed the evidence of Cajal, van Gehuchten, and Melland, as reviewed earlier in Chapter 10, and strongly opposed it, upholding the view that the striations reflected the essential contractile apparatus of the muscle fiber rather than the "universal" intracellular reticulum. Kölliker must therefore initially have had little reason to put particular stock in the Spaniard's new venture into the even more treacherous terrain of the nervous system; Cajal, for his part, chastened by his muscle fiasco, must have been even more apprehensive in placing his offerings on nerve cells before the master.

Cajal was in no doubt, however, that it was above all Kölliker whose stamp of approval was critical. He (Cajal, 1989) records their first meeting through the eyes of van Gehuchten, who made the following observation:

> Cajal . . . found himself alone, exciting around him only smiles of incredulity. I can still see him taking aside Kölliker, who was then the unquestioned master of German histology, and drawing him into a corner of the demonstration hall to show him under the microscope his admirable preparations, and to convince him at the same time of the reality of the facts which he claimed to have discovered. The demonstration was so decisive that a few months later the Wurzburg histologist confirmed all the facts stated by Cajal.

It was characteristic of the clear-eyed Kölliker that he was able to separate Cajal's flawed concept of the muscle cell from his accurate concept of the nerve cell. As indicated in the citation above, within a few months he had confirmed for himself Cajal's findings, and published them (Kölliker, 1890a,b).

Kölliker's immediate conversion to Cajal's view is the more amazing in that, as we have seen (Chapter 5), Kölliker was at that time a supporter, albeit reluctantly, of the reticular theory of nervous connections. It was as if all the frustrations of wanting to believe what he intuitively felt must be right were swept away on viewing Cajal's stained preparations, with their sharply etched fibers and bluntly terminating fiber endings. He literally could be said to have waited a half century for that moment of revelation. No wonder, as Cajal (1989) recalls, he exulted, "I have discovered you, and I wish to make my discovery known in Germany." According to Cajal, Kölliker set about learning Spanish in order to read Cajal's early publications, and later did translations for him into German. Cajal (1989), for his part, records his "ineffaceable recollections of and profound gratitude towards the glorious master . . . it was due to the great authority of Kölliker that my ideas were rapidly disseminated and appreciated by the scientific world."

His Introduces a New Term: "Dendrite"

We have seen (Chapter 9) that His already referred to Golgi's work in his paper of 1886. Although he did not carry out studies himself with the method, he was well aware of its advantages and potential by the time of the Berlin Congress. We do not have a record of his reaction to Cajal's new evidence against anastomoses between nerve cells, but may assume that he was pleased to have his view of the nerve cell as a separate entity upheld. Cajal was always careful to credit His and Forel with the first formulation of this fundamental idea.

In 1889, His published a paper entitled "Die Neuroblasten und deren Entstehung im embryonalen Mark" ("The neuroblasts and their development in the embryonic spinal cord"), which contained further observations on the way that the nerve cell gives rise to its different processes. In this paper he suggested a new term that is of special interest for the neuron concept:

> As a particularly meaningful result I consider the initial one-sided [unipolar] development of all central nerve cells. Each neuroblast gives rise to an axis cylinder [axon] which from its cell of origin pushes out toward a certain target

> area. Considerably later it begins the generation of new extensions which with increasing branching spread out in the region of the cell. Dendrite-fibers, or dendrites, we can call them, in contrast to the axis fibers, in order not to need an adjective each time to describe them.

Thus was introduced the term "dendrite" in place of the cumbersome phrase "protoplasmic prolongation," which had been used, in one form or another, ever since the 1840s to refer to all those processes arising from a nerve cell body that are distinct from the single axis cylinder. As we shall see, several years of debate over terminology ensued before its acceptance, but "dendrite" has endured since then as the general term used for non-axonal branches from a nerve cell body.

Retzius

One of the authorities Cajal was eager to meet at the Berlin Congress was the Swedish anatomist, Gustav Retzius, who made important contributions to studies of the nerve cell throughout this period (see his judgments on Nansen, Chapter 9; Waldeyer's review, Chapter 12; Schafer's reference to his work, Chapter 16; also Chapter 19).

Retzius was born in Stockholm in 1842, of a distinguished academic family; his father, Anders, was professor of anatomy at the Karolinska Institute, and contributed much to establishing the Institute as a leading medical school (Larsell, 1953). Retzius thus grew up in scholarly surroundings; during his gymnasium years he accompanied his father on trips to Germany, France, and Switzerland, where he met such luminaries as Johannes Müller, Ernst Weber, Rudolph Wagner, and Justus Liebig.

The young student set his sights on emulating his father's career, studying medicine at the Karolinska Institute and at Lund between 1860 and 1872. During his studies he took time out to collect and edit his deceased father's papers and letters, publish a volume of poetry, and start research on the anatomy of the nervous system. He joined the faculty of anatomy at the Karolinska in 1871, becoming professor there in 1877. His microscopical studies included descriptions of the membranes of the brain (with Axel Key), the inner ear, the spinal cord, and the ganglia of the invertebrate nervous system. He also developed an interest in anthropological studies of the human brain and cranium of different races, a popular subject in the late nineteenth century. His work, published mostly in German, gave him a solid reputation in the fields of histology and anatomy.

Retzius' main contribution to the study of the nerve cell began with his use of the method of Ehrlich for staining cells with the dye methylene blue.

Paul Ehrlich (1854–1915) was one of the great biologists of all time. His early work, in the 1870s and 1880s, was focused on the mechanisms by which different dyes, especially aniline dyes, stain animal cells. This work was of fundamental importance for clinical medicine, for in it he worked out the classification of blood cells that is the basis for modern hematology, and for the staining of bacteria that is the basis of modern bacteriology. He then went on to analyze the mechanisms of toxin-antitoxin interactions and drug-receptor interactions that helped to found the fields of modern immunology and chemotherapy.

In 1886, Ehrlich reported that methylene blue could be used to stain living nervous tissue, that is, without the need for previous fixation and hardening. This was the first "vital stain" to come into general use. Retzius experimented with this new tool; as he later was to describe (Retzius, 1908):

> In the higher animals, the vertebrata, the method could be well applied to the peripheral nervous system, but to the central one only with the utmost difficulty. I then determined to try and find some *lower* animals which admitted of having their whole nervous system, or, at any rate, the principal parts of it stained, *so that by experimenting with them one might obtain a comprehensive idea of their entire construction* [italics added]. At last in 1890, I found, with a certain modification, that the method gave excellent pictures in the ganglions of the ordinary crawfish [*sic*] (Astacus). A general survey was obtianed [*sic*] of their construction. One could clearly perceive that their so-called "Punktsubstanz" of Leydig was formed of the lateral twigs of the processes of the unipolar nerve-cells, which twigs could be traced in the substance in their most delicate ramifications, where they did *not* unite with each other, and on the whole did *not* form a *network* (reticulum), but a twist-work (plexus). One could also trace the stem-processes of the nerve-cells even in their various courses through the ganglions towards the periphery [Fig. 22].

It may be noted that the use of smaller, more primitive, species in order to analyze their "entire construction" has become a very modern mode of attack in neuroscience.

Retzius applied the methylene blue method to a number of invertebrate and lower vertebrate species. After the Berlin Congress, where Cajal passed on the secrets of his techniques, von Lenhossék (see later) and then Retzius applied those Golgi techniques to the nerve ganglia of the earthworm, and were able to confirm the methylene blue results: both the neurites (dendrites) of the ganglion cells and the branches of incoming sensory fibers end freely without anastomoses. This work was therefore important in extending the principles elucidated in the vertebrates to the invertebrates as well. It may be noted that Retzius' beautiful drawings of the large

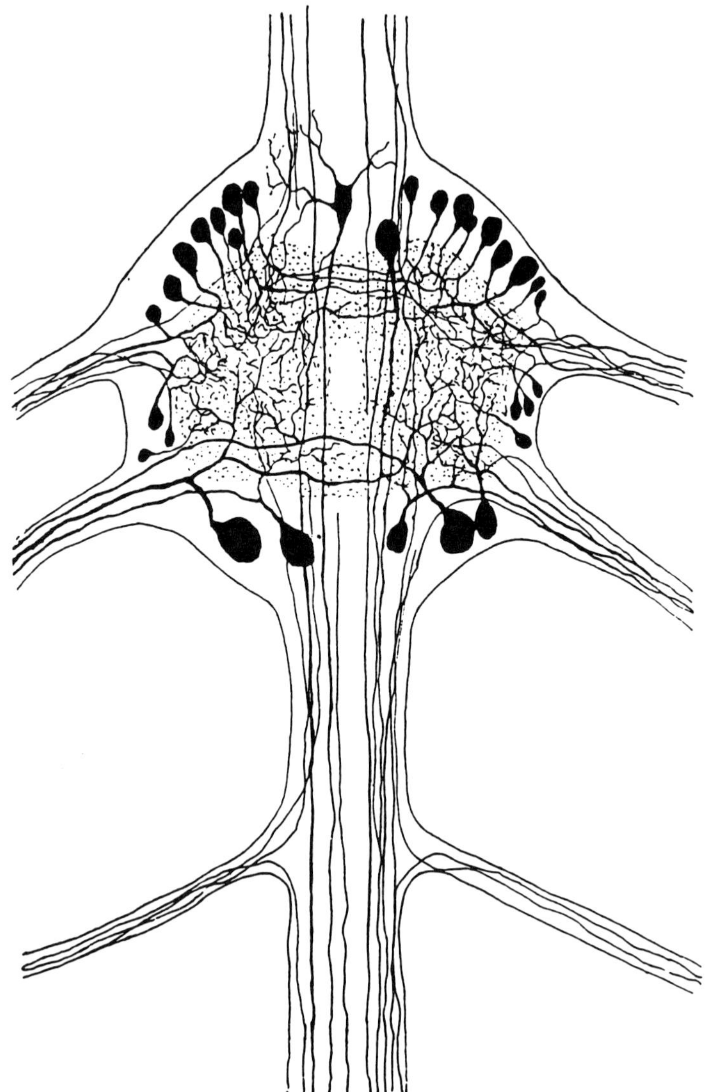

Fig. 22. "A Part of the Ventral Nervous Chain of the common Crawfish (Astacus), showing a ganglion with coloured (black) nerve cells and their processes." (Retzius, 1908; from Retzius, 1890)

identifiable cells in the ganglia of the leech and the spinal cords of Amphioxus stood well the test of time, and have served as reliable guides for modern studies of these systems (cf. Muller et al., 1981).

Retzius displayed an astonishing range of abilities, aided by independent means through marriage. From 1884 to 1887 he was editor-in-chief of a leading Swedish newspaper, *Aftonbladet,* owned by his father-in-law. After briefly succeeding to his father's chair in anatomy in 1888, he resigned to devote himself to his research. He published the results of his investigations privately (using *Aftonbladet's* printing presses) in 19 successive volumes entitled *Biologische Untersuchungen* (*Biological Investigations*) from 1890 to 1920. Besides his scientific, editorial, and administrative abilities, he was an artist, illustrating most of the volumes of the *Biologische Untersuchungen* with his own drawings; a poet; and a composer of cantatas (see Larsell, 1953). A remarkable individual, who, like Kölliker, maintained a sure grasp of the important issues surrounding the controversies about the nerve cell (see also Chapter 19).

14
The Neuron Doctrine

Good news travels fast in science, as Cajal's demonstration at the Berlin Congress showed; in the months that followed, his adaptations of the Golgi method were quickly adopted and modified, the results tested, confirmed, and extended. Cajal (1989) noted and appreciated each one of his supporters: His, Waldeyer, Kölliker, and Edinger in Germany; Lugaro and Tanzi in Italy; van Gehuchten in Belgium; von Lenhossék in Switzerland; Retzius in Sweden; Azoulay, Dejerine and Duval in France. As van Gehuchten (in Cajal, 1989) recalled:

> It was the time . . . when the method of Golgi at last received practical application. The new facts revealed by this procedure were to revolutionize the anatomy of the nervous system. The laboratories of Europe were in a ferment. We all wished to carry our stones for the new edifice which, under the brilliant direction of Cajal, became so magnificent. Not only had the technique of the method been simplified, but the results procured were more constant and more decisive.

In those critical years of 1890 and 1891, Kölliker's published confirmation of the results, and his rigorous championing of his new friend, comrade, and, in some ways, savior from the purgatory of unseen anastomoses, were the most decisive. The His–Forel theory of the individuality of the nerve cell became, for Kölliker, the theory of His–Forel–Cajal. So eloquent an advocate was he that others even began to refer to the theory of His–Forel–Cajal–Kölliker!

But what exactly was this theory? The new results illustrated vividly how variable nerve cells are in the branching forms of their dendritic trees, the lengths of their axons, the profuseness of their axon collaterals and terminations. What did this imply about nerve cells as cells? What did it imply about the ways that nerve cells, in all their variety, could serve as the basis for nervous function? Where did this leave the reticular theory? With so much new data pouring forth, a new synthesis was needed. To be persuasive, it required someone who could speak to the great traditions of the field of histology as it had developed in central Europe, starting with the cell theory of a half century before; who could master the outpouring of knowledge that had occurred in the preceding half-dozen years; and who could give the imprimature of the authorities in the field, perhaps with a perspective a bit removed from the heat of battle.

Waldeyer

Wilhelm von Waldeyer was born in 1836 in the village of Hehlen, to the east of Hannover in Germany, to a family of aristocratic extraction. He had an early love of music, and entered *hochschule* in Göttingen in 1856 intending to study mathematics, but was drawn to medicine after hearing lectures in anatomy by Jacob Henle. While pursuing his medical studies in Berlin, he began his research training in anatomy in Königsberg and in Breslau under Heidenhain. After receiving his medical degree in 1862, he stayed in Breslau as an assistant to Heidenhain, quickly rising to a personal chair (*extraordinarius*) and then full professor (*ordinarius*) of pathological anatomy in 1867. During these years he worked on topics as varied as the development of the crayfish, the histology of the ovum and the ovary, and the fine structure of nerve endings in sensory organs and in muscle. In Stricker's *Handbook* of 1872, he contributed the chapters on the teeth, the auditory nerve, and cochlea; to other handbooks of the time he wrote on the cornea, dermis, eyelids, sperm cells, and development.

In 1872, Waldeyer was named professor of normal anatomy in the German *hochschule* in Strassburg, which had come under German rule in the aftermath of the Franco–Prussian War of 1870 (see Fig. 11). Here he spent the happiest time of his life (Fick, 1921). He continued his broad interests in anatomy and histology, and published a definite text on the topographical anatomy of the pelvis.

In 1883, Waldeyer became director of the Anatomical Institute at the University of Berlin. To his catholic interests he added there comparative anatomical and anthropological studies on the brains and crania of different human races and different higher primate species such as the gorilla and gibbon. As we noted for Retzius, this was a popular topic in the latter part of the nineteenth century, when it seemed only a logical requirement of Darwin's "survival of the fittest" to search for evidence that the brains of Europeans represented the pinnacle of human evolution.

Thus, by 1891, Waldeyer, at the age of 55, was an anatomist of broad expertise and acknowledged reputation. He had made a number of solid contributions to the progress of anatomy and histology. As an administrator, organizer, writer of reviews, member of committees and participant at congresses, he appears to have become the kind of public figure who is a highly respectable representative of his academic field.

New Times, New Terms

New discoveries demand new terms, and the 1880s were etymologically especially fecund. *Cytology,* as the study of the microscopic organization within cells, emerged during the 1880s as a new discipline within *histology,* the study of how cells form tissues, owing largely to the systematic application of new types of stains derived from the German chemical industry. During this period were introduced many of the basic terms we use today for describing and understanding the cell. In 1882, in plants, Edward Strasberger of Bonn coined the terms "cytoplasm" and "nucleoplasm," and, in 1884, "prophase," "metaphase," and "anaphase" for the sequence of stages in mitosis of the cell. "Mitosis" itself had been introduced by Walter Flemming of Prague and Kiel in 1882, in a book entitled *Cell Substance, Nucleus, and Cell Division,* which was a seminal work in founding the new discipline (see Singer, 1951).

Waldeyer had in fact a talent for terminology. After Flemming, in 1879, had suggested "chromatin" for the substance within the nucleus that stains most intensely, Waldeyer, in 1888, suggested the term "chromosome" for the individual stained bodies. His role as an arbiter in these matters was described by his biographer (Fick, 1921) as follows:

> Waldeyer was also a member of a committee established by the Society of Anatomy to simplify anatomical terminology. . . . He was the right man in the right place to do this, combining considerable teaching experience with a particularly fine feeling for the requirements and suitability of individual terms. Waldeyer showed a remarkable knack for coining striking, suitable technical terms.

Scientists are in fact quite ambivalent about introducing or accepting new terms. Old terms acquire a patina of convenience and shared understanding, and there is a deep suspicion of attempts to be jarred loose from them. This suspicion is only heightened by the many clever neologisms that dazzle and disappear like roman candles in the night. A new term must have a sober logic to it, must fit the needs of a field in promoting understanding and facilitating discourse, enabling people to get on with their work more effectively.

We have considered Waldeyer's qualifications for this role in order to place in a better perspective his contribution to the neuron doctrine. But instead of being appreciated for his role, he has been regarded as an interloper, even the villain of the piece, gaining credit that should have gone to Cajal. We have seen that, in fact, by virtue of his wide experience, high regard, and acknowledged skill in matters of histological and cytological terminology, he was admirably suited to bring together the new work on the nerve cell and interpret it in the light of the long history of the cell theory, the recent developments in cytology, and the relations between nerve cell structure and nervous function.

This Waldeyer did in a lengthy review written for the *Deutsche medicinische Wochenschrift* (German Medical Weekly), a publication then in its seventeenth year, which carried the subtitle: "Serving the German medical profession with communications for the counties, public health authorities, and in the interest of medical practitioners." The review was entitled "Über einige neuere Forschungen im Gebiete der Anatomie des Centralnervensystems" ("On the newer research on the subject of the anatomy of the central nervous system"). It was divided into six parts, which ran in the issues from October 29 to December 10, 1891. We will summarize briefly the gist of the early, more detailed, articles before considering the concluding summary article in full.

Waldeyer's Review Articles

First article (October 29). This begins with a quotation of Jacob Henle from his textbook of anatomy just 50 years before, in 1841, "Regarding the extensions of ganglion cells, little is known." Waldeyer summarizes the history of this problem, tracing most of the actors and issues we have covered, focusing mainly on the spinal cord. He discusses the terminology for the axis cylinder (axon): "The older name 'axis cylinder prolongation' is awkward, 'Deiters' prolongation' is not precise, 'nervous prolongation' can be misleading since the protoplasmic prolongation is most likely nervous as well; my judgement is that 'nerve prolongation' is the best." He then summarizes the findings and conclusions of Golgi, and contrasts them with those of Cajal, using, in passing, His' new term "dendrite" for the "protoplasmic prolongations" of the nerve cell.

Second article (November 5). Waldeyer quotes extensively from a review of Kölliker in 1890, incorporating the latest findings in the spinal cord. He gives particular emphasis to the "nervous nature of the dendrites." He summarizes recent findings of Cajal, von Lenhossék, and others on the sources of fibers in the anterior (motor) and posterior (sensory) roots of the cord, mentioning also his own recent study of the gorilla spinal cord. In addition to "dendrite," he uses "collaterals" and "terminal arborizations" in referring to the axis cylinders and their branches.

Third article (November 12). Waldeyer again begins with Kölliker's review of the spinal cord; he includes Freud's anatomical work among the references. A large part of the article is concerned with an extensive summary of the organization of the cerebellum based on Cajal's reports and on another review by Kölliker in 1890 of Cajal's results and of Kölliker's confirmation of those results. It is clear that much of Waldeyer's summary is refracted through the lens of Kölliker's recent writings. The article ends with a summary of the cellular and fibrous elements of the grey matter of the cerebral cortex. Cajal's studies of the cerebral cortex had only just begun, so the account draws heavily on work of others, including Golgi, Martinotti, Sala, Flechsig, and Retzius.

Fourth article (November 19). The first part deals with invertebrates, summarizing evidence regarding the origin of axis cylinders from the monopolar ganglion cells. The studies of Retzius, Nansen, and others do not support the idea of a dotted substance composed of anastomosing processes. The second part deals with sensory cells in the vertebrate, including especially olfactory sensory cells in the nasal mucosa and dorsal root ganglion cells. He discusses the development of the peripheral process of the ganglion cell from a protoplasmic prolongation (the "dendrite of His"). The article ends by stating that the work of Cajal on histogenesis supports Forel's work in opposing the idea of a nerve net.

Fifth article (December 3). This is mostly concerned with a review of work by many authors on neuroglial cells in the central nervous system.

Sixth article (December 10).

A REVIEW OF NEW RESEARCH ON THE ANATOMY OF THE CENTRAL NERVOUS SYSTEM

Summary and physiological remarks.

The following main conclusions can be drawn from the findings as communicated above:

I. *The axis cylinders of all nerve fibers (motor, secretory, sensitive and sensory; centrifugally or centripetally conducting) have been shown to originate directly from cells. There is no connection with a network of fibers or any origin from such a network.*

Examples have been given in earlier discussions:

a) Motor root fibers

b) Centrifugally-transmitting pyramidal pathways

c) Fibers originating from Purkyne cells (according to Golgi, Ramón y Cajal, Kölliker; loc. cit.)

d) Centripetal first-order sensory fibers (connected with spinal ganglion cells)

e) Centripetal second-order sensory pathways which lead upward from the spinal cord to the brain, e.g. the spino-cerebellar pathway originating from cells of the Stilling-Clarke columns consisting of anterior primary tract and lateral secondary tract, equivalent to Ramón y Cajal's cord cells.

f) First-order sensory pathways arising from the sense organs, such as: 1a) the origin of the olfactory nerves from olfactory cells; 2b) the relationships in the retina; these still need further investigation, though there we have not learned of any fiber origins other than from cells (cf. the connection of optic fibers with ganglion cells, as shown by Corti and Kölliker); 3) the connection of the fibers of the *cochlear nerve* with the bipolar cells of the cochlear spiral ganglion of Corti. When citing the origin of the *olfactory nerves* from olfactory sensory cells, and of ampullar and vestibular nerve fibers from the hair cells of the acusticae maculae (see Retzius, 1881) re: one must also mention, as I found (Stricker, 1872), the inner hair cells of the organ of Corti; 4) the connection of taste cells with taste fibers, a connection which the discoverers of the taste cells, Loven and Schwalbe (1868) already described as very probable. Now, after the research of Fusari and Panasci, it is to be considered as established.

II. *All these nerve fibers terminate freely with "end arborizations" (Kölliker) without a network or anastomotic formation.*

Examples: The end arborizations of motor fibers on muscle fibers; the terminal arborizations of pyramidal fibers in the spinal cord; the endings of ganglion sensory fibers at the periphery (free nerve endings in the cornea, free nerve endings in the small terminal bodies of the membrane of the skin (see Schwalbe, Retzius among others; the free-lying tacticle disk of the small Grandry bodies) as well as in central organs (terminal arborizations of sensory collaterals). Therefore, communication does not occur by *continuity,* but at most by *contiguity,* through contact and emission of one free ending to another. For example, in the olfactory glomeruli, as we have seen, two terminal arborizations are directed toward one another [i.e., axonal terminals toward dendritic terminal branches]. Alternatively, the terminal arborizations may be directed to cells, as are the terminal arborizations of pyramidal fibers, or the sensory collaterals to the motor cells of the anterior horn, or of the fibers entwining Purkyne cells (Kölliker).

Certain difficulties exist, however, for sensory nerves in relation to points I and II when we get into a more exact definition of the concept of "origin" and "ending" of a nerve. In so doing, one must be governed by three determining factors: a) physiological, b) topographical-anatomical, and c) genetic. *Physiologically,* the origin of a nerve is apparently that place from which, in a normal fashion, the nerve activity begins; the ending is where it ceases proceeding in this direction. Topographic and descriptive *anatomy* would place the origin in the central organs, the ending in the periphery. *Genetically*, the site from which a nerve fiber develops is the origin, and the place where it stops at the end of its development is the ending. For motor and psychomotor fibers it is now simple and clear, for in these instances all three factors are in agreement.

If we accept the above criteria in ascertaining the origins of sensory fibers, great disparities arise, because it appears that, physiologically, some sensory fibers have peripheral cells of origin, while others, e.g. those of the cornea and the other mucous membranes, and those of the senses of touch, temperature and pressure, arise with free fiber ramifications. These latter have terminal arborizations in the brain and spinal cord; at a particular place during their course, they are connected with an interpolated cell, the spinal dorsal root ganglion cell, which, embryologically and anatomically, acts as a cell of origin. Thus, the physiological conduct does not agree with the embryological direction of growth and the anatomical levels for the distance from the body periphery to the spinal ganglion cell. Physiology and embryology again correspond for the stretch between the spinal ganglion cell and the grey matter of the spinal cord as well as for the second order pathway (see I e above), but not the anatomy. Anatomy and embryology finally agree for the psycho-sensory cells, but for the speech area they are incompatible with the physiological orientation.

Due consideration must be given to these matters in all questions hereto related. If we for now set aside the unsettled concepts of "origin and ending", then all those authors who do not accept a network formation of the nerve fibers inside the central organ (Ramón y Cajal, Kölliker, His, Nansen, Lenhossek, Retzius) can easily unite points I and II above into one common brief fundamental law of wider range. It would sound thus:

"*The nervous system consists of numerous nerve units (neurons), anatomically and genetically independent. Each nerve unit consists of three parts: the nerve cell, the nerve fiber and the fiber arborizations (terminal arborizations). The physiological orientation of conduction may be either from cell to fiber arborization or the reverse. Motor orientation is in the direction from cell to fiber arborization; sensory orientation may be in one or the other direction.*"

When we now consider the nature of the pathway which leads from the seat of conscious perception and will to the periphery, we find—in so far as these matters are known to us—still more neurons—at least two—along this stretch. Presumably, only two can be present in the pyramidal pathway: one nerve unit stretches from a ganglion cell of the cerebral cortex to the terminal arborizations in the grey matter of the spinal cord, the second from a motor anterior horn cell to the terminal arborizations in a muscle fiber [see Fig. 23, tracts 15, 17–21, 23]. Presumably, all sensory nerve transmissions consist of more than two neurons. This relationship is easily illustrated in Kölliker's diagrams [Fig. 24*A*,*B*,*C*] and in two of my own [Figs. 23, 25]. In Kölliker's diagrams [Fig. 24], *A* represents transmission through the pyramidal tracts and anterior roots; (1) describes the pyramidal anterior primary pathway, (2) the pyramidal collateral pathways with their various crossings, the repeated crossings in the anterior commissure for (1) and the large, single crossing in the decussatio pyramidum for (2). The longitudinal pyramidal fibers either

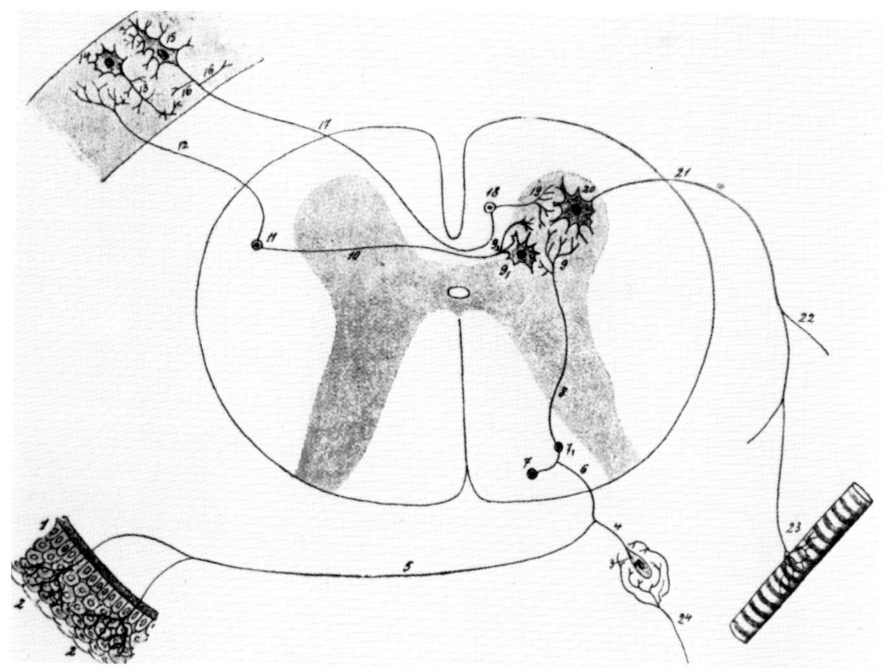

Fig. 23. (Waldeyer, 1891, Fig. 9)

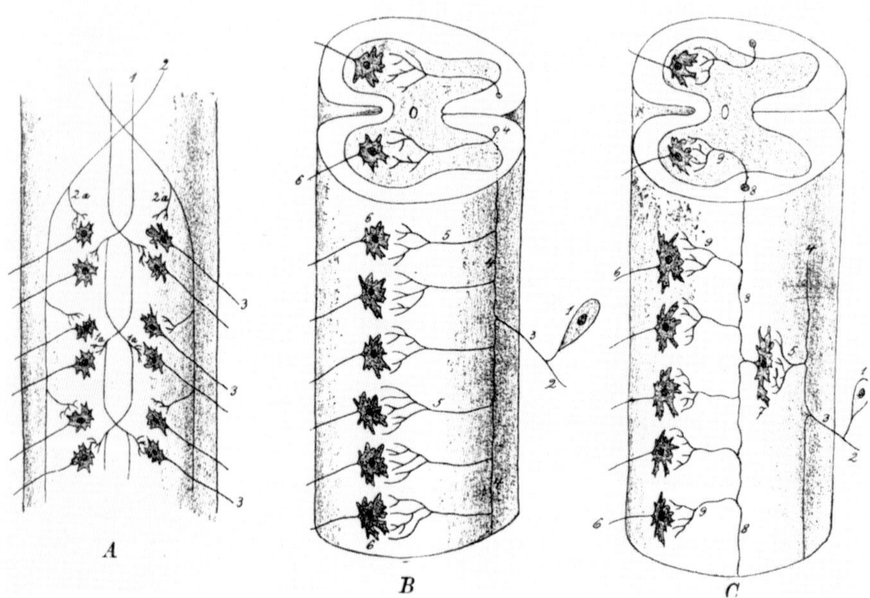

Fig. 24. (Waldeyer, 1891, Fig. 4)

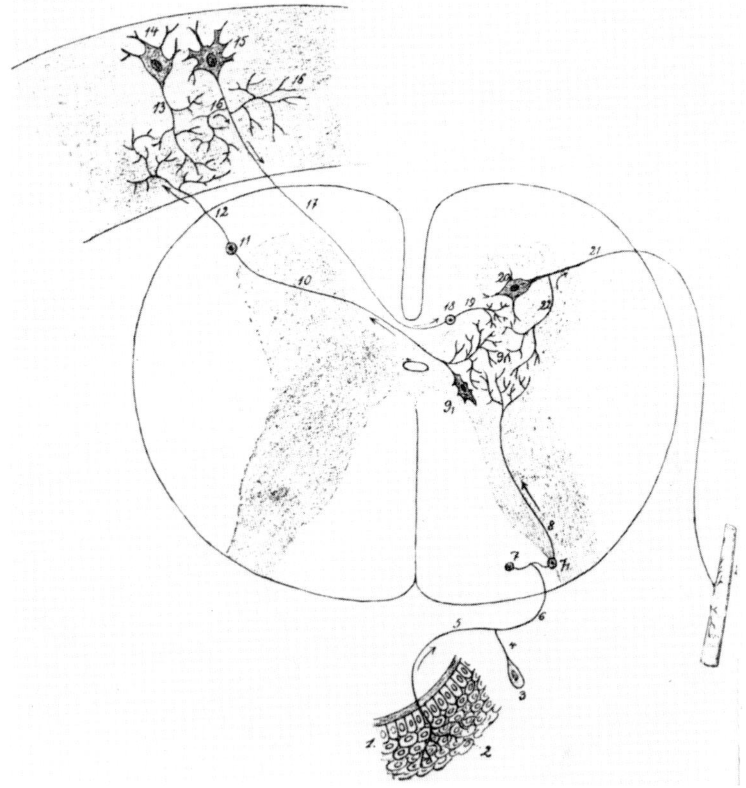

Fig. 25. (Waldeyer, 1891, Fig. 10)

turn back completely into the grey substance, or send out collaterals. The latter, like the main fibers, end in small terminal arborizations (1a and 2a) from which the excitation of the ganglion-cells of the anterior horns and their extensions is transmitted to the anterior motor root fibers (3). This pathway, which includes two neurons, is described in more detail in my schematic Figure [23], where (15) represents a pyramidal cell of the cerebral cortex from which the pyramidal fibers are shown to originate. As we know, the course of the pyramidal fibers is unbroken and crossed (17–18, Fig. [23]). The turning of the fiber in the longitudinal direction of the anterior column (we are using the direct pyramidal tract as an example) is indicated by a circle (18). From here the collateral with terminal arborizations (19) goes to the grey matter in the vicinity of an anterior ganglion cell (20) and transmits onto this the psycho-motor impulse, which through the nerve fiber (21) is transmitted to the motor terminal arborizations in the muscle fiber (23). In (22) a collateral of the motor nerve fiber is shown as it has been identified in many animals by f. ex. Golgi and Ramón y Cajal. We would like to know how to ascertain (Kölliker) whether they occur everywhere. In (22) is shown the branching which occurs repeatedly to the motor fibers in their path.

The diagram of a sensory reflex pathway is represented in Kölliker's Fig. [24] *B*; (1) is the spinal ganglion cell; (2) is the conducting fiber, coming from the periphery; (3) is the [dorsal] root fiber rising towards the brain; these divide into an ascending and descending branch (4,4) from which arise collaterals (5,5) with terminal arborizations which in turn transmit the impulse to the anterior horn cells 6,6 etc. Here we thus find three neurons, the first from the periphery to the spinal gangion cell, the second from there to the sensory terminal arborizations, the third from the motor ganglion cell to the muscle fiber.

In Fig. [23], this reflex is presented in more detail. (1) is the dermal epithelium, in which, as we know, the sensory nerves with terminal arborizations (2,2) "terminate" and "originate," respectively. The impulse is transmitted further through fiber (5) to the connection with the spinal [dorsal root] ganglion cell (3)—it is questionable whether it actually must touch it—then, through the posterior root fiber (6), which divides into an ascending (7) and descending (7_1) ramus, it reaches the spinal cord and medulla oblongata, and, through a collateral, marked (7_1) here, to the grey matter to terminal arborization (9), from where the relay to motor transmission takes place, which (in order to relate to a reflex example familiar to everyone) we may consider to be on a muscle fiber of the orbicularis oculi muscle (23). For this example to be of value, we must now suppose that Fig. [23] belongs to the medulla oblongata and that the spinal [dorsal root] ganglion cell specified as (3) is a cell of the gasserion ganglion equivalent to a spinal ganglion, and the motor cell (20) is such a cell of the facial nerve. In this diagram, the psycho-sensory transmission is also shown. It gives from terminal arborization (9) to ganglion cell (19)—a commissural cell, as I have chosen it at random here, in order to indicate crossed transmission in the simplest way—then the nerve continuation (10) to the longitudinal fiber (11) and from there upwards to the brain. We do not know how often it is interrupted on this stretch, or, in other words, how many neurons there are here. For reasons of simplicity, unbroken transmission is indicated here, which ceases with a terminal arborization in the cerebral cortex. Perhaps this [arborization] transmits the impulse—this is entirely hypothetical—to a sensory ganglion cell of the second Golgi type, and can perhaps therefore be regarded as the seat of conscious perception.

In Fig. [23] is shown also, with no. (24), the fiber-basket with the centrifugal (or centripetal ?) fiber, which, according to Ehrlich and S. Ramón's findings, surrounds the spinal ganglion cell. Further is the commissural cell (9), joined to another collateral (9_2), which ends with a terminal arborization in the grey matter. Such collaterals appear frequently (here compare, for example, Kölliker, Zeitschrift für w. Zool., vol. 51, p. 28, paragraph 4). In explaining Fig. [25] we shall later find use for this.

In Kölliker's diagram Fig. [24] *C* we have a picture of a much extended reflex conduction. The sensory conduction (2,1,3,4,5) influences an intermediate cell (7), passing there through a T-shaped division into two longitudinal fibers so that the influence is carried at the same time to many motor transmissions through many collaterals.

These concepts of the course of conduction depend, however, on the assumption that in fact no anastomosing nerve net is present, but only a neuropil (the neuropilema of His). If, with Golgi and B. Haller, we accept nerve nets, our interpretation is somewhat modified, but even so we can retain the nerve units. Then the boundary between two nerve units would always lie in a nerve network, and—at least anatomically—would not be sufficiently definable with our present methods.

Concerning the question of neuropil or nerve net, it must again be stressed briefly here, that most researchers who have recently concerned themselves thoroughly with this matter have discarded the nerve net. Indeed, Kölliker gave the important and surprising report at the Munich Anatomy Meeting that Golgi, both in writing and orally, had told him that it was a misunderstanding to attribute the assumption of a genuine anastomotic nerve net to him. Golgi must then have changed his opinion, as his denunciation, as far as I can see, sounds very determined in anatomical publications (loc. cit.) and likewise the denunciations of his pupil L. Sala (loc. cit.) appearing in recent weeks. It is also evident from Golgi's latest communication (loc. cit.: Rendiconti dell' R. Istituto Lombardo di Sc. e Lettere, vol. 24, Milano, 1891) that he no longer stresses a network so strongly. As the matter stands at present, one can at any rate assert that sure evidence of an anastomotic nerve net has not been produced and that most evidence speaks for a neuropil of discontinuous fine processes.

III. Hitherto unexplained in their physiological and anatomical relations are two types of cell, one of which was discovered by Golgi and the other by S. Ramón y Cajal (see above). I am referring to the cells of the second Golgi type, whose axis cylinder prolongation, after a brief course, branches out into free end fibers; and the Ramón cell of the cerebral cortex (shown in young rabbits) from which two axis cylinder prolongations extend in a bipolar fashion, in the manner of protoplasmic-prolongations. Further research, especially in embryos and lower vertebrates, should produce more information about these types; meanwhile we are not able to explain their meaning.

IV. Equally unknown is the meaning as well as the anatomic relationship of the protoplasmic prolongations (Deiters), or dendrites (His). I refer the reader to Kölliker's earlier thorough discussions of this question. It will only be noted here that Nansen, Sala, Martinotti, and Gad favor Golgi, according to whom these prolongations were not of a nervous kind, or more strongly put, not transmitting; whereas S. Ramón y Cajal, His, and Lawdowsky (in a manuscript recently submitted, see discussions of the X. International Congress in Berlin, Section for Anatomy, p. 92–93) favor the older view that we are dealing with nervous structures. Also, Kölliker, to judge from his communication to the Munich Anatomy Meeting, where he presented a number of new reasons for and against the nervous nature of the dendrites, is apparently inclined to side with the latter named authors.

For me this question is decided on the basis of the answers to the following question:

V. *What importance do the nerve cells have? Are they a nerve-functioning apparatus, or do they only have a subordinate, somewhat supporting, function?*

Besides Nansen [1887] nobody has yet dared to challenge the concept of the ganglion cells as a nervous-functioning apparatus. He does it with a bold hand, and not without some basis. He conceives of the nerve cells only as a supporting body of the whole nerve apparatus. According to him the psycho-motor and psycho-sensory functions would exist only in the nerve fiber terminations of the brain cortex; in the spinal cord, the transmission of a motor impulse would happen, for example, from a pyramidal fiber to a motor axis cylinder in the fiber network there and would be transmitted from there to the motor root fiber. Conversely, sensory centripetal conduction would progress in continuity from the peripheral receiving station to the spinal cord feltwork; there it would be transmitted to a centripetal path of the second order and from there be conducted further to the brain-feltwork, where the conscious sensation occurs. The cells need not be immediately involved in the transmission. Fig. [25] illustrates this and needs no further explanation, since Fig. [23], which shows nearly the same thing, has just been thoroughly explained. Hereby the earlier mentioned collaterals (9_1) and 20 (d.i.22) also come into their rights. At the Munich Anatomy Meeting, Kölliker spoke out decidedly against this concept of Nansen's. He then stressed that side branches (collaterals), as Nansen's hypothesis requires, do appear at the motor roots (see above) but so rarely that they cannot be taken into consideration. Further, we must remember the olfactory fibers which arise from cells in the periphery, as well as instances where ends of nerve fibers weave around nerve cells (spiral fibers of the sympathetic ganglion cells), and whose tract weaves around the spinal ganglion cells, as discovered by Ehrlich and Ramón y Cajal (see Figs. [23], [24]);—and further we must remember the fiber baskets around the Purkyne cells which were shown by S. Ramón y Cajal and Kölliker. . . . In favor of Nansen appear to be the majority of unipolar cells of invertebrates, which nearly all lie outside of the nerve feltwork and where no entwining fiber baskets appear. But Kölliker points to Gad's assertion that every impulse which meets a motor fiber is transmitted further to both sides and thus also comes to the motor cells; it is thus not impossible that these divide when the reflex occurs.

At present it appears to me too early, because of these difficulties, to deny to cells this role in nerve function, and I think we must therefore also grant the protoplasmic prolongations (which, indeed, are only ramifications of the vital substance of the cells) the same function, by simple inference. The previous assertion that nervous prolongations extend from dendrites at long distances from cell bodies agrees with this. We shall not deny that assuming a nervous function for the dendrites creates an unusual difficulty and complication for the physiological and pathological use of this finding. Here we cannot dispense with help from physiologists and pathologists; the work of anatomists finds its limit here.

VI. Connected to these problems is a further question: *Are there no transmissions from fiber to fiber—without requiring the cells?* I believe that the glomeruli olfactorii supply affirmative proof. The terminal arborizations of the olfactory nerves here meet with S. Ramón's tufted cells without interpolation of cells, certainly no nerve cells.

VII. According to recent findings it appears that side branches (the collaterals of S. Ramón y Cajal) originate from all nervous prolongations. As we have seen, these have been identified in all spinal cord pathways, in the corresponding fibers of the medulla oblongata (Kölliker's demonstration) at the Munich Anatomy Meeting and anatomical publications 1891, loc. cit., in the cerebellum and cerebral cortex and in the corpus collosum (see above). The development of our knowledge of collaterals started with Golgi's original evidence that nerve prolongations give off branches; it was then carried much further and made common knowledge by Ramón y Cajal. From the existence of such numerous collaterals follows—whether we now assume a nerve net or not—the fundamental principle, i.e., that *an isolated transmission in the central organs does not exist, or at any rate does not need to exist,* as the collaterals everywhere command exits to neighboring pathways. (see among others, Golgi, 1890.) On the other hand, however, an isolated transmission is also consistent with these findings, as the collaterals need not be taken to have any significance.

Finally, I will add a summary of the evidence which the above mentioned studies, in particular those of Kölliker, have rendered for the best known and most studied part of the nervous central organ, the spinal cord. I will give these results essentially from Kölliker's own excellent synopsis (Zeitschr. f. wissensch. Zool., vol. 51, loc. cit., p. 40), but must advise anyone who wants to study these things in further detail to consult the original work, as I can here give only a brief exposition of the facts and conclusions without thorough description and substantiation.

1. The anterolateral columns consist in part of fibers which are transferred from nerve cells (cord cells) from all parts of the grey horns [. . . Fig. (24) *C*].

2. These root fibers send collaterals to the grey matter . . . as do the nerve prolongations of the cord cells themselves, as far as they proceed into the grey matter [Fig. (23) (9,2), Fig. (25) (9,1)]. The root fibers themselves also bend in part towards the grey matter, so as to end there with terminal arborizations:

3. The posterior columns consist of dividing root fibers running longitudinally. . . . From the latter, as from the posterior column fibers, collaterals run everywhere to the grey matter, ending freely with terminal arborizations [. . . Fig. (24) 4 (*B, C,* 1–5)].

4. The motor roots proceed invariably from anterior horn cells as their nervous prolongations. . . . According to Golgi, these invariably give off collaterals [Fig. (23), (25) (22)]; according to Kölliker, only in certain cases.

5. The sensory roots come from the spinal dorsal root ganglion cells [. . . Fig. (24) (*B, C,* 1–5), . . . Fig. (23), (25) (3,4,6,)]; several fibers (Lenhossek, S. Ramón) also come as axis cylinder prolongations from anterior horn cells. . . .

6. Into the anterior commissure run:

a) Nerve prolongations from cells of all the grey matter which pass over to the contralateral anterolateral columns. . . .

b) Crossing collaterals from the anterior columns. . . .

c) Crossing dendrites of the medial anterior horn cells.

7. To the posterior commissure belong the crossing collaterals of the sensory dorsal root fibers. . . .

Anything else here, especially matters covered in Kölliker's thorough presentation, is at present uncertain.

The following is quoted from Kölliker's review of the physiological functions of the spinal cord.

1. Voluntary movements [cf. Figs. (23) and (25) (15–23) and Fig. (24)*A* ac-

cording to Kölliker]. I repeat briefly, for the sake of completeness and clarity, what was presented earlier in detail on this matter. Voluntary movements are mediated through the pyramidal pathways, in Kölliker's view, in such a way that the impulse goes from a pyramidal cell of origin in the brain to a pyramidal [corticospinal] anterior or lateral tract fiber, crosses there to the contralateral side and then passes through a collateral to the terminal arborization from which it is transmitted to a motor cell and from there to a motor fiber and its terminal arborizations on a muscle fiber.

In Kölliker's Fig. [24]*A* and in my diagram (Figs. [23] and [25]) it is assumed that the pyramidal [corticospinal] anterior tracts cross in the anterior commissure, which, however, is not yet certain for all the fibers in this pathway.

Motor cells lie, as pointed out by Schwalbe (Textbook of Neurology) in particular, in metameral segments (segmental nuclei). Each pyramidal fiber can now send collaterals to one or more segmental nuclei. If one muscle is supplied from several nerve roots, the question remains whether one is to assume the influence of one pyramidal fiber on several [ventral] root nuclei, or whether we think that at the same time several pyramidal fibers are influenced in the psycho-motor center.

2. Conscious sensations [Figs. (24)*B* and (23) and (25) (1–14)]. These are certainly transmitted from the periphery through the posterior [dorsal] roots to the posterior columns and in these further to the cerebrum. All posterior column fibers may end once in the medulla oblongata, but where and how is still uncertain (since Deiters, the nuclei graciles and cuneatis have been named). We expect Kölliker to carry out further research in these matters. From this ending in the (medulla) oblongata, which we must think of in the same way as a terminal arborization (in my diagrams, of Figs. [23] and [25], no consideration has been made for this discontinuity) a second and often a third nerve unit goes further to the end-station, which we assume to be in the psycho-sensory zone of the cerebral cortex. Part of the posterior column fibers does not go the medulla oblongata, but proceeds beyond in short pathways. The influence of spinal [dorsal root] ganglion cells on sensory transmission is completely unknown; we only know from Waller's transection experiments that they have a trophic influence. More cannot be said with certainty about the transmission of conscious sensations. Concerning the assertion that pain and heat sensations are transmitted through the grey substance, but sensations of touch and cold through the posterior columns, Kölliker's opinion is that transmission takes place through the grey substance by means of collaterals. These stimulate tract cells of the grey substance with their terminal arborizations, then fibers of the antero-lateral tracts which then lead upwards to the brain [see Fig. (24)*C* (2,3,4,5,7,8)].

3. Reflex pathways. We must distinguish between: a) short reflex arcs, and b) long reflex arcs. The short arcs lie between the sensory and motor fibers of the same spinal cord segment of the same side, or to the opposite side. Transmission from the sensory to the motor pathway of the same side is easily explained [cf. Fig. [24]*B* (2,3,4,5,6) or also Figs. [23] and [25] (1–9 from 9 to 20 etc.)]. Transmission to the other side happens in the following way: A tract cell on the right side, for example, is stimulated through a sensory collateral of the same side [Fig. (24)*C* (2,3,4,5,7)]; the stimulation goes through the nerve

prolongations in the anterior commissure to the other side . . . and here through the collaterals of this nerve prolongation to a motor cell of the contralateral grey substance. The known dampening of the reflex through the cerebrum cortex is, according to Kölliker, and probably rightly so, due to the influence of the pyramidal collaterals on the motor cells, under the assumption that this influence is stronger than that of the sensory pathway. This is explained in Figs. [23] and [25].

If we assume a network of anastomotic nerve fibers in the spinal cord, it is not difficult to explain the spreading out of the long reflexes; but if one assumes S. Ramón's and Kölliker's viewpoint, it arises by means of the so-called "short pathways", under the assumption that each sensory fiber of the posterior columns in its whole course gives off collaterals from interval to interval (as must be assumed, following S. Ramón). These can pass the impulses together, and their impulses can be transmitted to the motor cells of a large spinal cord area. See Fig. [24]*B* (2,6). The so-called short pathways are presented in the diagram of Fig. [24]*C*. When a wider reflex is induced through these, a circuitous path is hereby followed. From the sensory fiber (2,3,4), the impulse goes through the collateral (5) to a [posterior] column cell (7), from there somehow to a fiber of the anterior [propriospinal] pathway, which, however, remains in the spinal cord (hence "short pathway"), also when traversing a larger area. These in turn send collaterals (9,9) to the grey substance of the same or other side whose terminal arborizations together influence numerous motor ganglion cells (6,6). Further research must reveal whether the simpler or more complex path, or both, can be commanded by nature.

4. Relationships of the sensory pathways in the spinal cord to the brain.

Since Foville and Flechsig, we have been familiar with the [spino] cerebellar lateral column pathway to the cerebellum. From my studies of the spinal cord of the gorilla, I can only corroborate the assumption of Kölliker and others that the fibers of this pathway originate as nerve prolongations from cells of the Stilling nucleus (I see no justification for the name "Clarke column", as Stilling knew of it long before Clarke. Kölliker himself earlier called it "Stilling nucleus", even though he used the name "Clarke column" in his last publication—see my publication on the spinal cord of the gorilla, p. 19 loc. cit.). To these cells come in turn a large number of fibers with terminal arborizations (in my experience easily found in the spinal cord of the dog, but also in all others) which originate in the posterior [dorsal] roots and now are to be interpreted as collaterals of those. The pathway transmits centripetally; it can also function by reflexes, long and short, as in turn collaterals go off from its fibers to the grey matter.

No direct sensory connections exist with the cerebral cortex. Here "the arc" from the sensory columns and gracilis-cuneate nuclei exists as a pathway of the second order.[1] Fibers have been described by Bechterew, Edinger, Auerbach and myself (see my *Anatomy of the Spinal Cord of the Gorilla*, p. 120) which pass from the posterior [dorsal] horns through the anterior commissure across to the antero-lateral column of the other side. Bechterew, Auerbach and Edinger saw them as continuations of posterior root fibers; I was satisfied with reporting the simple evidence as I had seen it, namely that the fibers came from the posterior [dorsal] horns. Edinger[2] changed his concept recently in that he lets certain sensory root fibers come into contact with cells in the posterior [dorsal] horn; and, from these cells arise sensory fibers which cross through the anterior commissure and ascend to the brain (medulla oblongata). According to S. Ramón's and Kölliker's studies, we should further assume that collaterals of the sensory root branches influence certain lateral cells with their terminal arborizations, from which nerve prolongations then proceed through the anterior commissure to the opposite side and there ascend in the anterior column. Kölliker still has some considerations against the significance of this pathway as continuing directly to the "arc", but I can not go further into that here.

5. Relationships of the spinal cord to unconscious movements. In these movements, Kölliker includes the a) tonic contractions of the vascular muscles and the sphincter, both actions of instinctive muscles which occur partly as reflexes, partly from the brain (muscle contraction, acceleration of the heart beat, peristalsis, urine evacuation and others) as well as restraint of these movements (muscle extension, heart relaxation after vagal-stimulation, etc.), c) the movement Gad calls "autochthonic" (e.g. respiratory movements).

If we disregard the vagal fibers involved here (for which similar conditions should exist), a large part of the nerve pathways under discussion occur in the spinal nerves. According to Gaskell's studies in the dog, these are fine medullated fibers of the anterior roots which run from the second thoracic nerve to the second lumbar nerve, and emerge in the second and third sacral nerve. Kölliker thinks that these are nerve prolongations of the small anterior [ventral] horn cells, and is doubtful (as opposed to Gaskell) as to whether also posterior [dorsal] horn cells, in particular the Stilling cells, participate here. By this means the terminal arborizations of the pyramidal fibers from the brain or those of the antero-lateral tract, as well as those of the sensory collaterals, can assert their influence on these cells.

Here also, in Kölliker's opinion (see note to p. 16 of his study in the spinal cord, loc. cit.), should be noted the fibers discovered by M. v. Lenhossek and S. Ramón y Cajal . . . which arise from anterior horn cells and emerge in the posterior [dorsal] root, which thus can be considered to be centrifugal fibers of the posterior root. (See above.)

If we consider what is most profitable in the above mentioned anatomical studies, it is, in my opinion, to have specified more precisely the anatomical and functional elements of the nervous system, which we must now consider to be the nerve units (neurons), as well as the discovery, by Golgi and S. Ramón y Cajal, of [axon] collaterals with their terminal arborizations. These findings enable us to understand isolated transmissions as well as—even though it remains an open question whether such in fact exist—the spreading of transmissions over wide areas. But new facts, new projects! This consoling and happy side of scientific research has once again, as I earlier indicated in the introduction, become evident to us step by step. To solve these problems, we must call on physiologists and pathologists as well as anatomists.[3]

[1]. By the term second order is meant the pathway from the periphery to the center.

[2]. From the course of the touch pathways in the central nervous system. This journal 1890, no. 20.

[3]. After I had finished proofreading the preceding work, I received, through the kindness of the authors, the following papers on the same subject: 1) van Gehuchten, A. Recent discoveries in the anatomy and histology of the central nervous system. Talk given at the Belgian Microscopical Society, 25 April 1891, Bruxelles, Manceaux. 2) van Gehuchten, A. The structure of nervous centers. The spinal cord and cerebellum. "La Cellule", T. VI, p. 81, 1891. 3) von Lenhossek, M. Recent research on the fine structure of nervous systems. From a talk on May 14, 1891. Journal of Swiss Medicine, vol. 21, 1891. Further: 4) The latest issue of the publication "La Cellule", edited by van Carnoy, contains, besides the previously mentioned work of Gehuchten (No 2) a new communication by S. Ramón y Cajal: On the structure of the cerebral cortex of some mammals (p. 125). Van Gehuchten confirms in every respect the findings of S. Ramón and Kölliker. The essentials of S. Ramón's work, from an earlier communication in Spanish, is given above.

The first cited work of v. Gehuchten and that of von Lenhossek have the same goal as my own summary. They are of an earlier date; then comes the lecture by v. Kölliker at this year's anatomy meeting in Munich. The publication of four works with the same objective shows clearly enough the high interest which this subject occasions.

15
The Law of Dynamic Polarization

With the introduction of the neuron doctrine, anatomists had succeeded in uniting nerve processes and nerve cell bodies into one anatomical unit. Although there was the strong implication that this anatomical unit was also the basic physiological unit of the nervous system, it was not at all clear what kinds of functions this meant in precise terms. As we have seen, especially in the writings of Cajal and of Waldeyer, there was a great deal of speculation about the direction of nervous conduction within the nerve process and between the nerve processes of different cells, but no immediate generalizations that could be applied to all cells, due in large part to the bewildering variety of forms of different types of nerve cells and their processes revealed by the Golgi stain.

The apparent resolution of this problem was called the "Law of Dynamic Polarization of the Neuron." It came to be widely regarded as the essential physiological corollary of the neuron doctrine. In order to trace how this law came about, we need to consider the concepts then current concerning the nature of nervous activity.

The Nerve Impulse and the Reflex Arc

By the 1860s, the central concept of the physiology of a nerve cell or nerve fiber was the nerve impulse. Building on the pioneering studies of Matteucci and du Bois-Reymond (see Chapter 3), physiologists obtained increasing evidence that the nerve impulse is accompanied by a wave of negative potential as it propagates through a peripheral nerve. Since Helmholtz (1850) it had been known that the impulse has a finite, only medium fast, velocity, consistent with some kind of physicochemical process. There were indications from work on skeletal muscle and heart muscle that the impulse in these tissues had an all-or-nothing character (Bowditch, 1871) and was followed by a refractory phase of inexcitability, but these properties were not demonstrated in peripheral nerve until much later (cf. Adrian and Lucas, 1912). Physiologists generally understood that the impulse was a property of the nerve membrane, but the evidence was not definitive until Bernstein (1902). Thus, during the 1880s and 1890s, it was accepted that in peripheral nerves the nerve impulse is a brief propagating electrical event, and there was a consensus that this must be the main type of activity within and between nerve cells in the central nervous system.

With regard to the question of the direction of impulse conduction within a nerve cell, the main clue came from the study of reflexes. Here, the "Law of Bell and Magendie," set forth early in the century on the basis of the work of Sir Charles Bell (1811) in England and Francois Magendie (1822, 1823) in France, stated that the nerves in the dorsal roots of the spinal cord carry sensory information from the periphery to the spinal cord, and the nerves in the ventral (anterior) roots carry motor signals from the spinal cord to the muscles. This was the pathway for the spinal reflex arc. We have seen that this physiological law was the framework for interpreting all the studies of the cellular structure and organization of the spinal cord, beginning in the 1840s. Once it became accepted that the axis cylinder (axon) of the ventral root arises from the anterior horn cell (motor neuron), it was obvious that this fiber conducts the impulse from the cell body in the spinal cord to the motor nerve terminals on the muscle (as outlined by Waldeyer in his article). The progression of nervous activity in a reflex arc, from the sensory input to the motor output, was recognized by William James, the American physiologist and psychologist, as the "Law of Forward Conduction" (James, 1880; see Sherrington, 1906).

A difficulty in understanding the cellular basis of this law was the fact, known since the 1850s, that a peripheral nerve fiber, when stimulated by an electric shock, conducts nerve impulses in both directions. Thus, although the normal direction of conduction in the motor nerve is from cell body to nerve fiber to nerve terminals, this cannot be a property of the nerve fiber itself. This meant that the direction of conduction in a reflex arc must be imparted to it by some property of the central grey matter. In the 1880s the physiologist J. Gad, suggested that this directionality is due to the protoplasmic prolongations (dendrites), which receive the influence of the sensory root fibers and conduct only in the direction toward the axis cylinder (see van Gehuchten, 1900; Sherrington, 1906). Although this was wrong—dendrites can conduct in both directions just as axons can—it was a prevalent idea in the late 1880s. Only later did Sherrington present persuasive evidence that the directionality of impulse transmission through a reflex center is due to the one-way valve-like action of the junctions (synapses) between the axon terminals and the cells (see next chapter).

Cajal's Early Concepts

From the very start of his work on nerve cells, from the first views of those sharply etched images, Cajal was obsessed with understanding how they functioned. It was as if, in his artist's mind, he could not imagine a form without it having an action.

We have seen that the outlines of a theory of the functional organization of the nerve cell had begun to form in Cajal's mind with his early publications in 1888. To his anatomical laws, that axis cylinder (axonal) ramifications end freely, and that contacts are formed between them and the cell bodies and protoplasmic prolongations (dendrites) of other nerve cells, he had added two functional laws: that cell bodies and dendrites must also conduct nervous activity, and that the impulse in the axon terminals must induce in some way the impulse in the cell bodies and dendrites. These laws were well expressed in the example of the descending fringes (basket cell endings) and their relation to the Purkinje cells. By this example, he was, in effect, deducing that the basket cell was like a ventral horn cell (motor neuron), and its endings on the Purkinje cell were like the motor nerve terminals on a muscle, an idea he later made explicit (see below).

The next step in Cajal's thinking was in his paper of 1889, where he stated simply his belief in the nervous function of protoplasmic extensions (dendrites) (see Chapter 12). His two primary examples were the olfactory glomeruli, where transmission from the terminal arborizations of olfactory receptor cell fibers is confined to the most distal tufts of the protoplasmic extensions (dendrites) of the mitral and tufted cells, and the connection of parallel fibers onto the protoplasmic ramifications (dendrites) of the Purkinje cells in the cerebellum. The example of the olfactory pathway is shown in Cajal's diagram of Figure 26 (right). Cajal also cited retinal ganglion cells (Fig. 26 left) and cortical pyramidal cells as likely instances of nervous conduction in the protoplasmic prolongations (dendrites).

Although these examples would seem to have been sufficient to derive a general law about the direction of conduction of nervous activity through nerve cells, the picture was confused by several factors. First, there were layers within certain nervous centers where only protoplasmic prolongations (dendrites) seemed to intermingle. Cajal agreed with Golgi that these processes were not continuous with each other, but he assumed they might pass nervous conduction between each other in some discontinous manner,

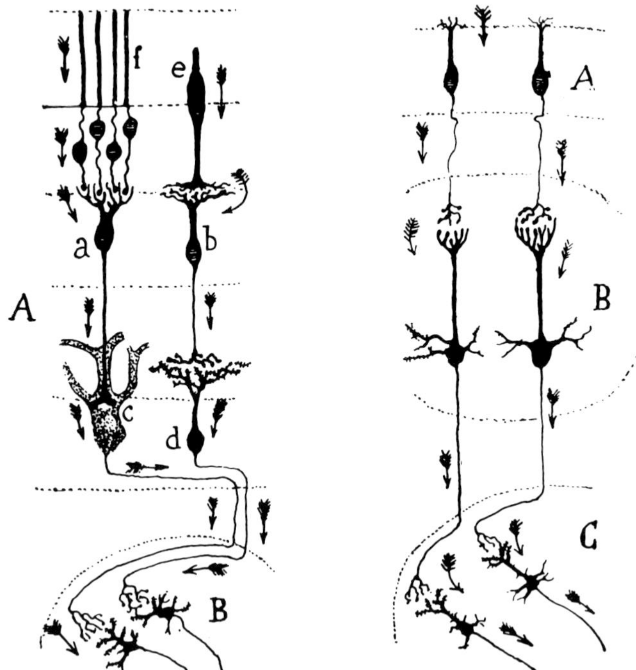

Fig. 26. Cajal's diagrams illustrating the direction of the nervous impulse in the vertebrate retina (left) and the olfactory pathway (right). Left: "*A*, retina; *B*, external geniculate body; *a*, rod bipolar cell; *b*, cone bipolar cell; *c*, *d*, ganglionic cells; *e*, cone; *f*, rods."

Right: "*A*, olfactory mucous membrane; *B*, olfactory bulb; *C*, pyriform lobe of the brain, to which the tracts from the bulb run." (Cajal, 1989)

by "induction." Cajal includes this as an explicit possibility in 1889, an example of what we would now call "dendro-dendritic interactions." In such a case, the dendrites would be presumed to support conduction in both directions, both to the site of intercellular "induction" and away from it.

A second problem was that certain types of cells seemed to have more than one axis cylinder (axon). This seemed to be true of a type of horizontal cell in the retina (cf. Cajal, 1889b; Piccolino, 1988), as well as a type of cell in the superficial layer of the cerebral cortex (Cajal, 1890b; cf. DeFelipe and Jones, 1989). A third, and contrasting problem, presented itself in the amacrine cells of the retina and the granule cells of the olfactory bulb, both of which lacked an axon altogether. These findings made it difficult to come up with generalizations about all activity being conducted out of a cell by means of a single axis cylinder (axon).

A final problem was the dorsal root ganglion cell. Cajal, drawing on the findings of Freud and His, could show that this cell started out develop-

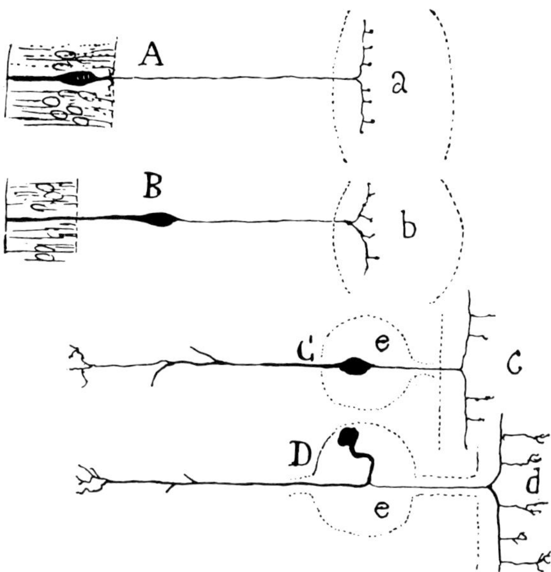

Fig. 27. "Diagrams showing the changes of situation and morphology undergone by the sensory cells in the animal series. *A,* sensory cell of the earthworm (the cell body, as demonstrated by Lenhossék, lies in the epidermis); *B,* sensory cell of a mollusc (after Retzius); *C,* sensory cell of a lower fish; *D,* sensory cell of amphibian, reptile, or mammal." (Cajal, 1989)

mentally as a bipolar cell, comparable to the bipolar sensory cell of the olfactory mucosa (cf. Fig. 26 right) or other bipolar sensory cells (see Fig. 27*A,B*). In fish, this bipolar form was retained into adult life, so it was easy to suppose that the peripheral process could still be considered a protoplasmic prolongation (dendrite), and the central process an axis cylinder (axon). Since Cajal believed that nervous conduction took place in a dendrite, and, most importantly, *dendritic conduction did not differ from conduction in an axon,* the bipolar dorsal root ganglion cell seemed to be quite similar in its functional organization to the other types of bipolar cells. However, in the mammal, the cell body is drawn off to the side in a stalk, and the peripheral process takes on a sheath of myelin, making it indistinguishable from a large axis cylinder (see Fig. 27*D*). Thus, the cell becomes a unipolar cell with a branched axis cylinder (axon). Cajal (1989) reasoned that the central and the peripheral expansions of these unipolar cells could still be considered as "functioning in the same manner as the two expansions of the . . . fish . . . so that this modification lacks significance."

Cajal (1989) wrote that he then abandoned the question as premature and perhaps insoluble. Two years later, the question was reopened by van Gehuchten in Belgium.

Van Gehuchten

Arthur van Gehuchten was an important but little remembered figure in our story; he is absent, for example, from Clarke and O'Malley's (1968) account.

He was born in 1861 in the Flemish city of Antwerp. He studied in Louvain (Leuven), which numbers Vesalius among its illustrious alumni. While there he began his training in microscopical anatomy under Jean-Baptiste Carnoy, a well-known anatomist, author of *Biologie Cellulaire* (*Cellular Biology*) and editor of the journal *La Cellule.* Van Gehuchten took further training in Berlin and Frankfort-am-Main in the 1880s, and then returned to Louvain in 1887, at the age of 26, to a chair of anatomy.

Van Gehuchten's first publications were on the microscopic structure of muscle. We have already had occasion to refer to this work in describing Cajal's own ill-fated venture into this same domain (see Chapter 10). To recapitulate briefly, the idea that in skeletal muscle the contractile apparatus resides in a diffuse intracellular reticulum, found in all cells that exhibit motility, rather than its distinctive striations, originated with Carnoy, van Gehuchten's teacher (Huxley, 1977). Van Gehuchten published two long papers in *La Cellule* supporting this idea, on invertebrate muscle (1886) and vertebrate muscle (1888). These papers influenced Cajal's own papers in 1887 and 1888, also supporting this idea. As we have seen, Kölliker (1888) quickly disposed of these excursions into the universal laws of nature.

Their muscle work led to correspondence between Cajal and van Gehuchten. Cajal (1989) quotes from van Gehuchten's remembrance of that time:

> It was in 1888. I was corresponding with Cajal in connection with papers which each of us had published upon the finer structure of the muscle cell. One day he wrote to me announcing that he was abandoning his investigations upon muscles in order to devote himself to the nerve centres, basing his decision upon the fact that he had obtained remarkable results from the application to embryos of one of the formulae of the method of Golgi, which had been discovered in 1875. I tested his statements and came to the conclusion that he was right. . . . The first step had been taken, other workers followed naturally.

Van Gehuchten immediately abandoned his previous work to follow Cajal in applying the Golgi method to the nervous system. When the two met at the Berlin Congress in late 1889, van Gehuchten had not yet published his first paper on the nervous system, but Cajal regarded him as the "young and already brilliant professor of anatomy from the University of Louvain" (he would have been 28 by then), and one whose approval he sought and valued.

Spinal Cord and Cerebellum

Van Gehuchten's first paper using the Golgi stain, and first on the nervous system, was: "La structure des centres nerveux: La moelle épinère et le cervelet" (1891a). Before dealing with the passages relating to the direction of nervous conduction, we cite two sections of the text that indicate how closely van Gehuchten agreed with His, Forel, Cajal, and Kölliker at this very early stage, and how lucidly he set forth the new ideas:

THE STRUCTURE OF NERVOUS CENTERS. THE SPINAL CORD AND CEREBELLUM

[*Spinal Cord*]

From this study of the structure of the spinal cord it obviously emerges that the nerve cells do not anastomose between themselves by their protoplasmic prolongations [dendrites], as Golgi proved a long time ago; that they do not take part either in the formation of an ordinary nerve network by their protoplasmic prolongations or by their cylindraxil prolongations [axons]. But all nerve cells with all these prolongations form an independent element, a whole autonomy, a kind of nerve unity.

This independence of the nerve elements from each other has moreover been proved embryologically by the beautiful reasearch of His. This learned man has shown that one nerve cell with all these prolongations comes solely from the transformation of a *neuroblast.*

This is a fact of the greatest importance.

When one researches in classical books which are the component elements of the nervous tissue, one ascertains that everywhere nerve cells and nerve fibers are considered as two absolutely distinct and completely independent structures. This is so true that, for many years, authors have been forced to search for the method of union and the method of action of the nerve fibers and the cell fibers. From new notions on the structure of the nerve centers, it clearly results that the nerve fibers and the nerve cells are not distinct elements: the nerve fiber considered by itself and in its essential part, the axis-cylinder, is not a nerve element, no more than the protoplasmic prolongations of the nerve cells: it is only a cylindraxil prolongation. The nerve cell in itself is not a nerve element either, one cannot separate it from either its protoplasmic prolongations, if these exist (this qualification is necessary because the nervous elements of the spinal ganglia are deprived of protoplasmic prolongations [dendrites]), or from its cylindraxil prolongation. *The sole nerve element is the nerve cell with all its prolongations* [italics added].

The nerve elements, thus composed, vary infinitely in their form, volume, and disposition and richness of the protoplasmic prolongations [dendrites]; only one of their characteristics seems constant and permits one to distinguish a nerve element from all other elements: it is the existence of a cylindraxil prolongation [axon].

This cylindraxil prolongation has particular characteristics which are rather difficult to describe, but which however permit one to recognize it at first sight, whatever may be the number of protoplasmic prolongations from the nerve cell. It springs directly from the cell body or arises, sometimes at a very great distance, from one or another of the protoplasmic prolongations. Before we carried out our own research with the Golgi method, we often asked ourselves, while examining the stained nerve cells in the work of Golgi and his students, why a given prolongation, colored in red by the author, was the cylindraxil prolongation, since it seemed not to differ by any of its characterizations from the neighboring prolongations, and since quite often one or the other of these, longer or more voluminous, deceived us at first. This same observation we have heard detailed many times by several of our colleagues.

It would be difficult for us to make a suitable answer to this. The cylindraxil prolongation, in our opinion, is distinguished from protoplasmic prolongations above all by the sharpness of its contours and by its regular trajectory. Whereas protoplasmic prolongations are most often irregular and sometimes jagged on their edges, and diminish imperceptibly in volume as one moves away from the cell body, the cylindraxil prolongation has clean and regular contours, as if it were made "ready-to-wear" (taillé a l'emporte-pièce). If it emits a collateral branch, or if it bifurcates, one always finds at the point of division a small triangular thickening with regular contours like the axis cylinder itself. In addition, it conserves for a long distance its original diameter. At any rate, the only way to familiarize oneself with the characteristics of the cylindraxil prolongation, in order to recognize it without any difficulty amidst the protoplasmic prolongations of a nerve cell and compare it at the same time with the drawings of other authors, is to make some attempts oneself with the Golgi method. A few good reductions [stains] will suffice to convince the most skeptical of the completely specific characteristics of the cylindraxil prolongation. It behaves everywhere in the same way, ending freely by one or several terminal branches. But here, again, one finds the greatest variety in the details. There are nerve cells whose cylindraxil prolongation is short and ends very near the cell body: there are others whose cylindraxil prolongation extends over a considerable length: such, for example, is the cyilndraxil prolongation of the radicular cell [motor neuron], which extends from the grey matter of the spinal cord to the peripheral muscle; but this morphological distinction is not clear enough to see, with Golgi, evidence for a physiological distinction; these are only two extreme forms between which one finds a whole series of intermediary forms.

All the central nervous system thus reduces itself, in the final analysis, to a superposition of independent nerve elements.

Among the nerve elements with long axis cylinder [axons], one can easily distinguish two types at first sight.

One type has its cell body in the superior parts of the cerebro-spinal axis, and its cylindraxil prolongation [axon] descends to end freely lower down. The other type has its cell body in the inferior regions of the central nervous system, and its cylindraxil prolongation, heading in an opposite direction from the first, ends freely in higher centers. To the first group belong, for example, the pyramidal cells of the cortical grey layer of the brain, whose cylindraxil prolongations constitute the pyramidal tracts and end freely at some point of the grey matter of the cerebro-spinal axis; or again radicular cells [motor neurons] of the anterior horn of the spinal cord, whose cylindraxil prolongations go to the peripheral organs. In these nerve elements the conduction is necessarily *centrifugal,* at the same time that it is *cellulifugal.*

In the second group are, without doubt, a certain number of *tract cells,* whose cylindraxil prolongation, arriving in the anterolateral cord, curves back to become an ascending fiber. The conduction thus is *centripetal* and *cellulifugal* at the same time. One can possibly also in a strict sense include in this group nerve elements of the spinal ganglia whose cylindraxil prolongations form the posterior roots. In birds these nerve elements are bipolar; they have a peripheral cylindraxil prolongation and a central cylindraxil prolongation. [Footnote on the spinal ganglion cell: see next section].

In mammals the nervous elements of the spinal ganglion have a single cylindraxil prolongation which bifurcates to give rise to a peripheral prolongation and a central prolongation. In both cases the central prolongation ends freely in the grey matter of the spinal cord. The conduction thus is *centripetal* and *cellulifugal.* In the peripheral prolongation on the contrary it is both *centripetal* and *cellulifugal* at the same time.

The sensorial nervous elements are equally a part of this group: such are the bipolar cells of the olfactory mucosa, whose nervous nature has been demonstrated, with the help of the Golgi method, by the observations of Grassi and Castranovo, of Ramón y Cajal and ourselves: the cylindraxil prolongation ends freely in the olfactory glomeruli; such are also the ganglion cells of the retina whose nervous prolongations, in birds, end freely in the optic layers (Ramón y Cajal). In all these elements the conduction is *centripetal.*

However, all nerve elements cannot be classified in these two categories. There exist, in fact, in the whole of the spinal cord, nervous elements (many tract fibers) whose cell body is situated in the grey matter of the spinal cord, and whose cylindraxil prolongation divides in the white matter into an ascending branch and a descending branch. When the excitation leaves the cell body, the conduction is necessarily *centripetal* in the ascending branch and *centrifugal* in the descending branch. If it were true that the nervous elements of *centrifugal* conduction must be considered as *motor* elements, and those where the conduction is *centripetal* as *sensitive* elements, these elements of the spinal cord which occupy our attention for the moment would be necessarily mixed elements, as they are neither exclusively motor nor exclusively sensitive.

But what obviously proves that this division of the nerve elements into *motor* elements and *sensitive* elements, according to the direction in which they transmit the nervous currents, is an erroneous division, resting on no positive evidence, is the fact that each central cylindraxil prolongation of a cell of a [dorsal root] spinal ganglion, an essentially sensitive element, divides, at its entry into the spinal cord, into an ascending branch of *centripetal* conduction and a descending branch of *centrifugal* conduction. And consider another fact no less convincing: that the fibers of the anterior [ventral] roots, which are obviously *motor,* of *centrifugal* conduction, sometimes emit, before leaving the spinal cord, collateral branches [recurrent axon collaterals] which reenter the grey matter, and whose conduction is necessarily *centripetal.* A final point is that in this grouping of nerve elements there is no place for the nerve cells with short axis cylinders.

Knowledge recently acquired on the structure of the nerve centers seems to bring forth again, quite obviously, this important fact, that, consistent with the ideas already established in physiology, the cylindraxil prolongation of a nervous element is an indifferent conductor, carrying excitation in whatever direction and transmitting it by its collateral or terminal ramifications to those elements with which it comes in contact.

This absolute independence of the nerve elements from one another is today accepted by HIS, FOREL, RAMÓN Y CAJAL and KÖLLIKER. Our observations on the structure of the nervous centers have led us to the same conclusion. It leaves room, regarding the mechanism by which nervous transmission takes place, for only one hypothesis: transmission is not made by continuity, but simply by contiguity or *by contact.* Ramón y Cajal and Kölliker have shown that certain physiological phenomena, such as a voluntary movement or a reflex movement, are explained by this hypothesis with no less ease than by accepting the direct continuity of nervous pathways.

This independence of nerve elements could moreover throw some light on other physiological phenomena hitherto unexplained, for example, the fact, that, for sensory reflexes, nerve transmission is much slower in [that part of the pathway in] the central nervous system than in the peripheral nerves. If it is true that the sensitive nerve fibers, at their entry into the spinal cord, *are continuous with* the motor nerve fibers by the interposition either of a nervous network or of one of several nerve cells, it is difficult to understand this great delay in conduction, because all in all there is no interruption anywhere in the conductor element. The recent researches have proved this interruption exists; it is perhaps the reason for the delay. Who knows if at the moment when the nerve current passes from a sensitive fiber to a radicular cell [motor neuron], there does not exist there a latent period analogous in some way to the latent period which precedes the whole muscular contraction? . . .

[*Cerebellum*]

. . . The study of the internal structure of the cortical grey layer leads to the same conclusions as that of the structure of the spinal cord: the true nervous element is the nerve cell with all its prolongations.

The nervous elements are independent of one another. The protoplasmic extensions [dendrites] always end freely; the cylindraxil prolongation [axon], whether long or short, has the same arrangement everywhere; it also ends freely, either as such, which seems to be the case for the small cells of the granular layer, or by a tuft of long and spindly branches, as we have acknowledged for the large cells of the molecular layer, the large cells of the granular layer, the mossy fibers, and the fibers ending in a plexus. The terminal branches of the cylindraxil prolongation always come in intimate contact with the neighboring nervous elements: the large cells of the molecular layer with the bodies of the Purkinje cells; the large cells of the granular layer with the granules of the same layer; the mossy fibers with the same granules; finally, the terminal fibers in a plexus with the bodies and the protoplasmic prolongations of the Purkinje cells.

In summary, the nervous elements of the cerebellum are independent elements. As a result, and this will be our final conclusion, nervous transmission takes place in the cerebellum as in the spinal cord and probably in the whole cerebro-spinal central nervous system, not continuously, but contiguously or by contact.

This paper was an important confirmation of the nerve cell as an independent unit; it was published too late to be a primary source for the enunciation of the neuron doctrine by Waldeyer later in 1891, but it was mentioned as strong supporting evidence in the final note in Waldeyer's review (see previous chapter).

Footnote on the Spinal Ganglion Cell

In the course of discussing the structure of the spinal cord and spinal roots, van Gehuchten (1891a) added a lengthy footnote on the problem of how to characterize the peripheral process of a dorsal root ganglion cell:

It is difficult for us to accept the hypothesis, otherwise quite ingenious, of Ramón y Cajal [1889c], in which the peripheral prolongment would be a protoplasmic prolongation [dendrite], whereas the central prolongation would represent the true nervous prolongation [axon]. Ramón y Cajal has arrived at this hypothesis by comparing, for example, the bipolar elements of the olfactory mucosa to the elements of the spinal [dorsal root] ganglia. But if this comparison is possible for the nervous elements of the spinal ganglia of birds, it is less so when one considers the nervous elements of the spinal ganglia of mammals. Here, we find a single cylindraxil prolongation [axon], as Ramón y Cajal seems to favor, but, in our opinion, it gives rise to two cylindraxil prolongations [axons], both of which go to form the axis cylinder [axon] of a peripheral nerve.

The notion of regarding the peripheral prolongation as a protoplasmic prolongation [dendrite] is ingenious in this sense, that one removes all difficulty in establishing a difference, if not morphological at least functional, between the protoplasmic prolongations [dendrites] and the cylindraxil prolongation [axon]. The protoplasmic prolongations [dendrites] would mediate *cellulipetal* conduction, and would serve to conduct to the cell body the nervous currents coming from neighboring elements, and the nervous prolongation [axon] would mediate *cellulifugal* conduction, serving to put the nervous element in which it occurs *en rapport* with the others. Apart from the protoplasmic prolongations [dendrites] the cell body itself can receive nervous currents directly by means of the collateral branches or terminals of a cylindraxil prolongation [axon]. These considerations are sufficiently persuasive that we do not attribute, as does Golgi, a different function to the pro-

> toplasmic prolongations [dendrites] and to the cylindraxil prolongation [axon]. For us, in accord with Ramón y Cajal, the nervous element [neuron] in all its parts is able to serve, and does serve, nervous conduction. But in order to accept this hypothesis, it will be necessary to change completely the [present] concept of a protoplasmic prolongation [dendrite], and accept that this prolongation is able to become the axis cylinder [axon] of a nerve fiber, which seems difficult [at present].

Toward a New Law

Cajal was never one to take criticism lightly, even when tucked into a footnote, and especially not when it touched on one of his own unresolved conceptual problems. As he recollects (Cajal, 1989):

> The reading of this incidental critique by the savant of Louvain attracted my attention and caused me to meditate anew upon the subject. . . . The precision with which [he] stated the problem altered the course of my thoughts, and the doubts and criticisms expressed by him, instead of deterring and dissuading me, produced the opposite effect. An obsession with the subject pursued me, and, full of hope and courage, I asked myself: "Why must not that formula be correct? Is it not plausible to think that with different morphological characters there correspond somewhat diverse functions? And could not this diversity, produced by physiological adaptation, be exclusively cellulifugal conduction for the dendrites and cellulipetal for the axons? Let us examine it again.

In order to resolve this issue, Cajal reconsidered the evidence that had stood in his way. As we have seen (Chapter 12), there were four problem areas, which he dealt with as follows.

The first problem was the zones and layers in which only protoplasmic prolongations (dendrites) came together. Reexamination (carried out largely, he writes, by his brother, Pedro) revealed in addition "rich plexuses" of axis cylinder (axon) terminations. In a stroke, this removed the need for transmission between dendrites, substituting for it transmission exclusively from the axon terminals to the dendrites, thereby reducing all impulse conduction within the cell to the direction from dendrites to cell body. However, we now know that intermingling of processes is not sufficient to guarantee contacts, which can only be proven by direct observation under the electronmicroscope. Furthermore, the electronmicroscope has demonstrated numerous instances of dendro-dendritic synaptic connections (see Chapter 20), even where axonal terminals are making connections onto the dendrites in the same area. So this conclusion of Cajal has not been borne out completely.

The second problem was the presence of more than one axis cylinder (axon) arising from retinal horizontal cells and cerebral cortical layer I cells. These cells are extremely amorphous in character, giving off many very fine processes, and when Cajal reexamined these he concluded that in all cases only one process qualified as a true axis cylinder (axon). Modern research has supported these interpretations (cf. Piccolino, 1988; DeFelipe and Jones, 1989), although it would be rash to rule out completely the possibility of multiple axons on some neurons.

The third problem was the retinal amacrine and olfactory granule cells that lack an axis cylinder (axon). Cajal was never able to account for them in his theory. There was no clear idea about their status as nerve cells or their possible functions until the modern era, when it was shown that the dendrites of these cells have both input and output functions (see Chapter 20).

The final problem was the dorsal root ganglion cell. Here Cajal (1989) returned to his comparative approach, both developmental and phylogenetic. He reasoned that

> the anatomical features of the processes of the neurons are not primary facts imposed of necessity by the law of evolution but are secondary conditions of an adaptive character and are related mainly to the length of the conductor. For example, the possession of an insulating myelin sheath in the dendrites (in the sensory cells of the ganglia) is related not so much to the direction of the nerve current as to the considerable length of the conductor. Fig. [27] shows the development of form and position which the sensory cell body has undergone during its phylogenetic history. It is seen that, as development progresses, this [cell] body first abandons the skin, confining itself to deeper organs, and when it is situated near the spinal cord (reptiles, amphibians, birds, and mammals) there begins another migration by virtue of which the nucleus lying between the two processes, central and peripheral, slips out towards the cortex of the ganglion while the processes thereafter rise from their pedicle of origin with the anatomical attributes of axons.
>
> This morphological evolution of the sensory neurons is reproduced during the embryonic development of the mammals and birds.
>
> These difficulties being surmounted, and a histological analysis of the structural plan of the sensory pathways more exact than any made up to that time having previously been carried out, I was led to the following pronouncement, which was received sympathetically by many neurologists and even by van Gehuchten himself. *The transmission of the nervous impulse is always from the dendritic branches and the cell body to the axon or functional process. Every neuron, then, possesses a receptor apparatus, the body and the dendritic prolongations, an apparatus of emission, the axon, and an apparatus of distribution, the terminal arborization of the nerve fiber.* And as this course of the nerve impulse through the protoplasm implies a certain constant orientation, something like a polar-

ization of the waves of excitation, I designated the foregoing principle: the theory of dynamic polarization.

The theory in this form seemed to explain how the three distinctive parts of the nerve cell—protoplasmic prolongations (dendrites), cell body, and axis cylinder (axon)—could function together as a physiological unit, this physiological unit fitting perfectly with the anatomical unity of the cell. However, Cajal was not yet satisfied, because he had not accounted for cases in which the axis cylinder (axon) arises, not from the cell body, but from a large dendrite, at some distance from the cell body; examples are many of the monopolar cells of invertebrates, and several types of vertebrate cells. As indicated in the diagram of Figure 28, activity in some of the protoplasmic prolongations (dendrites) could be conducted to the axis cylinder (axon) without passing through the cell body (Cajal, 1989).

Only later, in 1897, did I hit upon the realization that, contrary to the general opinion, the soma, or cell body does not always take part in the conduction

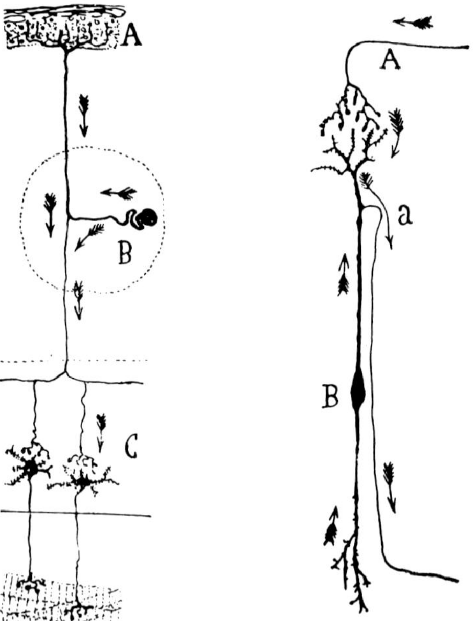

Fig. 28. Left. "*Scheme of the Course Followed by the Currents in Sensory-Motor Pathways.* While the formula of the axipetal polarization is conformed with, the supposition that the stalk of the sensory cell, contrary to the theory, conducts in both cellulipetal and cellulifugal direction is avoided. *A*, skin; *B*, spinal ganglion; *C*, spinal cord. Right. *The Course of the Currents in the Crosier Cells of the Optic Lobe of Fishes, Amphibians, and Reptiles,* where the axon originates from a dendrite far from the cell body. This is well explained by the theory of axipetal polarization." (Cajal, 1989)

> of the nerve impulses which are received [In this instance he was, in fact, adopting Golgi's and Nansen's view!]. The afferent wave is sometimes propagated directly from the dendrites to the axon. I had then to substitute for the preceding incorrect formula this other, which I designated *Theory of axipetal polarization: The soma and the dendrites conduct in an axipetal direction, that is, they transmit the waves of nervous excitation towards the axon. Inversely, the axon or axis cylinder conducts in a somatofugal or dendrifugal direction, carrying the impulses received by the soma or by the dendrites towards the terminal arborizations of the nerve fibre.* Consequently the currents flowing into the axon do not pass through the soma except when the latter is between the dendritic and the axonic apparatus.
>
> This formula is applicable to all cases without exception, as well of vertebrates as of invertebrates, as well in the adult as in the embryo. Thanks to its complete generality, it constitutes a valuable key to the interpretation of the courses of the currents in neurons of the nerve centres. This fact was recognized by distinguished scientists, who did me the honour of accepting it without reservations.

Well, perhaps a few reservations. Barker (1899) accords to von Lenhossék the first suggestion that "the impulses in dendrites . . . [are] . . . *axopetal* rather than cellulipetal." However, von Lenhossék (1895) also suggested that the unmedullated side branches of axis cylinders (axon collaterals) conduct activity *toward* the axis cylinder (axon), and only the medullated (myelinated) side branches conduct activity away (see also Barker, 1899). This suggestion has never seemed very likely. Von Bechterew (1896), on the other hand, emphasized the likelihood of transmission of impulses between intermingled dendrites, in which case "it is obvious that with a given impulse the direction of the conduction in one of the sets of dendrites must be cellulifugal and axofugal [away from the cell body and axis cylinder]" (see also Barker, 1899). As examples, von Bechterew cited the intermingling of protoplasmic prolongations (dendrites) in the ventral commissure of the spinal cord; of the dendrites of the granule cells and mitral cells of the olfactory bulb; those in layer I of the cerebral cortex; and those of the granule layer of the cerebellum. This suggestion of interactions between dendrites essentially disappeared without a trace, but it has turned out to be remarkably prescient in the light of modern research on dendrites in the olfactory bulb and elsewhere (see Chapter 20).

Cajal was quite proud of his theory of the dynamic polarization of the neuron, considering it the key to understanding the neuron as a functional unit. The enormous amount of mental energy he invested in it came at a price. For one thing, he only grudgingly admitted van Gehuchten's contribution to the theory. Despite their high regard for each other, the two sniped politely at each other for many years over priority (see van Gehuchten, 1900; Cajal, 1989). Van Gehuchten (1900) noted that, by removing the cell body from an obligatory role in nervous conduction, "Cajal abandoned what one refers to as the physiological unity of the neuron."

Far more serious was the problem that the theory gave Cajal's judgment what Piccolino (1988) has called a "neuron doctrine bias." Certain facts or possibilities difficult to account for under the theory were discounted or ignored. These included the issues we noted before: multiple axons; connections between dendrites; and the axonless retinal amacrine cells and olfactory granule cells. In addition was the possibility of anastomoses between dendrites to form syncytial networks, particularly in the retina (cf. Piccolino, 1988). Cajal would have none of it. In his defense we should note that the idea behind the theory, that nerve cells receive signals in their dendrites and send signals through their axons, seemed so obvious for most large neurons, and so reasonable for most small ones, that it hardly mattered to most anatomists and physiologists that there might be occasional exceptions to the rule. The theory provided a simple key for facilitating analysis of the cellular basis of nervous centers and pathways. That it concealed several critical levels of complexity in the organization of nerve cells would only be revealed by modern work.

16
Controversy

Waldeyer's review in 1891 did not establish the neuron doctrine with one wave of a master's wand. At the time of its appearance, it was regarded as an authoritative summary of what was known about the structure of nerve cells and nerve fibers. It gave clear expression to the point of view that all fibers arise directly from cells, and that a cell and its fibers form a unit, so that nervous transmission must take place from unit to unit. But the greatest influence of this review came from the new term "neuron" introduced for the unit. It was a quintessential example of the power of the word in science: a symbol for a new concept. Waldeyer forced his readers to judge not only the accumulated evidence for the varieties of nerve cells and their fibers as independent interacting units, but also whether the term "neuron" was acceptable, unambiguous, and useful in the light of this evidence.

Many of Waldeyer's readers of course had considerable personal stakes in this issue, as leading players in gathering the evidence, or as practitioners in the fields of the anatomy and physiology of the nervous system, so it should hardly be surprising that a period of controversy followed. In fact, Waldeyer's review served the important function of focusing all the different strands of debate that had grown out of the study of the nerve cell over the preceding half century on the essential issues. Out of this controversy, which lasted for about a decade until the turn of the century, was fashioned the consensus that came to be called the "neuron theory" or "neuron doctrine," and that has served as the central organizing concept of neuroscience to the present day.

To cover all aspects of this debate, even for the limited period of the 1890s, would embrace most of the history of research on the nervous system during that time. We will keep our focus specifically on the issues most directly involved in the acceptance of the neuron doctrine. First was the problem of agreeing on the term "neuron," and on related terms for describing the varieties of nerve cells and their processes (this chapter). Second was how to incorporate into the concept of the neuron a new idea, of the "synapse" as the junction between neurons (Chapter 17). Third was the gradual refinement of the neuron concept in the light of the greatly expanded research on the cytological and cellular composition of the nervous system following 1891 (Chapters 17, 18). Lastly, there were the final skirmishes between the neuron theory and the reticular theory, in its old form and in new incarnations (Chapter 19). Let us consider each of these issues in turn.

Hammering Out New Terms

The new term "neuron" threw the field into considerable etymological agitation. Opinions were expressed on every conceivable aspect, from its grammatical correctness to a variety of related terms and alternatives. We will sample the richness of this debate with citations from several of the key participants.

Edward Schafer

Edward Schafer (changed to Sharpey-Schafer in later life) was one of the leading anatomists and physiologists in Great Britain in the period 1880–1930. He was among the earliest and best known in Great Britain to respond to the new ideas set forth in Waldeyer's review.

He was born in London in 1850 and educated at University College, London. There he trained in physiology under William Sharpey, who was also the teacher of Joseph Lister. Schafer published his first microscopical studies in 1873. His biographer comments on the status of this field in Great Britain at the time (Sherrington, 1935c):

> What was called "general anatomy" was then customarily, more than it is today, considered in this country a discipline belonging to physiology. This state of affairs was doubtless related, part as cause, part as effect, to the lack of equipment of the laboratories for pursuit of experimental physiology in the modern sense. In this respect our country was quite behind France, Germany and Italy and some other of its European neighbours.

In the light of our previous comparisons of medical science in central Europe compared with Italy, Spain and the United States, this passage testifies to the fact that through the nineteenth century Great Britain also lagged behind Germany in this respect, a state of affairs that continued to the First World War of 1914–1918.

Schafer made an important experimental contribution to the study of the nerve cell in 1877 when he published his observations on the microscopic structure of the nerve plexus situated under the umbrella of the swimming bell of the jelly fish *Medusa*. Nervous activity in this plexus is responsible for the undulatory swimming motions of the bell. Whereas it had been believed that this plexus consisted of a nervous syncytium, in which all the cells were confluent, Schafer concluded that the nerve cells in it were separate, with "points of mutual contact" between them (Sherrington, 1935b). He suggested that fiber-to-fiber transmission could take place by some kind of electrical "inductive action," "the result being the same as if there were a real network" (Taylor, 1975). Subsequent work on this plexus favored the idea of an anatomical continuum, throwing some doubt on Schafer's study, though he was eventually vindicated.

Schafer had an extremely productive and varied career. In 1876 (at the age of 26), he was one of 12 founding members of The Physiological Society. He was a Fellow of the Royal Society by 1878 and Jodrell Professor of Physiology at University College, London, in 1883. In 1885, he published *The Essentials of Histology*, which was to see 16 editions. In the years 1884–1891 he studied cerebral localization.

Schafer thus had reason to follow developments bearing on the structure and organization of nerve cells. In his Presidential Address to the annual meeting of the Neurological Society in London, on January 19, 1893, he made a concerted effort to deal with problems of terminology:

> **THE NERVE CELL CONSIDERED AS THE BASIS OF NEUROLOGY**
>
> It is obvious that the nerve-cell must always form the basis of the science of Neurology in all its branches. But although this cell has been studied for a great number of years it is only now that we are beginning to arrive at a definite understanding regarding its structure, functions and relation to other nerve-cells. This has seemed to me therefore a suitable occasion for gathering up such threads of knowledge as we at present possess, and laying them before the members of this Society. . . .
>
> We may most naturally begin with the structure of the nerve-cell. I do not know why one should restrict the term "nerve-cell" to the body of the cell and thus exclude from that term the cell-processes. This is not done for any other kind of cell, and it appears to me that the custom which has hitherto prevailed with regard to nerve-cells in this matter is not only inadvisable but even misleading. Waldeyer [1891] has used the term "neuron" in this way to denote the whole nerve-cell, including all its processes. It is better, however, and simpler, to include under the term "cell", as is done with every cell of the body, the processes as well as the body of the cell. It will therefore be understood that by the term "nerve-cell" I shall denote not only, as has hitherto for the

most part been the case, the body of the cell or the part immediately enclosing the nucleus, but all the several processes of the cell, and in that sense the word "nerve-cell" will be here used as identical with Waldeyer's term "neuron." The term "neuron" is short and convenient, but I shall employ it in a different sense, as will hereafter be seen, and I adopt this course the more readily because it has not yet come into very general use in Waldeyer's sense, and it is, I think, undesirable that it should do so. . . .

We may next consider the processes of the cell. Every nerve-cell has one or more; it is an absolute characteristic of nerve-cells to possess processes. The processes are of two kinds. The first and the only essential kind is that which has long been known as the axis-cylinder or nerve-fibre process (Deiters). It is also the first kind to show itself in the course of development of the nerve-cell [His, 1889]. The other kind is that which was distinguished by Deiters as the protoplasmic process. This is not so essential, for we find many nerve-cells entirely destitute of it. A word is here again necessary with regard to nomenclature. The above terms have been long in use to indicate these two kinds of processses, but they are obviously inconvenient from their length and from the assumptions which they appear to imply. I propose therefore to term the axis-cylinder or nerve-fibre processes *neurons*; and the protoplasmic processses *dendrons*. And combined processes, such as occur in the motor nerve-cells of arthropods [Retzius, 1890] can conveniently be known as *neurodendrons*. It must clearly be understood however that all processes of nerve-cells are ultimately dendritic. Almost without exception the neuron or nerve-fibre process, although it may have a course of several feet without giving off a branch, finally ends in a terminal arborisation. . . .

There can be little doubt that this distinction into motor and sensory cells which was drawn by Golgi, can no longer be accepted. At the same time there may still be a functional difference between the two kinds of cell, but this functional difference may perhaps better be expressed by using the term *projection-cell* for the cell of Golgi's first type with long axis-cylinder process, and the term *intermediary cell* for the cell belonging to Golgi's second type, with relatively short axis-cylinder process. By the latter term is implied that the cell in question offers an intermediary link between centripetal impressions which may be brought to a nerve-centre by the neuron of a sensory projection-cell, and the centrifugal impressions which pass away from the nerve-centre by the neurons of motor projection-cells. . . .

In fact we may regard the basis of the grey matter of the nervous sytem—the granular-looking substance in which the nerve-cells are embedded—as an extremely fine interlacement of ramified processes, not only of the nerve-cells, which actually lie in that particular grey matter, but also of nerve-cells which lie in other parts of the nerve-centres or even in the peripheral parts of the nervous system, and which on arriving at the grey matter similarly break up into a fine arborescence of nerve-fibrils. This view is extremely probable by reason of the numerous observations which have recently accumulated on the disposition of nerve-fibres and nerve-cells within the grey matter of the vertebrate nerve-centres and it is rendered still more probable by what we now know regarding the granular-looking substance which forms a large portion of the ganglia of the central nervous system of invertebrates

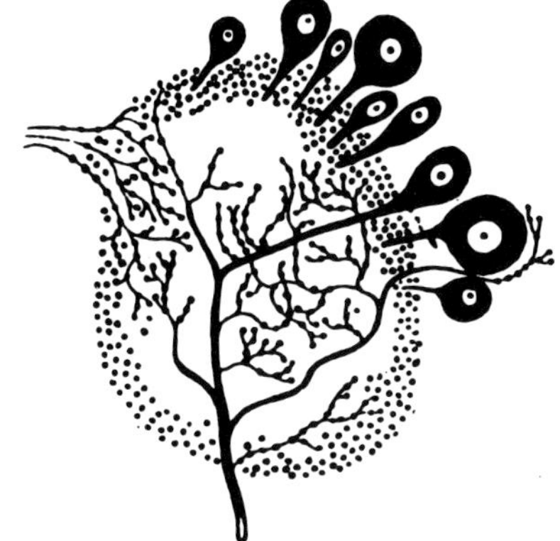

Fig. 29. Diagram illustrating how the "dotted substance" of Leydig in the crayfish (Astacus) is actually composed of the terminal branches of collaterals of axons from the unipolar ganglion cells (cell bodies on the right) and the terminal branches of incoming nerve fibers (on the left). (Schafer, 1893; modified from a drawing by G. Retzius)

and which was termed by Leydig, who first carefully described, it the *punktsubstanz.* Within this "Punktsubstanz" (dotted substance) it has long been known that many of the processes of the nerve-cells terminate, and it is now recognised by the employment of new methods, and particularly the method of Ehrlich, and the method of Golgi, that the Punktsubstanz is entirely made up of the finely ramified and somewhat varicose terminations, not only of the processes of the nerve-cells of the ganglia which constitute the central nervous system in these animals, but also of processes which arrive at those ganglia from nerve-cells at the periphery. I would refer you, in substantiation of this fact, to the accompanying figure [Fig. 29], after Retzius [1890]; showing the dotted substance in one of the ganglia of Astacus. In this it will be seen that the so-called Punktsubstanz is mainly made up of ramifications of fibres derived from the neuro-dendrons of the large motor nerve-cells. . . .

And in the case of invertebrates, such as the earth-worm, the structure of whose nervous system has recently been elucidated by Lenhossék . . . and Retzius . . . , it is clear that sensory impulses which are brought by the fibres from the integument to the central nervous system may perfectly well become converted into motor impulses within the Punktsubstanz without necessarily traversing the motor nerve-cells at all; the latter being only connected with the Punktsubstanz by dendritic collaterals, which pass off from their large neuro-dendritic processes. . . .

Although it seemed to make sense to Schafer to call the axon a neuron, one can feel grateful that this suggestion died quietly! Apart from this, the paper is notable in giving support to the new ideas; also, the term "projection cell" came into general use to refer to long-axon cells.

A curious aspect of this review is that Schafer does not cite his own earlier contribution to the subject. Except for a passing reference to bipolar cells in *Aurelia* (Schafer, 1893), there is no mention of Schafer's early demonstration that cells in the umbrella network are independent, or his notion that impulses might be transmitted between the cells by some kind of inductive interaction. Liddell (1960) notes that neither of these contributions is acknowledged by later workers. The explanation may lie in the fact that Schafer himself did not acknowledge them when he had the chance to do it. Why this is so is not clear. Perhaps he felt the issue in *Aurelia* was still in doubt. Or perhaps it was simply that his interests by then were leading him in other directions. Scarcely a year later (1894), he demonstrated for the first time the action of an extract of the adrenal gland in raising the blood pressure, and subsequently gave the name "endocrinology" to the new field he helped to found.

Michael von Lenhossék

By way of contrast, we turn to the views of Michael von Lenhossék. He is representative of the microscopical anatomists who devoted their full attention to the study of the nervous system, and were establishing neuroanatomy as a separate discipline. They thus had the greatest expertise in assessing the evidence, and the greatest stake in developing the central concepts and vetting the new terms for their field.

Von Lenhossék was born in 1863 in Budapest, where his father (Josef) was professor of anatomy, as was his grandfather before him (Michael the elder) (Huzella, 1937/38). Young Michael kept up this tradition, studying medicine and training in microscopic anatomy in Budapest. His father was an authority on the anatomy of the spinal cord, and his professor at the Second Anatomical Institute, Miholkoviecs, on brain development (Környey, 1937), so it is not surprising that his interests gravitated toward the nervous system. After his father died, in 1888, von Lenhossék took a series of posts abroad, including Basel (1889–1893) under the embryologist Kollman; Würzburg (1893–1895) with Kölliker; and Tübingen (1895–1899) with Froriep. He finally returned to Budapest as head of the First Anatomical Institute in 1899. These moves are recounted to indicate how much von Lenhossék moved within, and represented in his thinking, the central European traditions of his field, and also to indicate the high standards of Hungarian neuroanatomy, which have lasted to the present.

During his career, von Lenhossék made many fundamental contributions to the microscopic anatomy of the nervous system; nor was he unpracticed in matters terminological: we owe to him the term "astrocyte" for one of the main types of neuroglial cells. With regard to the neuron doctrine, his early contributions have been summarized as follows (Huzella, 1937/38):

> Stimulated by the impressive presentation given by Cajal at the 1889 Anatomy Congress in Berlin, where Lenhossék was in attendance, the insight came to

him that the foundation for research on the elementary structure of nervous systems lay in knowledge of the histogenesis of the nervous elements. Since he had already initiated a series of neurohistological studies in 1886, he decided to join the Spanish master [Cajal] in the use of the simplified chrome silver stain. He was one of the first in the early 1890s to pursue the research which, under Cajal's leadership, through workers in many countries, enriched knowledge and led to an enormous change in research on the nervous system.

In 1891, von Lenhossék studied, at the same time as Cajal and completely independently of him, the earliest development of the nerve cell and nerve fiber in the spinal cord of the chick. Through clear and striking histological sections he was able to verify with uncontestable observations the concepts of early development and interneuronal contacts that had been put forth by His on the basis of insufficient normal staining methods.

Von Lenhossék was thus closely involved in establishing the neuron doctrine. He was certainly so regarded by his contemporaries. Waldeyer (1891) includes him along with Cajal, Kölliker, His, Nansen, and Retzius as one of the founders (see Chapter 13). Cajal (1989) acknowledges his contribution profusely. Von Lenhossék's later work on the outgrowth of nerve fibers was also acknowledged by Harrison (1907).

In 1895, von Lenhossék published his monograph, *Der feinere Bau des Nervensystems* (*The Fine Structure of Nervous Systems*). In it, he discussed at some length the issues surrounding the new terminology of the neuron. At the time he was in Würzburg with Kölliker; the passage reflects the balanced view characteristic of Kölliker, but von Lenhossék was not afraid to point a gentle criticism or two at the old master:

1. THE HISTOLOGY OF THE NEURON

An extraordinarily simple concept of the nervous system follows from the important observations explained here. The nervous system appears to us to be comprised of a great mass of independent units, which are independent of one another in their first primordial structure, in the condition of a prolongationless neuroblast; later as well, after they are subjected to the most complicated developments by means of diverse outgrowths of their protoplasm, they display only contact relationships with one another. This entire confused complex, seemingly so intimately linked together, whose elements compose the compact central organs through their close union, whence peripheral nerve fibers pass to all parts of the body, is divided into a mass of specific separate "individuals" (Edinger), into nervous units, in light of our new way of thinking.

The concept of the nervous unit encompasses the most essential contents of the results to which the newer research has led in its most important points. The theory, which finds its most succinct expression in these words: that the *nerve cells, including their prolongations and their branches, form isolated monads* [italics added] *in themselves,* will naturally always remain linked with the names of the men who established the current views, such as *Cajal, His, v. Kölliker* et al., but one cannot pass on without mentioning that it was Waldeyer, who, in his critical review article, first emphasized the "nervous unit" as the salient point (punctum saliens) of the new explanations of the structure of the nervous system; and indeed, *the popularity of this concept originates from Waldeyer's summary* [italics added]. The emphasis of this basic principle in the structural relationships of the nervous system turned out to be an entirely fortunate concept; because now, the most essential, characteristic catch-word for the new theory had been found, and such a unifying term is, after all, absolutely necessary, in order to bring a theory which encompasses a greater number of facts into the consciousness of wider circles, and in order to make possible its further progress.

Another fortunate idea of Waldeyer's was also to point out the importance of the concept of the nervous unit through a short, convenient, Greek technical term (Terminus technicus). Waldeyer suggested the word "neuron" for this purpose (ὁ νευρω'ν or Neurōn [in German] in the plural Neurōne [German]) a designation, which to be sure, should not be spared the justified reproach (v. Kölliker) that it would mean more an assembly point of many nerves than a single nervous element. Von Kölliker calls the nerve unit (Handbook, 6th edition, vol. II, p. 1) a "neurodendron" or "neurodendridion", a word which is indeed much more complete, since in it a characteristic quality of the nerve element, the tree-like branching of the prolongation, also finds its expression; however, the word seems to us to be a bit too long for use in daily language, namely, when one considers that the theory of nervous units, thanks to the work of *von Leube, Struempell, Goldscheider,* et al., has already begun to penetrate powerfully into medical language usage, which requires a convenient terminology, as much as we would like to see the word preserved for us anatomists. It almost seems to us that here the old word (νεῦον) suggests itself to us as the most suitable and convenient. "Neuron" means, in any case, in its original sense, "tendon or sinew", and, already somewhat figuratively, "nerve"; however, one could risk a small alteration in meaning, without having to fear misunderstandings, because, strangely enough, this exact old original word remains unused in its original un-Latinized form outside of Greece, except in compound words. It would be called [in German]: [. . . das Neuron, die Nerveneinheit, im Plural die Neuren ("Neurenlehre")]. Rauber's word, "Neure" (ἡ νευρά) is short and also established in ancient Greek usage, but it does not sound nearly as appealing as "neuron".

Fundamentally, to be sure, the nervous unit is nothing other than the modified nerve cell itself. Schaefer [*sic*] sees therefore no reason why the whole thing, after as well as before, could not be designated simply as a nerve cell, even when the various prolongations have positioned themselves around the neuroblast, and have begun to extend themselves into an enormous expansion. In this he refers to the notion that it is otherwise unconventional to give a cell structure another name besides "cell", even if its parts have changed in such a complicated manner. This objection surely cannot be considered justified; a lens fiber, for example, is conceived of not as a cell, but rather as a fiber, although it demonstrates its cellular character clearly through its nucleus, etc. Moreover, there exist unique circumstances with the nervous unit which do not easily allow comparisons with other cells. Nowhere else do we find such an enormous extension, such an intervening inner transformation of a component of a cell; it is for this reason unquestionably justified, if one reserves the designation "cell" only for the nucleus-containing protoplasmic mass, and conceives the transformed part, the fiber, which has already evidenced its independence by the fact that to all appearances it is not fed with nourishing fluids from the cell but rather acquires its own nourishment locally, as a derivation of the cell, acquiring its special name according to its difference from the cell itself.

Only in the simplest form of the neuron do nerve cell and nervous unit coincide completely: [e.g.] in those elements which lack a prolongation. Such a simple form is certainly not fictitious. All neuroblasts belong in this category, up to the instant in which they produce a process; to be sure, this stage is of extremely short duration, because it is likely that a neuroblast anticipates the formation of the prolongation already at the moment of its origin. But later as well, in definitive [mature] forms, we encounter such elements, not perhaps as "apolar spinal ganglia cells", because such cells, where often as they have been described, do not indeed exist, but probably at the periphery of the body as sensory epithelial cells, where we encounter them as hair cells in the auditory organs, taste cells in the circumvallate papillae of the tongue, rod cells in the end buds and side organs of amphibians and fish. All of these elements lack direct connection to the nerve fibers; this has been ascertained by [numerous] recent investigations. They represent small modified prolongationless epithelial cells, and all terminate bluntly, without ending in a prolongation. Nevertheless, they can be identified decisively, at least with respect to their function, through their whole appearance, their characteristic reaction to staining (namely with regard to the relationships to the nerve fibers) as nerve cells, as elements, which, through a unique composition of their protoplasm, possess the capability to be in a certain condition of arousal in reaction to certain outer stimuli. Here the simplest circumstances exist; an axon [on this early use of the new term "axon," see later] is lacking, and the cell body as well remains free from peripheral processes. At its basal end, the axons of other nerve cells approach and take care of the task which would otherwise be carried out by its own prolongation: the conduction of the stimulus stored in the cell body to the center. Perhaps it would be simplest to consider some of the elements of the retina in this category, above all the rods and cones, whose basal section gives more of the impression of a cell stricture than of a true prolongation.

In all other nervous units, one can distinguish two major components: the actual nerve cell (neurocyte), and the nervous prolongation that histogenetically emerges from it: the neuroaxon, or simply *the axon* (Kölliker), *neurite* (Rauber) [italics added]. The appearance of this prolongation can be various: in one case it grows, while maintaining its independence, into a true nerve fiber, in which case we designate it as an inaxon or as an inoneurite (from ἴς [the Greek word] for "fiber"); in the other case, it has another fate: from its origin on, it progressively gives off fibers until it becomes an irregular mass of branches which finally exhausts itself. For this reason, it is also known as a dendraxon (dendroneurite). One can use both names for both the cells in question without hesitation, that is, one can call the cells of the first kind inaxons, of the second kind, dendraxons.

In the inaxons, the one component, the prolongation, can be multiple, and this multiplication can occur in such a manner that the prolongation, in its course, divides itself into two or more equally strong stems (schizaxons) long before its termination. To each of these stems is attributed the character of a true nerve fiber; each forms its particular end-tree. Or the unit can establish itself so, that from its very beginning two or more separate nervous prolongations spring forth from the cell (diaxons, polyaxons). Spinal ganglia cells in fish, for example, are definitely diaxons. We encounter polyaxons most beautifully in the visceral ganglia of the Sympathicus [sympathetic nervous system] (Cajal, v. Kölliker). But both these forms are in a small minority compared with the typical monaxons (mononeurites). They represent exceptional forms; the actual prototype of a nervous unit is given in the monaxons.

The nervous prolongation ends freely in one as well as in the other type. Sometimes this free ending consists of a simple undivided point. Such a manner of ending appears to exist in some Vater bodies; according to the discovery of R. y Cajal, the parallel fibers of the molecular layer of the cerebellar cortex, that is, the nervous prolongations of the small granule cells, end in such a way; the epidermal sensory nerves of the earthworm have such a simple ending, which, proceeding outward from the sensory nerve cells of the skin, penetrate into the tissue of the nerve cord, in order to end freely there, in any case in the form of a forked division, in one ascending and descending branch, branching out only slightly within its profusion of dendrites [note this early use of the term "dendrite"] (Lenhossék, Retzius).

This simple manner of ending remains, however, in the great minority in comparison with the other form, where the ending branches in a treelike manner, and with this a third element enters into the formation of the nerve unit: the end branches or end bush, the telodendrion (Rauber).

The peripheral sensory nerve cell offers itself as the simplest example of an inaxon, as it is found in vertebrates in a single place: in the olfactory membranes. In invertebrates, it is more widely found. It distinguishes itself from the sensory epithelial cell by the possession of a prolongation. The spindle-shaped cell body of the olfactory cell, for example, passes smoothly underneath into the olfactory fiber; this passes, united with others of its kind, in small bundles through the holes of the cribriform plate upwards towards the base of the brain, plunges deeply into the olfactory nerve layer, in order to elaborate itself in its end branches in the formation of the olfactory glomeruli. Here we encounter in a completely typical fashion, without secondary structures, the three segments of the neuron: cell, fiber, and end branches.

Most cells, especially all central cells, are, to be sure, not of this simple type. Branched prolongations connect as secondary structures to the first two parts of the nervous unit; the dendrites to the nerve cell, which truly correspond only to the fibrous peripheral areas of the cell body, the collaterals or paraxons to the prolongation, delicate small threads, which soon branch out to similar little trees, as we see them on the prolongation itself, to paradendrien. All of these adnexa have to be sure an extensive distribution throughout the nervous system, but are not to be designated as indispensable attributes of the nervous unit, because just as there exist on the one hand adendritic nerve cells (e.g. the cells of the spinal ganglia, the aforementioned sensory nerve cells), on the other hand there are also inaxons, whose prolongation lacks collaterals completely, as do e.g. cells of origin of the anterior roots, optic fibers, olfactory fibers, etc.

In the invertebrates as well, the nervous system is comprised of neurons, and there as well the nervous unit consists of those three parts. The difference with respect to the vertebrates consists in the fact that, on the one hand, here adendritic cells occur to a much greater extent, and represent the prevalent type; on the other hand, the paraxons gain a much greater significance as "secondary prolongations".

The nerve cell together with its dendrites appears without a doubt to be the most essential of the three parts, the perceiving and impulsive element; the nerve fiber, terminal branches, and side branches represent conducting media, outgrowths of the cell body, which develop according to its needs, in order to enter into relationships with elements near to and remote from it, to encompass other nerve cells, to extend into sensory end regions, or to attach itself to contractile elements. These relationships consist of an intimate contact. In this lies an important organizational law, not only for higher organisms, but also for invertebrate animals, down to the level of life where the first nerve cell and nerve fiber appear.

Albrecht Kölliker

During the 1890s, Kölliker was still a vigorous participant in his field. As the guardian of truth and reason, he was busy during these years putting out brushfires of overzealous speculation. Most of these matters lie outside our province. We will only note two of the theories that exercised him. One was the idea of Duval (1895) and Rabl-Rückhard (1890) that amoeboid movements of the "neurodendrons" (dendrites) might be responsible for various behavioral states, such as sleep or hysteria. The other was the related idea of Cajal (1890a) that contractions and relaxations of glial cell processes could control the spread of currents in the neuronal processes and the amount of contact between cells, and thus the amount of nervous transmission between them. Recalling our previous discussion of the abortive speculations on the basis of muscle contractility (Chapter 9), we can see that these theories carried forward the idea of contractility as a universal cellular property to the processes of neurons and glia. Kölliker (1896) would have none of it, calling both theories flights of imagination that lacked any experimental basis. This was true; yet both theories carried the seeds of modern evidence for the widespread occurrence of contractile proteins and the dynamic activity-related molding of axonal and dendritic processes. In Cajal's case, this view was also a natural extension of his discovery of the growth cone of a developing axon (Cajal, 1890a), and the way he imagined that it would ram through obstacles in its path as it elongated (see Chapter 19).

In 1896, in his eightieth year, Kölliker published the sixth edition of his *Handbuch der Gewebelehre des Menschen* (*Handbook of Human Histology*). The fifth edition, nearly 30 years before, had appeared just after Deiters' monograph, and had assimilated Deiters' findings to the field; this edition did the same for the neuron doctrine. Here he stated his conclusion that the question of the nerve cell as an independent anatomical unit was settled. However, the new terminology that had been introduced was not entirely to his liking. He makes his own suggestions as follows:

> **THE NERVOUS SYSTEM**
>
> The essential elements of the nervous system are the nerve bodies or nerve cells, which, together with their prolongations, which have the significance of conducting apparatuses or nerve fibers, as the most recent investigations show, form anatomical units in themselves, which are not directly connected with one another, but rather, affect one another only through contiguity or contact. *Waldeyer* suggested the word "*Neuron*" . . . as a designation for such a unit, but the word does not imply what it should; I allow myself to replace it with the words "small nerve tree", "neurodendron" or "neurodendridien". Each of these neurodendrons consists of at least two parts, the nerve cell and its extensions; the latter are divided, in many cases, into two special groups, the protoplasmic prolongations of *Deiters*, or the *dendrite* of *His*, and the axis cylinder prolongation or nervous prolongation, for which I will employ the word *neuraxon* or *axon*—prolongations which in the later course of things often become "myelin bearing nerve fibers." . . .
>
> The word *neuron*, though it sounds good, cannot be employed grammatically, as has been suggested, because [in Greek] it means a point of assembly of many neurons or nerves. Of the words neurodendron and neurodendridien, the latter, although longer, is perhaps more appropriate as a translation of "small nerve tree."

Although "neurodendron" was never popular for the protoplasmic prolongations, the term "axon" for the axis cylinder quickly caught on. Since then we have had the three basic terms for the nerve cell: "neuron" from Waldeyer (1891), "dendrite" from His (1890), and "axon" from Kölliker (1896).

In his textbook, Kölliker discussed at length the various types of neurons with their characteristic axons and dendrites as visualized by the Golgi stain. Typically, most of the new examples were from his own laboratory. However, he also included several figures from earlier editions, such as Figure 6 (Chapter 5), and even examples of nerve cell bodies similar to those in Figure 3 (Chapter 3) from the first edition 45 years earlier, perhaps to give a perspective on how far he, and the field to which he had devoted his whole life, had come.

In addition to covering specific details of neuron morphology, Kölliker (1896) also discussed more general questions of the neuron as a unit underlying nervous function (e.g., his paragraph 199). A critical question concerned the relation between neuronal structure and function. As we have seen, there was an interesting proclivity of anatomists to discount the incredible variety of shapes and sizes and try to view all neurons as essentially similar. Kölliker (1896) ascribed to this view:

> . . . all nerve cells when they originate possess essentially the same function . . . [the development to their final form] depends solely on the many external influences or stimuli which affect them, and the many possibilities for responding to those stimuli.

This "epitome of his belief" (Haymaker, 1953) conceives that neuronal form and function are dependent on the mechanisms of development; this consists of the basic plan, expressed by the genes, which is molded by the interaction of the developing cell with its environment, a very modern view.

With this, we leave Kölliker. He dominated the work leading to the neuron doctrine, from the beginnings in the 1840s to its introduction and acceptance in the 1890s. He died in 1905 at the age of 88, universally remembered for his "enchanting modesty and exceptional rectitude and calmness of judgement" (Cajal, 1989). His many well-deserved honors "never spoiled his personal charm" (von Bonin, 1953).

17
The Synapse and the Growth Cone

Although anatomists by the 1890s could agree that nerve cells are separate units and interact by contacts, it left many unanswered questions. Two questions in particular aroused great interest. One was the nature of the contacts between neurons made by axons and dendrites. Another was proof that the axon and dendrites of a neuron grow out from the cell body during development. It was recognized that these questions were not only important for understanding the nature of the nerve cell as a unit and the way nerve cells interact but also constituted critical tests of the validity of the theory itself.

Kühne and the End-Plate

The first clue to the nature of the junctions made by nerve processes came from the neuromuscular junction, where the motor nerve terminates on the muscle surface.

Willy Kühne, a physiologist who worked in Berlin, Amsterdam, and, from 1871, in Heidelberg, studied the neuromuscular junction intensively for most of his career. In a series of papers from the 1860s to the 1890s he showed that the branches of the motor nerve terminate blindly in "end-bulbs" in the specialized area of the end-plate. From this, Kühne (1888; see Clarke and O'Malley, 1968) concluded that "it appears that contact of the muscle substance with the non-medullated nerve suffices to allow the transfer of the excitation from the latter to the former." This work was very well known to anatomists, and was often cited in favor of the idea of interaction between nerve cells by contact and not continuity. However, it did not play the decisive role it might have in the final formulaton of the neuron doctrine because it was never certain whether the arrangement at this special contact of nerve onto muscle could be generalized to apply to contacts between the very different kinds of processes of nerve cells in the central nervous system.

Held and the Bouton

What was needed was the demonstration of nerve endings and cell-to-cell contacts actually made in the central nervous system. Since the Golgi stain rendered a dendrite or axon completely black, it did not reveal very much about their structure, other than that they ended freely, either in simple terminals, or in more complicated terminals such as the mossy endings in the cerebellum. Moreover, since the Golgi stain has the mysterious property (still not understood to the present) of selectively impregnating individual cells in a random manner, it never revealed how the terminals of one cell actually ended on the branches of another; this had to be inferred in order to interpret how cells are connected together, as in the diagrams of Cajal, Kölliker, and Waldeyer.

In the late 1890s, new kinds of stains, combined with high-magnification microscopy, began to reveal more precise cellular details that seemed to shed light on this problem. The most striking evidence came from Hans Held (1866–1942), who studied under Flechsig and His in Leipzig, and remained there for his entire career. In 1897, he reported that in the embryo he could see that the axon terminates by an "end-foot" on the cell with which it comes in contact. In some regions these end-feet are large and quite distinct; in the auditory pathway, these are now termed the "end-bulbs of Held."

This was a promising beginning toward identifying what we now call "synaptic terminals" or "synaptic boutons." Unfortunately, Held went on to report that, in the adult, the "end-foot" of an axon fused with the target cell, so that there was continuity of the protoplasm between them. In so doing, he explicitly compared this arrangement to the connections between the second system of small fibers and the "protoplasmic prolongations" described 30 years before by Deiters (Held, 1897; see Clarke and O'Malley, 1968, see also van der Loos, 1967, and Chapters 4, 10 this volume). Thus, Held came to espouse the concept of nervous transmission between neurons by continuity rather than by contact. To make matters worse, Istvan Apáthy (1863–1922), a Hungarian working at the Naples Marine Laboratory, claimed that, using special staining methods, he could visualize extremely fine "neuro-fibrils within neurons which are continuous between neurons through the 'end-feet'" (Apáthy, 1897). Neurofibrils have turned out to be an important constituent of nerve cells, but the idea of their continuity between cells was quite erroneous. Held and Apáthy, together with Albrecht Bethe (1872–1954), nonetheless doggedly promoted their belief in interneuronal continuity through neurofibrils at the sites of contacts. They were a tiny resolute band of holdouts, still keeping alive the idea of a nervous reticulum.

Sherrington and the Synapse

If anatomists were unable to produce satisfactory evidence for the nature of the contacts between neurons, physiologists still had to explain how such contacts could function. This was particularly needed in order to account for transmission in a reflex arc, in which the impulses travelling in the sensory fiber from the skin into the spinal cord have to be transferred through the cord to the motor fiber that innervates the muscle.

We have seen that physiologists had adduced increasing evidence that the central pathway for the reflex, involving the connection between the sensory nerve terminals and the motor neuron within the ventral horn, had different properties from those of the peripheral nerves. These included a delay in speed of transmission, a "resistance" to transmission requiring the summation of impulses; a persistence of activity beyond the time for a single brief impulse; and a one-way direction of impulse transmission, from sensory nerve to motor neuron. There was much speculation on whether some of these properties might reside in the sensory nerve terminals or in the motor neuron dendrites, or whether some might be due to the actual contacts themselves.

One of the leading physiologists studying these properties was Charles Sherrington in England. Sherrington was born in 1857, and studied medicine at Cambridge University, where he began laboratory research under one of the leading British physiologists, Michael Foster. Sherrington first worked on the descending pathways from the motor area of the brain to the spinal cord. By around 1890, he had fixed his attention on the spinal cord itself and launched into an exhaustive study of the contribution of specific sensory nerves to carefully characterized spinal reflexes. These studies led to a revolution in understanding the reflex organization of the spinal cord.

In the course of this work Sherrington began to speculate on how the special properties of reflex transmission, as noted above, might relate to the new anatomical evidence on spinal pathways that had been brought to light by the microscopical work on nerve cells. The opportunity to put his thoughts on paper came with the 1897 revision that Michael Foster was carrying out of his well-known textbook of physiology. He asked Sherrington to contribute the chapters on the spinal cord. In phrases that are by now well known, Sherrington (in Foster, 1897) wrote:

> So far as our present knowledge goes, we are led to think that the tip of a twig of the arborescence is not continuous with but merely in contact with the substance of the dendrite or cell body on which it impinges. Such a special connection of one nerve cell with another might be called a synapse.

This new term "synapse" was derived, like most other scientific terms in biology, from the Greek, and meant to clasp, connect, or join. Sherrington considered the synapse as a "surface of separation," but did not discuss further its structural basis; for himself, as a physiologist, he always considered the synapse as a functional connection, which might have various properties. Almost 10 years later, in his great work, *The Integrative Action of the Nervous System,* Sherrington (1906) elaborated on what some of those functions might be:

> Such a surface might restrain diffusion, bank up osmotic pressure, restrict the movement of ions, accumulate electric charges, support a double electric layer, alter in shape and surface tension with changes in difference of potential . . . or intervene as a membrane between dilute solutions of electrolytes of different concentration or colloidal suspensions with different sign of charge.

In those early years it was not at all clear how this physiological concept of the connections between neurons would be related to the anatomical concepts of the contacts between neurons. Perhaps this explains why the concept of the synapse was at first only slowly incorporated within the framework of the neuron doctrine as formulated by neuroanatomists. In Cajal's (1989) entire massive autobiography of 638 pages the word "synapse" does not appear. Barker, in his exhaustive review of the work establishing the neuron doctrine, makes only passing reference to it: "The anatomical relation of one cell with another is spoken of by Foster and Sherrington as a *synapsis*" (Barker, 1899). Neurophysiologists, on the other hand, more readily accepted the anatomical basis of the neuron doctrine and incorporated it into their thinking, as is evident in this passage in which Sherrington (1906) discussed the neuronal basis for summation of reflexes:

> As to the intimate nature of the mechanism which . . . by summation or by interference, gives co-ordination where neurones converge upon a common path [in a reflex path] it is difficult to surmise. . . .

The work of Ramón-y-Cajal, van Gehuchten, v. Lenhossék, and others with the methods of Golgi and Ehrlich, establishes as a concept of the neuron in general that it is a conductive unit wherein a number of branches (dendrites) converge toward, meet at, and coalesce in a single out-going stem (axone). Through this tree-shaped structure the nervous impulses flow, like the water in a tree, from roots to stem. The conduction does not normally run in the reverse direction. The place of junction of the dendrites with one another and with the axone is commonly the perikaryon. This last is therefore a nodal point in the conductive system. But it is a nodal point of particular quality. It is not a nodal point where lines meet to cross one another, nor one where one line splits into many. It is a nodal point where conductive lines run together into one which is the continuation of them all. It is a reduction point in the system of lines. The perikaryon with its convergent dendrites is therefore just such a structure as spatial summation and immediate induction would demand. The neurone . . . may well, therefore, be the field of coalition, and the organ where the summational and inductive processes occur. And the morphology of the neurone as a whole is seen to be just such as we should expect, arguing from the principal of the common path.

The Growth Cone

Ramón y Cajal

We have seen that one of the keys that led to the neuron doctrine was the embryological approach, pioneered by His. Both von Lenhossék and Cajal took up this strategy in 1890; as Cajal (1989) noted:

> Since the silver chromate yields more instructive and more constant pictures in embryos than in the adult, "why" I asked myself, "should I not explore how the nerve cell develops its form and complexity by degrees, from its germinal phase without processes, as His demonstrated, to its adult or definitive condition?"

These studies quickly led to one of Cajal's most important discoveries. In his Golgi-stained sections, he could see that the growing axis cylinder had a club-like ending (Fig. 30). His imagination immediately endowed it with motile properties. This idea may have come from his muscle work of 1888, which had been based on the idea of the universality of a motile reticulum in all cells (see Chapter 10), so that, to him (Cajal, 1989),

> this ending appeared as a concentration of protoplasm of conical form, endowed with amoeboid movements. It could be compared to a living battering-ram, soft and flexible, which advances, pushing aside mechanically the obstacles which it finds in its way, until it reaches the area of its peripheral distribution. This curious terminal club, I christened the growth cone. Confirmed

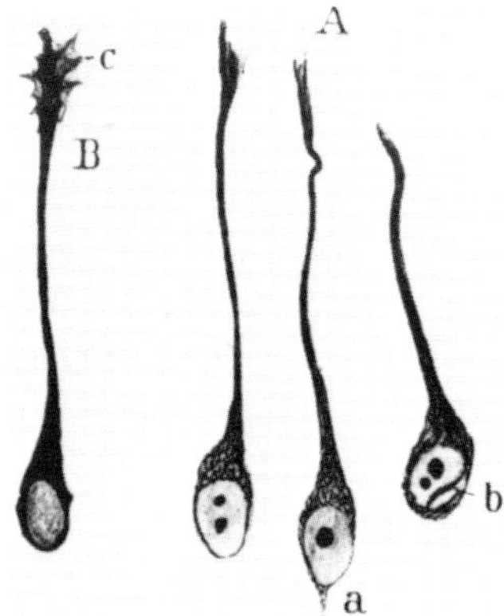

Fig. 30. Illustrations by Cajal of embryonic nerve cells giving off processes ending in growth cones (c). (Cajal, 1967; reproduced in Harrison, 1908)

> by Lenhossék, Retzius, Kölliker, and Athias, and later by Held, Harrison, and others, it is to-day one of the common facts of nervous development.

The growth cone was an important contribution to the neuron doctrine, because it showed that the axon (and, by implication, all processes of a nerve cell) grows out from the cell body and ends bluntly and freely at all times during its development. Note that Cajal could actually claim no more than that the ending "appeared" to move; once again, his powerful imagination gave dynamic properties to the static forms under the microscope.

Ross Harrison

The actual observation of the forward movement of a growth cone at the end of an axon had to wait for the work of Ross G. Harrison. Harrison was born in 1870 in Germantown, Pennsylvania. He entered Johns Hopkins University at 16, receiving his A.B. degree in 1889, at 19, some three years earlier than the normal graduation age at an American university. He was attracted to biology, first as an outdoor naturalist and then in the laboratory (Nicholas, 1959).

Harrison started graduate studies at Johns Hopkins in biology and mathematics. The first summer (1890) he worked on the embryology of the oyster in the laboratory of the United States Fish Commission at Woods Hole, Massachusetts. The Marine Biological Laboratory had been founded at Woods Hole in 1888. In 1892, Harrison travelled to the University of Bonn, where he studied the fins of teleost fish, under Moritz Nussbaum. This became the basis of his Ph.D., which he received from Johns Hopkins in 1894. During the years 1892–1896 he alternated between faculty positions in anatomy at Johns Hopkins and further studies in Bonn toward an M.D. degree, which he received from Bonn in 1899.

Harrison exemplified the bridge between the scientific traditions of central Europe and the transplantation of those traditions to the United States. The chairman of the department of anatomy at Hopkins was none other than Franklin P. Mall, the student of His, who felt so keenly the disparities between German and American universities (Chapter 8). Harrison's own devotion to German ideals was deep; with a German wife, he spoke German as fluently as English, and many of his early papers (5 of his first 12 full papers in the years 1893–1904) were in German (Oppenheimer, 1972; Wilens, in Nicholas, 1961).

Harrison's work for his medical degree, on the development of the fins of bony fish, directed his interests toward experimental embryology. His first important work was with the new techniques of embryonic grafting, introduced in 1896 by Gustav Born. Born showed in amphibians that one could graft parts of one embryo to another, and that the graft took even between different species. Harrison adopted and perfected this technique of *heteroplastic grafting*. He could graft successfully the head of one larva onto the body of another; furthermore, by using species with different pigmentation in their cells, he could easily identify the cells as they migrated into the host body from the graft. The results of these experiments were important for the theories of embryonic induction of Hans Spemann, who received the Nobel Prize for this work in 1935.

In the course of this work Harrison became interested in the question of how a nerve innervates a muscle, and this brought him to the question of how a peripheral nerve is formed. The prevailing idea was based on the evidence of His, Cajal, Retzius, and von Lenhossék, that the axon grows out from the nerve cells, but because no one had actually seen this happening in a living cell there was plenty of room for other theories. One was the "chain" theory, in which it was suggested that strings of neuroblasts formed short segments, which became the axon by fusing with each other and with a central cell body. Another was the "protoplasmic bridge" theory, which presumed that a simple neuroblast underwent a series of divisions in which bridges of protoplasm between the dividing nuclei persisted to form the elongated axon. The fact that adult skeletal muscle cells are multinucleated, being formed by fusion of myoblasts, gave some credence to these theories, as did the syncytial nature of other types of excitable cells, such as cardiac muscle fibers (and, as later work showed, certain giant axons in invertebrates).

Harrison realized that he could test these theories if he could grow the nerve cells under the microscope. For this purpose he devised a technique in which he placed pieces of primitive nerve tube in a nutrient drop of clear lymph fluid on a glass slide; he let the lymph clot, which protected the cells from drying out, and then placed the inverted slide on the microscope stage and observed the cells. By this "hanging drop" technique he was able to observe the axon growing out of the nerve cell; at its tip was a growth cone with tiny slender spicules probing the space in front. These observations were reported first as a brief note entitled "Observations on the living developing nerve fiber" (Harrison, 1907), and at length in a paper read before the Harvey Society and published in 1908. The main conclusions were as follows:

EMBRYONIC TRANSPLANTATION AND THE DEVELOPMENT OF THE NERVOUS SYSTEM

We may next inquire into the question as to how the nerve fiber extends from the ganglion cell to its peripheral ending. Is this process a mere differentiation of protoplasmic connections already *in situ*, as Hensen first maintained, or is it an actual outflow of substance from the ganglion cell towards the periphery?

In the past few years the trend of opinion has been unmistakenly toward the support of Hensen's theory, according to which protoplasmic bridges are supposed to be left everywhere between dividing cells of the embryo, so that at the time when the nerves begin to differentiate there is already a complex system of protoplasmic connections between various parts of the body; those which function as conduction paths are supposed to differentiate into nerve fibers, while the rest ultimately disappear. There has ever been something insinuating about this theory, putting, as it does, the whole question of the development of nerve paths upon the physiological basis of functional adaptation; but, brilliant and attractive as it seems, very little real evidence has ever been brought forth to support it. In fact, its mainstay has been the imaginary difficulty of conceiving how the alternative view could be true. "How can it be possible," it has often been asked, "that a nerve fiber can grow out for a long distance from its ganglion cell and always reach the right place? . . ."

In order to reach a final settlement of this question it thus became necessary to devise a method by which to test the ability of a nerve fiber to grow outside the body of the embryo, where it would be independent of protoplasmic bridges. At first a number of futile attempts were made to cultivate pieces of embryonic nerve tissue in various physiological salt solutions and within the cavities of the normal embryonic body. It then seemed that the outgrowing nerve might be stereotropic, and hence unable to leave a solid mass of cells to grow in a perfectly fluid medium. As the most suitable solid medium in which it would be possible to envelop embryonic tissue and observe its subsequent development, fresh lymph was chosen, first, because the fibrin threads which are formed on clotting might simulate mechanically Held's "plasmodesmata," though they could not be supposed to actually transform themselves into the nerve fiber; and, secondly, because the serum of the lymph would presumably afford a natural culture medium for the embryonic cells. Small portions of various tissues of the embryo were dissected out and removed by a fine pipette to a cover slip upon which was a drop of lymph freshly drawn from one of the lymph sacs of an adult frog. The cover slip was then inverted over a hollow slide and sealed on with paraffine. These manipulations were carried out as far as possible under aseptic precautions. The lymph clots almost immediately and holds the transplanted tissue in place. The specimen can then be readily observed under high powers of the microscope from day to day.

It has been found possible to keep such preparations alive for more than five weeks, and during the first week at least, differentiation takes place in a manner characteristic of each tissue. Cells taken from the muscle plate differentiate into muscle fibers with striated fibrillae, and when small pieces of spinal cord with portions of the muscle plates attached are taken, twitching movements of the muscle fibers may often be observed on the following days.

In order to understand the behavior of nervous tissue under the conditions just described, it will be well to examine for a moment the appearance of the end of a growing nerve fiber as pictured by various authors from normal preserved specimens. In the figure by Held . . . the nerve fiber is seen to run out into a number of fine filaments, which are supposedly the protoplasmic bridges (plasmodesmata) between the cells. According to Ramón y Cajal we find at the end of the growing fiber a swelling (cône d'accroissement), which has a few short processes extending out from it; such endings have been demonstrated both by the Golgi and the silver reduction methods. . . . [here Harrison reproduces Cajal's illustration shown in Fig. 30]. In the regenerating fiber, as shown by Ramón y Cajal and Perroncito, there is found a somewhat similar structure at the end of the axis-cylinder.

Let us now observe how the nerve tissue under cultivation in the lymph behaves. It must be borne in mind that when this is taken from the embryo it consists entirely of rounded cells without any signs of differentiation into fibers. Examined after a day or two of cultivation, fibres are found in a considerable number of cases extending out from the mass of tissue into the lymph clot. An early stage of this development is shown [in the Figure], which represents a cell that has become detached from the main mass of tissue. This cell is still gorged with food yolk, but at one pole it has sent out a hyaline protoplasmic process, which was observed to undergo distinct changes in form. [The Figure] shows another case. Here the fiber proceeds from a mass of cells and its own particular cell of origin can not be distinguished. The figure represents two stages of the same fiber sketched at an interval of twenty-five minutes, during which time the fiber has lengthened twenty microns. The case shown in [Fig. 31] is a much larger fiber, about 3 microns in diameter, with much more protoplasm at the end. The movements of this fiber were extremely active, and the change of form with accompanying lengthening is well shown by comparing the two sketches, which were made fifty minutes apart. . . .

The foregoing observations show beyond question that the nerve fiber begins as an outline of hyaline protoplasm from cells situated within the central nervous system. This protoplasm is very actively amoeboid, and as a result of this activity it extends farther and farther from its cell of origin. Retaining its pseudopodia at its distal end, the protoplasm is drawn out into a thread, which becomes the axis-cylinder of a nerve fiber. The early development of this structure is thus but a manifestation in a marked degree of one of the primitive properties of protoplasm, ameboid activity. We have in the forego-

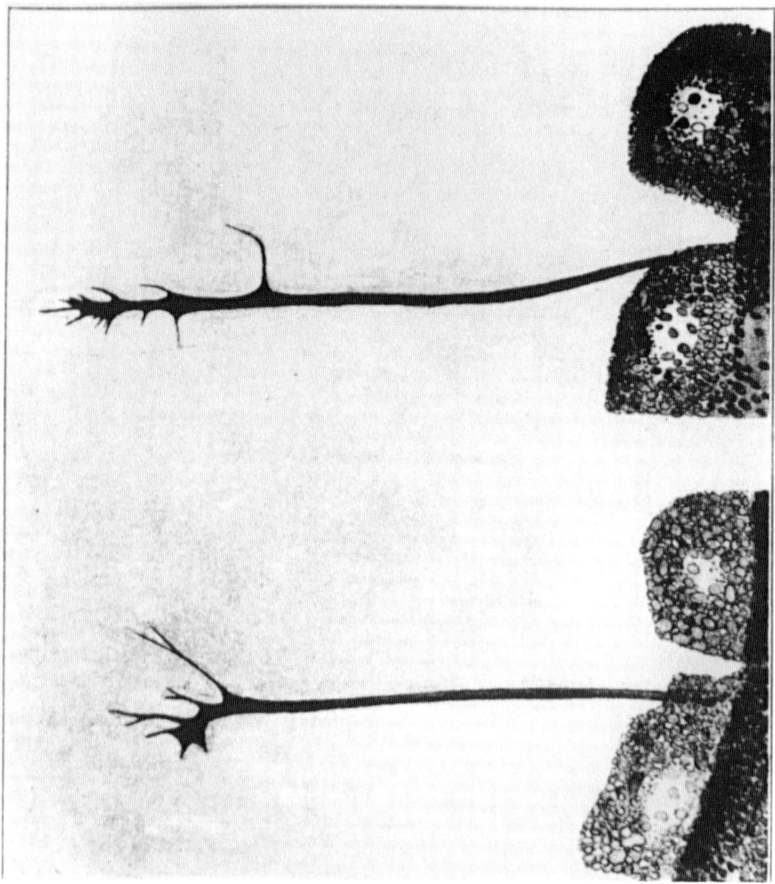

Fig. 31. Microscopical observations by Harrison of nerve fibers growing in tissue culture. "Two views of the same nerve fiber, taken fifty minutes apart." (Harrison, 1908)

ing a positive proof of the hypothesis first put forward by Ramón y Cajal and von Lenhossék, who based it upon the consideration of the cones of growth found by the Golgi method at the end of the growing fiber.

At present we have but little evidence regarding the influences which bear upon the growing nerve, though *now that its mode of growth is known with certainty* [italics added], we may hope that further experiments will soon throw light upon the problem. From the fact that the nerve fiber is capable of growing out into a lymph clot, and from other facts touched upon in the above discussion, it seems to be established that the mere act of extension is independent of external stimuli, or in other words, that it is due to properties that lie within the cell itself. On the other hand, we cannot escape the conclusion that within the body of the developing embryo there are many influences, exerted by the various organs and tissues, that guide the moving protoplasm at the end of the fiber and ultimately bring about the contact with the proper end organ. The experiments in transplanting limbs show, for instance, that we must seek in the limb itself for the factors which influence the distribution of the ingrowing nerve; for any nerve at all, in whose way a limb may be implanted, may enter the latter and become distributed in a manner normal for that limb. The shifting of parts during development is another factor of importance, as Hensen originally pointed out. For example, the lateral line nerve grows out and establishes its connection with the rudiment of its end organs at a time when its ganglion and the latter are very close together; and the enormous length that the nerve attains in the full-grown tadpole is due solely to the shifting of the sensory rudiment during development. Still, such crude mechanical factors are by no means sufficient to explain the intricacies of the nervous system of a higher animal, and we must seek farther for more subtile influences, possibly such as tropisms, as originally suggested by Ramón y Cajal. Very convincing evidence of chemotropic influences has already been found in the case of regenerating nerves by Forssmann, who showed in a most ingenious manner that degenerating nerve tissue would attract the regenerating fibers. How far such influences, and how far mechanical stimuli determine the course of the nerve fiber in embryonic development, can only be determined by experiment. It is to be hoped that the method of isolation as described above, will here yield results of value.

As regards the theories of nerve development that have been the subject of the foregoing argument, I need scarcely point out that the experiments now place the outgrowth theory of His upon the firmest possible basis—that of direct observation. The attractive idea of Hensen must be abandoned as untenable. *The embryological basis of the neurone concept thus becomes more firmly established than ever* [italics added]

So Cajal had been right after all! The idea that nerve processes are capable of amoeboid movement finally was vindicated; in fact, it was a necessary property for the growth of the nerve processes to their destined targets.

This was one of the most revolutionary results in experimental biology. The observations indicated that all nerve cell processes, whether axons or dendrites, are formed as outgrowths from the cell body. As Harrison makes clear, the experiments removed any doubts that the nerve cell belonged in the cell theory. This was the last critical experimental confirmation of the neuron doctrine in the classical period. It was also the main contribution to come from an investigator working in the United States. The work was of even wider significance for biology, because "it was a first step in establishing that the cell is the primary developmental unit of the multicellular organism" (Oppenheimer, 1966). The "hanging drop" technique was the forerunner of cell and tissue culture methods that have become indispensable tools for research in embryology, oncology, urology, genetics, and molecular biology.

In 1907, Harrison was named professor of comparative anatomy at Yale University, and remained there the rest of his life. He first lived near the campus on York Street in a house that, in 1912, became Mory's, a historic Yale undergraduate club. Though a man with a difficult personality, he was widely respected and honored, and continued to make fundamental contributions to experimental embryology well into the 1940s. He was "an important bridge between the old morphology of the nineteenth century and the new molecular biology of the twentieth" (Oppenheimer, 1966).

18
Forging a Consensus

The direct observation of the outgrowth of nerve cell fibers from nerve cell bodies under the microscope ended the classical period of experimental studies that established that the cell theory applies to the nervous system. The parallel debate over the theoretical framework within which the experimental results would be fashioned into the neuron doctrine ended about the same time with the awarding of the Nobel Prize jointly to Golgi and Cajal in 1906. In their formal lectures of acceptance, the two protagonists defended their beliefs in the reticular and neuronal concepts, respectively, of nervous organization. We will briefly sketch the background for this historic confrontation.

Development of Cajal's Ideas

In early 1892, the chair of Normal Histology and Pathological Anatomy fell vacant at the University of Madrid. Cajal, soon to be 40, with over 60 publications (Cajal, 1989), entered into several months of competitive examinations, and was unanimously elected.

The move from Barcelona to Madrid hardly interrupted the flow of his work. He began an ambitious extension of his earlier studies of the retina to embrace a wide range of vertebrate species. This led to the publication of a long paper on "The vertebrate retina," which was published as a monograph by *La Cellule* in 1892, and is still considered "a point of departure for any anatomical studies of retinal circuitry" (Piccolino, 1988). The German translation appeared in 1894. During this period, Cajal (1989) also started his work on the hippocampus and dentate, two structures that fascinated him because of the artistic beauty of their neuronal forms and arrangements: "Their pyramidal cells, like the plants in a garden—as it were, a series of hyacinths—are lined up in hedges which describe graceful curves."

Here, as in many other brain regions, Cajal had to acknowledge that much of the structure and arrangement of the cells had already been described by Golgi, the "celebrated savant of Pavia." However, Cajal's drawings and descriptions were much clearer and, in addition, had the benefit of being interpreted within the context of the neuron doctrine, so that they immediately were accepted as definitive representations of the basic types of neurons and their interrelations in the different brain regions.

During his last year in Barcelona, Cajal gave a series of lectures summarizing his research. For this he prepared "large wall plates in colours, representing diagrammatically the structural plan of the nerve centres and sense organs." In his autobiography, Cajal (1989) relates that the students who had asked him to give the lectures were so enthusiastic that they copied his drawings and transcribed their notes into a series of articles; Cajal revised the text and retouched the drawings, and the articles were published in the *Revista de Ciencias Medicas de Barcelona* (*Medical Science Review of Barcelona*) in 1892. By then Waldeyer's review had appeared announcing the neuron doctrine, so that any publications by Cajal, even in Spanish, did not go entirely unnoticed. These articles summarizing his views were therefore an instant hit. Wilhelm His supported their translation into German (carried out by none other than Hans Held, then his assistant, later his successor in the chair, who became a voluble proponent of the continuity theory opposing Cajal, as we discovered in the previous chapter). These articles appeared in the *Archiv für Anatomie und Physiologie* in 1893. Although Cajal did not speak German, he read it well enough to discover that the translation was "full of errors and misunderstandings" (Cajal, 1989). Much more satisfactory was the French translation, made by Leon Azoulay, published in 1894 as *Les Nouvelles Idées sur la Structure du Système Nerveux chez l'Homme et chez les Vertébré's* (*New Ideas on the Structure of the Nervous System in Man and Vertebrates;* English translation by Swanson and Swanson, Cajal, 1990).

This French translation was the first book on the new subject. Coming in the aftermath of Waldeyer's articles, and during the period of controversies and debates that we have summarized in the previous chapter, it was eagerly and widely read as a definitive statement of the new concepts by one acknowledged to have been the *primum movem.* So clear were Cajal's diagrams, so forceful his deductions from them, so vivid and elegantly simple his functional interpretations of the pathways formed by the neurons and their connections, that an entirely new concept of the organization of the nervous system was immediately evident. The substance of this new concept was summarized in his Croonian lectures (see below). It became the foundation for his later great two-volume opus on the neuronal structure of the nervous system (Cajal, 1909, 1911; see below), for which an English translation is now in preparation.

Cajal's Croonian Lecture

In early 1894, Cajal received an invitation from the Royal Society of London to deliver the Croonian lecture for that year. In his autobiography, Cajal (1989) describes how "confounded," "abashed," "flattered," and "hesitant" he was over this invitation. It seemed to rock his whole perception of himself, as the humble scientist in the far-off backward provinces, compared with the famous scientists in the centers of learning. Cajal's trip to Germany had been a premeditated, urgent, and practical matter of setting out his research results in the hurly-burly of a convention of his peers, in a country, Germany, that had only recently emerged as a nation. The invitation from the Royal Society, on the other hand, came from the oldest scientific society in the world, founded in 1660, and numbering most of the illustrious scientists of modern history among its native and foreign members.

Cajal made the trip with some doubts as to whether he was up to the honor, and in some awe and apprehension about how he might be received. He was quickly put at ease by the cordiality of his hosts. In the comfortable club atmosphere of the society there was little of the pomp that had accompanied his recognition at the Berlin meeting five years before. Cajal stayed in Charles Sherrington's home during his visit in London, and Sherrington provided assistance in preparing the lantern slides and large-scale colored diagrams for Cajal's lecture (Cajal, 1989).

The lecture was entitled "La fine structure des centres nerveux" (Cajal, 1894). Lacking confidence in his command of English, Cajal read it in French, having consulted on the text with Azoulay on his way through Paris. Kölliker, who had given the Croonian lecture in 1862, advised Cajal to give his lecture a "physiological slant" (Cajal, 1989). Cajal did just that, summarizing the broader account contained in "Les Nouvelles Idées . . . ," and emphasizing the physiological implications. The first half of the lecture is reproduced here in its entirety; the second half, dealing specifically with the organization of the cerebral cortex, is reproduced in its entirety in DeFelipe and Jones (1988):

THE FINE STRUCTURE OF THE NERVOUS CENTERS

At the gracious invitation made to me by the honorable members of this learned society to come to this meeting and give an account of my work on the structure of the nervous centers, my first intention, I cannot deny, was to turn down an honor which I judged to be too disproportionate to my merits; but I then imagined that your willingness to hear me would not be less than the generosity of your invitation, and I resigned myself to the role, little flattered at that, to interrupt for a moment the harmonious concert of your beautiful work. I have all the more need of your indulgence as I am going to engage you in a subject you know to perfection. All that I am going to tell you has already been published and summarized in an almost irreproachable manner by masters as eminent as His, Kölliker, Waldeyer, von Lenhossék, and van Gehuchten. However I shall try to give you my own perception of the structure of the central nervous system, for which I shall above all draw inspiration, as I have been asked to do, from my own research.

The nervous centers of mammals, especially those of man, represent the true masterpiece of nature, the most subtly complicated machine that life can give us. In spite of this complication, capable of discouraging the boldest minds, there has been no lack of patient anatomists who, using the technique of their era, have attempted to unravel the delicate framework of the encephalo-spinal axis. They were guided, no doubt, by the hope that the discovery of the structural key of the nervous centers would throw a keen light on the important activities of these organs. The first positive facts, though incomplete, relative to the fine anatomy of the grey and white matter, we owe to Ehrenberg, who in 1833 discovered the nerve fibers; and to Rémak, Hannover, Helmholtz, and Wagner, who in the same era, or a few years later, discovered multipolar corpuscles, and believed that the ramified expansions of these cells were continuous with nerve fibers. In 1865, Deiters, one of the wisest observers that anatomy has ever had, took us a big step forward in knowledge of nerve cell morphology; he demonstrated that in all nerve cells there were always two kinds of expansions; that is to say, beside the ramified or protoplasmic expansions, he found a non-ramified axis cylinder, continuing directly with a nerve tube. This important discovery was already anticipated by the work of Wagner, who in 1847 had called the attention of scholars to the existence of two kinds of prolongations in the cells of the torpedo encephalon, and by Rémak, who in 1854 found in bovine spinal grey matter a similar arrangement.

The work of Gerlach extended further the ideas of Deiters. They served as a basis, as you well know, for the theoretical conception of the structure of the grey matter which has ruled in our science almost up to our time. Gerlach imagined that these nervous expansions of the cells of the anterior horn of the spinal grey were continuous with the motor roots, whereas the sensory roots had their origin in an interstitial nervous network formed by anastomoses of the protoplasmic expansions.

I will not elaborate further on this conception, nor on the physiological deductions which have been drawn from it. Suffice it to say that the theory of the interstitial protoplasmic network is an anatomical hypothesis which does not rest on any positive observation. One has to realize that, in fact, the methods used by Gerlach and his successors to establish the theory of the interstitial network—thin sections cut in series, colored in carmine, hematoxyline, nigrosine or gold chloride—are absolutely inadequate to resolve a problem of this difficulty, permitting one to discern in the grey matter only a pale, very complicated, plexus, in which it would by rash to suppose any particular mode of termination of the fibers.

As for the more modern methods of Weigert-Pal and Freud, and the methods based on secondary degeneration developed by Charcot, Gudden, Türk and Bouchard, they can only show us the trajectory of the myelinated fibers and the location of the cellular stations to which they are linked; they are not in any way able to instruct us on the method of union between cells and fibers or between the cells themselves.

At this juncture, Camillo Golgi, an Italian scholar of great merit, well known for his discovery of the musculo-tendinous terminal organs and by the light which he has thrown on the biology of the *plasmodium malariae*, announced in 1875 a method of coloration which permits one to dye and observe perfectly the finest nervous expansions, a method which gave hope of a near and definitive solution of the difficult problem of intercellular connections. This method, in its essence, consists of submitting pieces of the nerve centers previously hardened in potassium bichromate or in a mixture of Mûller's liquid and osmic acid to the activity of silver nitrate. Under the influence of a bath of silver it forms an opaque red precipitate of silver chromate, which deposits itself exclusively within the thickness of some of the cells and fibers. The latter stand out in a very clear and almost schematic manner against a transparent yellowish background. Thanks to this important innovation in microscopical technique, Mr. Golgi was able to bring to the fore the following facts:-

First, the protoplasmic expansions of nerve cells end freely in the thickness of the grey matter.

Second, the functional prolongations of the nerve cells emit, in their trajectory across the grey matter, collateral twigs, which are very fine and which branch several times.

Thirdly, regarding the manner in which the functional prolongations behave, one can distinguish two kinds of cells: a *motor* type characterized by the presence of an axis cylinder which does not lose its individuality and is continuous with a fiber of the white matter; and a *sensory* type, characterized by the existence of an axis cylinder which, almost from its origin in the grey matter divides a great number of times and loses its individuality without leaving the grey matter itself.

In the fourth place, there exists within this substance a network of fibers formed by the ramifications and anastomoses of the following three types of nerve fibers: the terminal twigs of the centripetal or sensory nerve fibers, the terminal branches of arborization of the axis cylinders of the corpuscles of the sensitive type, and the collaterals of the nervous expansions of the corpuscles of the motor type.

Finally, Mr. Golgi believed he could state with the help of his observations that the protoplasmic prolongations play a nutritive role, since they place themselves preferentially in contact with blood vessels and with neuroglial cells.

The research that we have undertaken over the past five years on the structure of nearly all the nerve centers—hindbrain, spinal grey, brain, olfactory bulb, sympathetic ganglia, optic centers, retina, etc.—has allowed us to confirm for the most part the facts put forth by Golgi, but they have brought us at the same time to substitute for the three anatomicophysiological hypotheses of the Italian scholar (existence of an interstitial nervous network, distinction between cells as sensory or motor, and nutritive role of the protoplasmic prolongations) the following propositions which we consider to be demonstrated completely:

The axis cylinder ends in the same way as the protoplasmic prolongations within the grey matter by perfectly free twigs.

The protoplasmic prolongations, as well as the bodies of the nerve cells, are able to serve in the conduction of nerve currents.

The two physiological types of nerve cells accepted by Golgi do not precisely have physiological or functional reality. Their morphological reality is on the contrary beyond doubt. In fact, in the grey matter, beside the elements which we have named cells of short axis cylinder, whose axis cylinder prolongation resolves itself in a terminal arborization around neighboring corpuscles, one encounters others which we call cells of long axis cylinder, abounding in organs essentially and undoubtedly sensory, like the retina and the olfactory bulb; hence the conclusion that they do not necessarily and exclusively have a motor role.

The same circumstance and the same reasoning applies to the corpuscles of short axis cylinder; one cannot really consider them as sensory cells since they are found indiscriminately in all nervous centers, such as the brain, cerebellum, striatum, retina, olfactory bulb, etc.

The connections established between the fibers and the nerve cells take place by means of contacts, that is to say, with the help of a veritable articulation between the varicose arborizations of the axis cylinders on one side and the body and the protoplasmic prolongations on the other. One is thus brought to conceive of the encephalo-spinal axis as an edifice composed of superimposed nervous units, of *neurones,* following the expression of Waldeyer.

From a morphological point of view our research has taught us other facts of some importance.

The functional expansions of the nervous cells can divide in a T at their arrival in the white matter, thus producing two or a greater number of myelinated nerve tubes.

The nerve tubes of the white matter of the brain, like those of the white matter of the spinal cord, olfactory bulb, Ammon's horn, the fibers of the great sympathetic chain, etc., emit at a right angle collateral twigs destined to ramify and end freely within the immediate grey matter. These collaterals, which Golgi had already mentioned briefly in the spinal cord, constitute a large part of the commissures of the central nervous organs, anterior and posterior commissure of the spinal cord, corpus callosum, hypocampal commissure, etc., and almost the entire dense plexus of fibrils that surround the nerve corpuscles.

Finally left to examine is the fundamental question of the ending of the axis cylinders in the grey matter. As early as 1886, His and Forel upheld, in opposition to Gerlach and Golgi himself, that the axis cylinders end in the grey matter not by forming networks, but solely by free extremities.

Here, briefly cited, are the reasons that His, in a recent work, advanced against the network theory: "Embryology demonstrates that nerve fibers represent the continuation of the expansions of neuroblasts; every fiber must, thus, during the long period of its development, advance freely. One does not see why this disposition should modify itself ulteriorly [i.e., after development has terminated]. Moreover, we have known for a long time of a series of completely free endings, including those in muscles, cornea and the corpuscle of Pacini, etc., which consist either of a rounded and thick extremity or of a completely free nervous arborization. It seems to us, then, unreasonable to admit any fundamental distinction between the peripheral endings and the central terminations."

For Forel, denial of the existence of networks is based on his never being able to recognize anastomoses of nerve fibrils in sections of grey matter impregnated by the Golgi method.

These were the arguments strongly in favor of the absolute independence of nerve corpuscles, yet the majority of neurologists stayed faithful to the old doctrine. This was because, in order to resolve this question definitively, it was necessary in fact not to content oneself with negative arguments or with reasonings by analogy; it was necessary to provide certain and absolute proof of the final ramifications of the axis cylinders and their collaterals in the grey matter and resolve, at the same time, the problem of intercellular connections. This is the work that we believe we have accomplished in applying the Golgi method, somewhat modified, to nervous regions along the path of evolution, or very close to their complete development. In a series of studies having as their subject the spinal cord, cerebellum, cerebrum, retina, great sympathetic chain, etc., we were able to demonstrate, without leaving room for any doubt, the terminal nervous arborizations which are formed around the cells of these organs, and the subsequent research of Kölliker, van Gehuchten, His, Waldeyer, Edinger, von Lenhossék, A. Sala, P. Ramón, G. Retzius, etc., has confirmed the existence of this terminal arrangement, while adding important discoveries. It is to Retzius that we owe the most convincing proof, as he has succeeded in demonstrating the free endings of nerve arborizations not only in the cerebro-spinal axis of vertebrates, but also in the ganglia of invertebrates, crustaceans, worms, etc., where he has used the Ehrlich method of methylene blue, which discoveries agree completely with those using the Golgi method.

The general principles of the morphology and connections of neurons being thus explained, we will now review succinctly the diverse kinds of relations or articulations displayed by the elements of various nerve centers.

Let us look first at the sensory roots [dorsal spinal roots] and the spinal cord.

The research of Ranvier, Retzius, and von Lenhossék has taught us that dorsal root ganglion cells have a single expansion divided into two branches; *one external,* generally thicker, oriented toward the periphery to end in the skin or in a sensory corpuscle; the *other internal,* which joins the sensory, posterior, root to enter the spinal cord. This latter branch, according to our observations in birds and mammals, does not penetrate directly into the grey matter, but bifurcates within the posterior column to give an ascending and

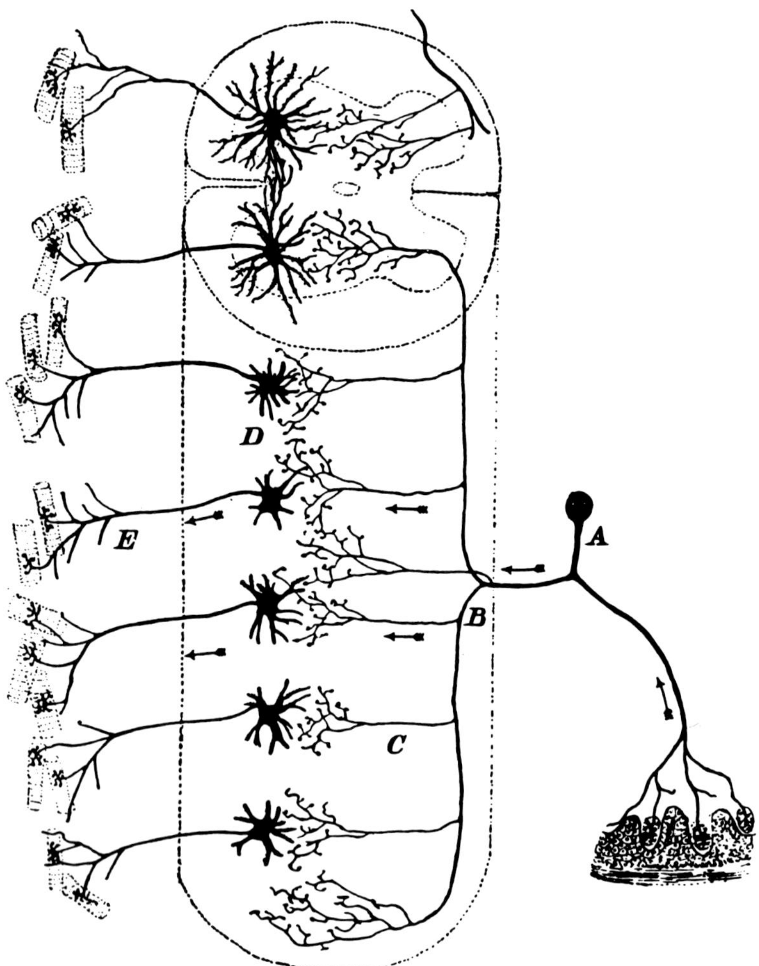

Fig. 32. "Schema of the relations between the dorsal root ganglion cells and the motor corpuscles of the anterior horn. A, Dorsal root ganglion cell; B, bifurcation of the fibers of the posterior root; C, long collaterals coming into relation with the cells of the anterior horn; D, radicular [motor] cells; E, fiber of the anterior root. Note. The arrows indicate the probable direction of the nervous currents and the dynamic relations between different cells." (Cajal, 1894)

descending branch [Fig. 32]. From this Y-shaped bifurcation the resulting fibers extend the length of the posterior column in an undeterminable path, but which can be observed for several centimeters; their terminations take place in the depth of the grey matter, by way of varicose and pericellular arborizations.

Beside these terminal arborizations, which often stain with difficulty, the dorsal root fibers possess an infinite number of collateral branchlets, arising at right angles, either from the trunk or from the ascending or descending branches, by which they put themselves in contiguous connection with the cells of the grey matter. From these collaterals one can distinguish some which are long, destined for the anterior [ventral] horn, and some short, destined for the posterior [dorsal] horn.

The *short collaterals,* joined in meridian bundles, cross the substance of Rolando, and resolve themselves in very complicated varicose arborizations which surround the cells of Clarke's column, as well as the cells located at the top of the posterior horn.

The *long collaterals* comprise a very thick antero-posterior bundle which, crossing the posterior horn, is disseminated in the depth of the anterior horn [Fig. 33]. These collaterals give rise to a great number of ramifications, the

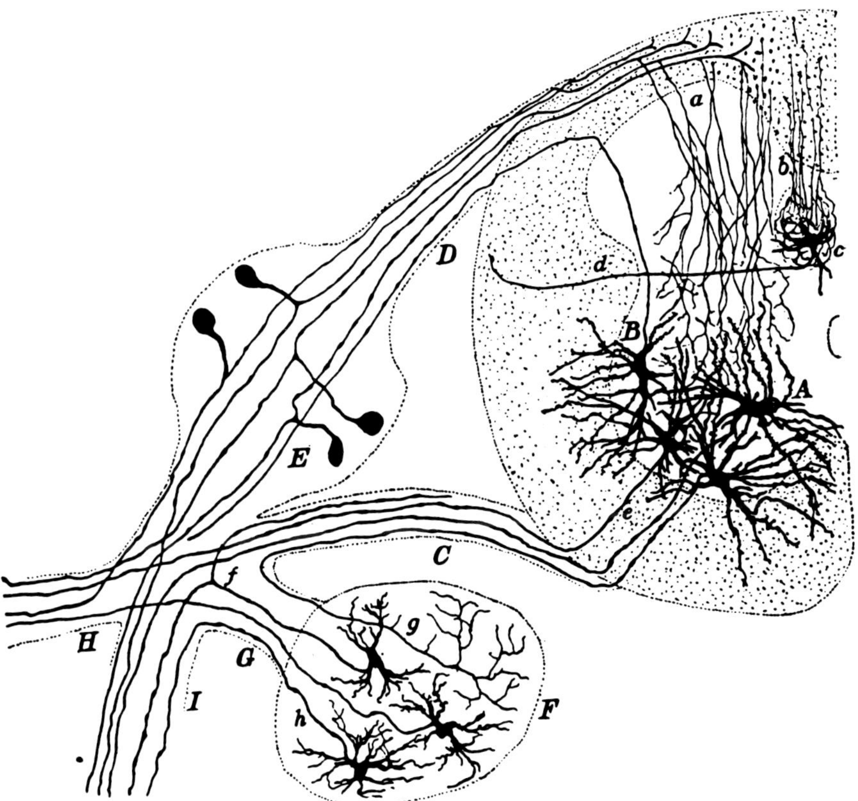

Fig. 33. "Schema of the spinal cord and the sensory and sympathetic ganglia. A, radicular [motor] cells; B, radicular [motor] cell whose axis cylinder goes to the posterior root; C, motor root; D, sensory root; E, dorsal root ganglion; F, sympathetic ganglion; G, *ramus communicans;* H, posterior branch of the root pair; I, anterior branch of this; a, long collaterals reaching up to the anterior horn; b, short collaterals directed toward the anterior horn; c, cells whose axis cylinder seems to go to the cerebellar pathway; e, anterior root fiber; f, sympathetic axis cylinder which gives rise to a branchlet penetrating into the anterior root; g, fiber of the anterior root seeming to terminate in the sympathetic ganglion; h, sympathetic fiber in the *ramus communicans,* and going to the periphery." (Cajal, 1894)

majority of which end in contact with the cell body or the protoplasmic expansions of the motor cells. Given that the long collaterals represent the only means of communication between the sensory [dorsal] roots and the cells of the anterior horn, it is necessary to consider them as the ordinary route for reflexes. This is why one currently calls these collaterals *reflexo-motor* fibers, following the example of Kölliker, or *sensory-motor,* the name which I have attributed to them. According to research we have undertaken very recently in the chick embryo, the long collaterals arise preferentially not along the vertical path of the ascending and descending branches, but from the portion neighboring the bifurcation. Along the remainder of their distance the bifurcating branches give rise mainly to short collaterals.

The fibers of the posterior root do not all bifurcate in the white matter; Lenhossék and ourselves have recognized that there also exists a small group of centrifugal fibers whose cells of origin are in the anterior horn.

The role of these sensory collaterals is considerable; they establish lines of contact with almost all the corpuscles of the grey matter which we are going to consider.

The corpuscles of the grey matter of the spinal cord can be classified in four categories: first, *commissural cells,* whose axis cylinder contributes to the formation of the anterior commissure in passing to the antero-lateral tract of the other side; second, the *tract cells,* whose axis cylinder is continuous, either as a single right-angle inflection or by means of a T-shaped bifurcation, with a fiber of the white matter of the same side (lateral and posterior/anterior cord); third, motor or *anterior root cells,* whose functional expansion comprises the anterior roots; fourth, the *pluritract cells,* or cells of complex axis cylinder, whose nervous expansion, at first simple, furnishes two, three, or a greater number of tubes to the tract of one or both sides.

We lack the time, certainly, to study the probable course of sensory excitation through the axis cylinders of all these elements; therefore, we will content ourselves to follow it in two pathways where the interpretation seems to us the simplest; the reflexo-motor path and the cerebellar path.

Carried by the posterior roots, sensory impressions divide at the level of the aforementioned bifurcations into two currents, ascending and descending. If the excitation is of weak intensity, it is diverted to the long or reflexo-motor collaterals, which arise, as we have just seen, from the first portion of the path of the ascending and descending branches, as well as from the trunk of origin, and are transmitted then to the motor cells of a restricted segment of the anterior horn; but if the excitation is stronger, extending beyond the reflexo-motor pathways, it will enter all of the ascending and descending branches, and the whole system of short collaterals will then be influenced. The movement will proceed in this manner to Clarke's column, a region where several short collaterals end, and, by the intermediation of the axis cylinders of the cells situated in this column, it will reach the ascending cerebellar tract of the spinal cord.

Let us add again that the short collaterals, as well as the terminal arborizations of the ascending and descending branches of the sensory roots, are in connection with the commissural cells of the posterior horn, whose axis cylinders pass either to the antero-lateral cord of the opposite side or to the fundamental bundle of the lateral tract of the same side, comprising there the short pathways, in great part ascending, apparently destined to carry the sensory currents to the motor cells of segments further away in the spinal cord.

Propagation of the sensory impression up to the cerebrum demands the mediation of certain intermediary neurons which one calls *central sensory cells.* These cells would be located in all the regions of the spinal cord and bulb [medulla oblongata] where the sensory root fibers terminate; their axis cylinders would have an ascending course, and would end after having crossed the mid-line, in the cerebral cortex of the other side. The crossing would be made mainly in the inferior part of the medulla oblongata, at the level of the ribbon of Reil [medial leminiscus]. But, according to van Gehuchten, it would also take place all along the spinal cord at the level of the anterior commissure.

It remains to note that the existence of central sensory cells is still very enigmatic. In the spinal cord, outside the cerebellar tract, one cannot distinguish, using anatomical methods, any special ascending pathway destined to receive the sensory excitations brought by the posterior root fibers. There are, however, two facts in favor of the existence of a central sensory pathway; first, the absence of crossing of the sensory root fibers, and then, the circumstance that the majority of the latter represent short pathways, ending in diverse segments of the spinal cord.

Let us study together the *connections of the olfactory nerve fibers* [Fig. 34].

Our research, in accordance with that of d'Airstein, Grassi and Castronuovo, van Gehuchten and Brunn, shows us the bipolar nerve cells of the olfactory mucosa emitting at their extreme depth a varicose fibril, or axis cylinder prolongation, which is continuous with a filament of the olfactory nerves. During their passage across the sub-epithelial conjunctive tissue, these filaments retain their individuality and do not give off ramifications; at their arrival at the olfactory bulb they penetrate into the thickness of the glomeruli, where they end by way of a short, varicose, and completely free arborization.

The component layers of olfactory bulb are: the zone of the olfactory nerve fibers, the zone of the glomeruli, the zone of cells with protoplasmic tuft [mitral cells] and the zone of granules and deep nerve fibers.

The layer of the tufted [mitral] cells is one of the most interesting, because it contains the elements destined to gather the olfactory excitation. These elements, which vary in shape and location but not in essential characteristics, distinguish themselves in possessing a long axis cylinder which goes to the external root of the olfactory bulb, and in giving rise to lateral protoplasmic expansions which spread out in a molecular layer, and, finally, in presenting one or two thick peripheral protoplasmic prolongations, which terminate in the thickness of the glomeruli by way of an elegant tuft of short and very varicose twigs. The glomeruli themselves are simply the result of the juxtaposition and interlacing of two kinds of terminal fibers: the varicose twigs of the olfactory fibers and the relatively robust branches of the protoplasmic tuft that we have just mentioned. Between these two kinds of ramifications there exists no anastomosis, but truly a very intimate contact. One never sees fibers other than the tufted trunks penetrating into the glomeruli; one can also

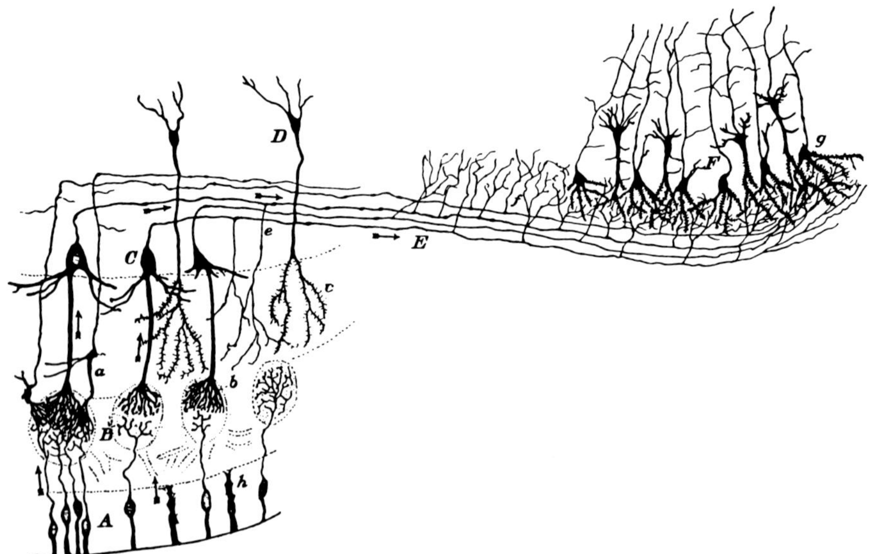

Fig. 34. "Schema of the ensemble of relations of the cells of the olfactory apparatus. A, bipolar cells of the olfactory mucosa; B, olfactory glomeruli; C, mitral cells; D, granule; E, external root of the olfactory nerve; F, cortical grey of the sphenoidal region of the brain [olfactory, or pyriform, cortex]; a, small tufted cell; b, protoplasmic tuft of a mitral cell; c, spiny tuft of a granule [cell]; e, collaterals of fibers coming from the mitral cells; f, collaterals terminating in the molecular layer of the frontal and sphenoidal cortex; g, superficial triangular cells of the cortex; h, epithelial cells of the olfactory mucosa." (Cajal, 1894)

affirm that no ramification of the olfactory fibers ever emerges from the glomeruli. Such an arrangement presents us with two facts whose importance will escape no one. First, the protoplasmic expansions have a conductive role, for they constitute the links in the chain of olfactory neurons; second, transmission operates by the contacts between the nervous ramifications [axis terminals] and the protoplasmic arborizations [dendrites].

To summarize, let us briefly indicate the route followed by olfactory excitation. It traverses successively the bipolar cells of the mucosa whose axis cylinders comprise the fibers of the olfactory nerve; the tufted [mitral] cells of the bulb, whose axis cylinders join to form the external root [lateral olfactory tract] of the bulb; finally, it ends at the pyramidal corpuscles of the frontal and sphenoid cerebral cortices where the axis cylinders of the mitral cells emit their free arborizations.

Concerning the termination of the fibers of the lateral olfactory tract we should focus our attention on a fact of some interest. These fibers, according to the results of my research and that of Mr. Calleja, furnish their terminal arborizations, as well as a great number of collateral ramifications, exclusively to the first cerebral layer or molecular zone, so that the olfactory excitation is received only by the peripheral tuft of the [dendritic] trunk of the pyramidal cells. We will soon come back to this fact, which one can also observe in

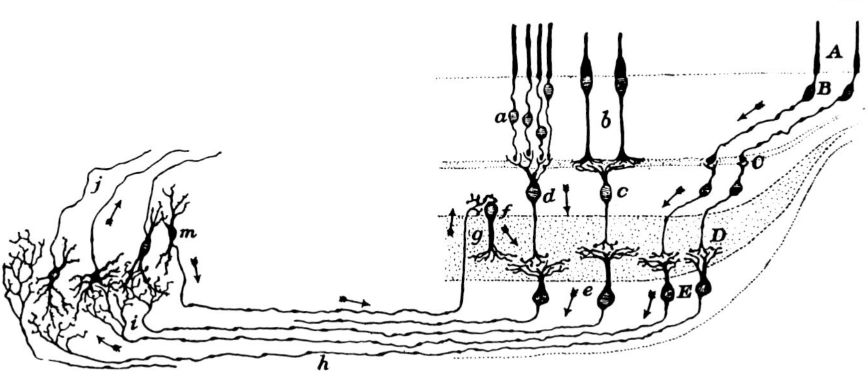

Fig. 35. "Schema of the ensemble of relations of the cells of the visual apparatus. A, cones of the region of the *fovea centralis;* B, external granules of this region; C, articulation between bipolars and cones; D, articulation between bipolar cells and ganglion cells. a and b, cones and rods of other regions of the retina; c, bipolar destined for cones; d, bipolar destined for rods; e, ganglion cells; f, spongioblast; g, centrifugal fiber; h, optic nerve; i, terminal arborizations of optic fibers in the geniculate bodies; j, cells which receive the visual impression; m, cells which probably give rise to the centrifugal fibers." (Cajal, 1894)

the optic lobe of birds; this seems to indicate that the molecular zone is the place where is established the transformation of the conscious sensory current arriving there into the voluntary motor impulse which leaves from it.

The *connections of visual fibers and of retinal cells* [Fig. 35] will in turn teach us a series of facts of great significance.

One can, despite many complications, consider the retina as a nerve ganglion formed by three rows of neurons or nerve corpuscles; the first row contains the cones and rods with their descending prolongations forming the layer of the external granules; the second is constituted by the bipolar cells, and the third is due to the grouping of ganglion cells. These three series of elements articulate between each other at the level of the layers called the molecular or reticular layer, and the internal layer.

The *external molecular layer* of the retina contains a multiple articulation whose elements are: outside, the terminal spherules of the rod fibers and the conic pedicles, equipped with lateral filamentous excrescences, of the cone fibers; inside, the external tufts or peripheral extensions of the bipolar cells, of which there exist two kinds: the bipolars of flattened tufts, destined for the cones, and the bipolars of ascending tufts, destined for the rods; the protoplasmic twigs and the nervous arborizations of certain horizontal cells constitute the stellate or sub-reticular cells of certain authors.

The *internal molecular layer* contains an articulation still more complicated, which one could break down into three or more levels. The principle factors [elements] are represented, outside, by the varicose terminal tufts of the descending prolongation of the bipolars and the terminal ramifications of the spongioblasts; inside, by the flattened protoplasmic arborizations of the cells of the ganglion cell layer.

Apart from certain elements whose role is still very obscure, such as spongioblasts and horizontal cells, here are the neurons which participate in visual transmission: cones and rods, bipolar cells, ganglion cells and the fibers of the optic nerve, pyramidal and fusiform cells of the geniculate bodies, and the tuberi [corpora] quadrigemina [also termed the superior and inferior colliculi, or, in birds, the optic lobes].

In birds, where we have succeeded in coloring very completely the elements of the optic lobe, one recognizes that the optic fibers first surround this organ, and that they end by way of arborizations which are very varicose, very rich and completely free. These ramifications, which are located in the most peripheral layers of the optic lobe, come into contact with the external protoplasmic expansions of certain fusiform cells whose axis cylinders penetrate more deeply. Each optic arborization is related to a group of cells; in this way the excitation carried by a fiber disseminates itself within the thickness of the grey matter, increasing the number of cells and axis cylinders which intervene in the conduction so that the visual excitation advances.

The optic nerve possesses additionally centrifugal fibers which terminate by very varicose free arborizations around the bodies of spongioblasts in the retina, to which they carry nervous excitation of central origin and whose significance is currently undetermined.

The very succinct and somewhat dry examination which we have just made of the progression of sensitive-sensory excitation in the retina, olfactory bulb and spinal cord, proves not only that protoplasmic expansions fulfill a conductive role, but also that the nervous movement is cellulipetal [toward the cell body] in these expansions, while it is cellulifugal [away from the cell body] in the axis cylinders. In other words, the nerve cell consists of an apparatus for *reception* of the [nervous] currents formed by the dendritic expansions and the cell body; an apparatus for *transmission* represented by the axis cylinder prolongation; and an apparatus for *repartition* or *distribution* represented by the terminal nerve arborization. In all the organs where the direction of the currents is sufficiently known, such as the spinal cord, pyramidal tract of the cerebrum, spiral ganglion of the cochlea, cutaneous sensory cells of worms, according to von Lenhossék, this dynamic orientation is easy to verify.

There is still another induction which it seems legitimate to us to draw from the facts that we have just enumerated, and that is the increasing diffusion of the currents as they reach the most central organs. For example: olfactory excitation brought to the glomeruli by olfactory fibers is conducted to the cerebrum by the intermediation of a few tufted [mitral] cells—recall that one encounters in the glomeruli a bundle of olfactory fibers and a group of trunks of tufted [mitral] cells—and this fact is repeated in the molecular zone of the brain [olfactory cortex], where each fiber of the lateral olfactory tract contacts, with the help of collateral and terminal ramifications, a considerable quantity of peripheral tufts [apical dendritic branches] of pyramids. One can say as much of the visual excitations and the sensory excitations of the spinal cord.

Let us now look at the *neurons and the connections of these neurons in a lamella of cerebellum* [Fig. 36]. A transverse section, for example, will show us three concentric layers of neurons.

The first, or molecular zone, is formed principally by small superficial stel-

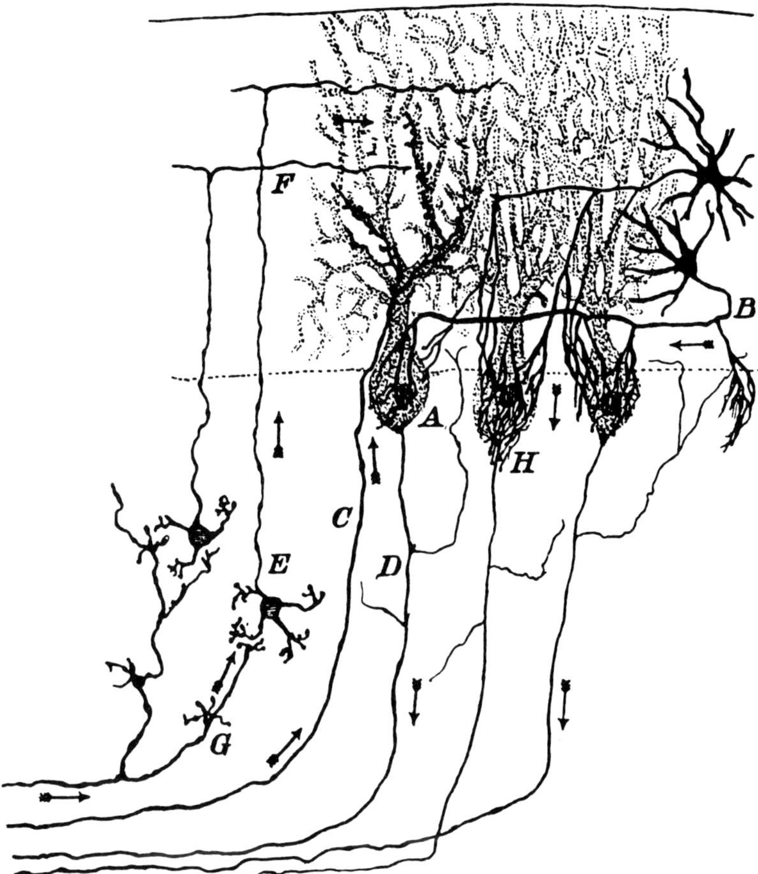

Fig. 36. "Schema of the connections of Purkinje cells of the cerebellum. A, Purkinje cells whose bodies appear surrounded by the nervous branchlets coming from the axis cylinder prolongations of the small stellate corpuscles of the molecular layer; B, axis cylinders of these corpuscles; C, climbing fibers; D, axis cylinder of a Purkinje cell; E, granules whose ascending axis cylinder bifurcates in the molecular layer; G, mossy fiber." (Cajal, 1894)

late cells. The second, or intermediary, is comprised of bodies of Purkinje cells. The third results from the agglomeration of granule cells.

All these elements display two kinds of relationships: intrinsic relationships, that is to say, those established between the cells of the three layers; and extrinsic connections, that is to say, those taking place between the neurons of the cerebellum and neurons belonging to other nervous organs.

Let us examine successively the intrinsic and extrinsic connections. First, the connections of the Purkinje cells with the small stellate elements of the molecular layer. The relationships established between these two orders of cells constitute the most classical example of pericellular nervous arborizations, and the most eloquent fact of transmission by contact, by contiguity, of nervous action.

The small stellate elements of the molecular layer are flattened in the same direction as the Purkinje cells; they have one divergent protoplasmic ramification, which never exceeds the thickness of the layer containing them, and a horizontal axis cylinder whose path is perpendicular to the longitudinal axis of the cerebellar lamellae. This axis cylinder prolongation emits several descending collaterals, and, after a variable distance, curves to arrive at the level of Purkinje cell bodies by means of a very rich and varicose arborization. These terminal arborizations, as well as the descending collateral twigs, branch several times and form around the Purkinje cells a very tight plexus ending in a point of a fringe in the inferior part of the bodies of these cells, at the same level as the origin of their axis cylinder. We have given to this arrangement the name *descending brushes*; Kölliker, Retzius and other authors have confirmed its existence, and prefer the term *terminal baskets*.

How can one not consider these pericellular plexuses as a means of connection between stellate [basket] cells of the molecular layer and Purkinje elements? And one should also know that this connection is not individual; it is collective; that is to say, every pericellular plexus contains ramifications coming from several stellate [basket] cells.

Let us look at *the relations between the granules and the Purkinje cells.* The granules of the cerebellum are small nervous elements located almost exclusively in the granular layer. They possess three or four very short protoplasmic appendices, ornamented at their extremity by a digitiform arborization, and an axis cylinder of extraordinary fineness. This climbs up to the molecular zone and there bifurcates at different heights, thus producing a longitudinal fibril which crosses in parallel all of the cerebellar lamellae. These interesting fibrils, which we have called *parallels* [parallel fibers], because they are arranged in parallel in relation to the cerebellar lamellae, come into very intimate contact, during their trajectory, with the spiny contours of the protoplasmic branches of Purkinje cells. As each parallel fibril travels the total length of the cerebellar convolution, and there ends by free and rounded extremities, it follows that a single granule can act on a multitude of Purkinje corpuscles. It is also very probable that each of the latter is under the influence of a considerable number of granules.

The *extrinsic relationships, between the cells of the cerebellum and of other nervous centers,* have been and are still the most difficult to establish. As Golgi first showed, Purkinje cells give birth to nervous prolongations of the long type whose termination is unknown; conversely, within the grey matter of the cerebellum terminate axis cylinders coming from other organs whose location is still very problematical. These are the *mossy fibers* and *climbing fibers.*

The *mossy fibers* are large medullated tubes which ramify and terminate in the granular layer, where they come into contact with the protoplasmic expansions of these small elements by means of certain excrescences or collateral efflorescences. The terminal twigs end by a varicosity or a small ramification in the form of a rosette.

The *climbing fibers* traverse the granular layer, run alongside the Purkinje cell bodies, and envelop the ascending trunk and the principal protoplasmic

> branches of these elements with a magnificent extended terminal arborization, completely comparable to that of motor fibers on muscle fascicles.
>
> It results from what we have just shown that granules and Purkinje cells can receive the nervous actions of other centers by way of either mossy fibers or climbing fibers, whereas small stellate cells of the molecular layer, as well as large stellate elements of the granular zone belonging to the second type of Golgi cells [this type has become known as Golgi cells], seem not to have any relationship with the extrinsic fibers. From this we have decided to characterize these two last types of cells as *association corpuscles,* since their exclusive role seems to be to associate Purkinje's elements, or the granules, in a dynamic ensemble whose meaning is currently undecipherable.

This is a landmark paper in the history of neuroscience, bringing to the world at large a succinct synthesis of the core of Cajal's experimental findings and his functional interpretations drawn from the glorious years of 1888–1894. Let us summarize it briefly.

In the first section, Cajal sketches the historical development of work on the fine structure of the nerve cell, giving due recognition to Deiters and Golgi, to the crucial insights of His and Forel, and finally to Kölliker and the many others who supported "the absolute independence" of nerve cells against the prevailing idea of a reticulum originating with Gerlach and carried forward by Golgi. Cajal, as always, was careful to differentiate Golgi's technical and factual advances from his speculative interpretations. Note that Cajal acknowledges Waldeyer's "neuron" but still generally uses the term "nerve cell"; similarly, he uses "protoplasmic prolongation" or "protoplasmic expansion" even though "dendrite" was introduced by His in 1890 (see Chapter 13). He also uses "axis cylinder"; "axon" awaits Kölliker's suggestion in 1896 (see Chapter 16).

Cajal then illustrates the new findings concerning the structure and modes of connection of nerve cells in three regions: spinal cord, olfactory bulb, and retina. We have seen that the spinal cord was, in fact, one of the later regions that Cajal attacked, but he probably put it first knowing that his audience included many, like Sherrington, whose main interests were in spinal reflexes. More innovative was his use of the olfactory bulb and the retina to illustrate most clearly the new principles of nervous organization: that protoplasmic prolongations (dendrites) have a conductive role in nervous function, and that transmission occurs by contact, not continuity, between neurons. Some 70 years later, the olfactory bulb and retina were paired again in furnishing new evidence on the roles of dendrites in nervous function (see Chapter 20).

From a consideration of these three regions, Cajal draws the conclusion that each nerve cell consists of three parts, each with a distinct function:

cell body and protoplasmic prolongations (dendrites) for reception, axis cylinder (axon) for transmission, and axis cylinder terminals (axon terminals) for distribution. He notes that this gives the nerve cell a "dynamic orientation," but it is significant that he stops short of pronouncing this his "Law of Dynamic Polarization," perhaps diffident in the face of such august company. He uses the olfactory bulb to illustrate the further principle that there is ever increasing "diffusion" of activity through the sequence of divergent terminal ramifications from one cell to the next. In this he recognizes the need to account not only for specific pathways but also for widespread activation of different parts of the nervous system.

Cajal ends this part of the lecture with a summary of the organization of the cerebellum. Here are used most of the terms employed today: "fringes" have become "baskets" (in deference to Kölliker), "parallels" (soon to become "parallel fibers"), mossy and climbing fibers, and the main types of nerve cells: stellate, granule, Golgi, and Purkinje cells. Sequences of activity in these cell populations are outlined (mossy fiber to granule cells, climbing fiber to Purkinje cells, granule and Golgi cells to Purkinje cells) that have stood the test of time.

A final important point concerns the illustrations accompanying this article. We have here the artistic conceptions of the Golgi-stained images in very nearly the final forms conceived by Cajal. All of Cajal's skills as an artist are here nearing fruition, all the hours bent over the microscope, meticulously drawing the different nerve cell shapes, carefully composing the composite drawings, deducing the connections between the different cell types, retouching and revising to account for new findings, adapting them for display as large wall charts or lantern slides. We have left behind the more tentative sketches of the first publication (cf. Chapter 11) and have here the products of Cajal's mature imagination and judgment. These are the images that, more than any others, have implanted themselves in the minds of succeeding generations of scientists concerning the structures of different nerve cell types and their interconnections in the nervous system.

Observations on Universities and Research

During his month in England, Cajal had time to learn about the institutions for higher learning and research and compare them with his impression of Germany. He surmises that "the educational institutions are admirably organized for the production of *men*, but not for the formation of scholars" (Cajal, 1989). Scholars nonetheless abound, achieving eminence by individuality and "energies of the spirit" despite the "defective and incomplete organization of the educational centres. . . . Many of the English scholars put the final touches to their technical preparation and theoretical instruction in the most renowned German state schools" (Cajal, 1989). His English hosts acknowledged "shocking deficiencies" in the theoretical foundations for medical studies:

> The didactic effort is inspired by utilitarianism, or professionalism, even to a point where important theoretical disciplines included in the plans of study of the French, German, Italian, and even the Spanish universities, are completely absent or receive insignificant attention. To this influence is to be attributed the relative scarcity of histologists, pathological anatomists, embryologists, and bacteriologists in England as compared with Germany or France. Such a state of affairs, however, is tending to disappear. . . . In (the) . . . new schools . . . (London, Liverpool, Manchester and elsewhere) . . . there has been conceded to pure or theoretical science—which fundamentally is the most perfectly practical of all, since it contains the germs of every future application to the purposes of life—its due place, in imitation of the schedules of similar educational centres in Germany.

In this passage Cajal astutely gathered many of the themes about the growth of educational structures during the nineteenth century that we have noted were crucial for the growth of science in general and the work on the cellular structure of the nervous system in particular. These themes include: the overriding importance of the pursuit of knowledge for its own sake; the fact that practical applications of knowledge all flow, directly or indirectly, from prior basic research; the necessity of grounding medical education on a theoretical foundation of the basic sciences. The deficiencies he notes in British science were precisely in those fields, based on microscopical investigations, where the advances in understanding the fine structure of the nerve cell were made, by Golgi in Italy, His and Kölliker in Germany, Forel in Switzerland, van Gehuchten in Belgium, Retzius in Stockholm, Cajal in Spain, and by the many others we have noted.

The foundations for the neuron doctrine were built within institutions that fostered the pursuit of the new knowledge for its own sake, gathered from as wide a range of living organisms, vertebrate and invertebrate, as possible, in order to test its universal validity. Cajal cared passionately for that ideal. His statement is no less true today than it was then.

From 1894 on, the recognition of Cajal's contributions grew steadily: memberships in virtually all the Spanish academies; medals, prizes, and plaques from most countries of Europe; and honorary degrees from many universities. These paraphernalia reflected widespread acknowledgment not only of Cajal's predominant role in the new field of the neuron and its connections but also of the fact that this subject and this achievement were sufficient to place him among the greatest scientists of his time.

Spreading the Word

The emerging consensus on the neuron doctrine soon found its way into the textbooks. We have already mentioned Kölliker's sixth edition in 1896. Needless to say, the new ideas figured prominently in van Gehuchten's *Anatomie du Système Nerveux de l'Homme* (*Anatomy of the Human Nervous System*). The first edition was published in 1893; according to Papez (1953), "the second edition, published in 1897, ranks with the greatest works of our time" and, according to Papez, "had a lasting influence on neurological teaching and research in other countries."

For the English-speaking world, particularly Americans, an important book was Lewellys Barker's *The Nervous System and its Constituent Neurons* (1899). The subtitle—"Designed for the use of practitioners of medicine and of students of medicine and psychology"—recalls the subtitle of the journal in which Waldeyer published his articles in 1891; both authors intended to bridge the gap between the laboratory findings and their application to clinical neurology and the psychology of human behavior. A brief consideration of Barker's life (see Barker, 1942, 1943) will indicate how his work depended on interrelations within the network of teachers and pupils that we have documented in previous chapters.

Barker was born in Canada in 1867; after medical school in Toronto, he was drawn like so many others to Johns Hopkins to take further training in medicine under Osler, beginning in 1890. His interests in laboratory research led him to join the faculty of anatomy under Franklin Mall from 1894 to 1897. This is the same Mall whose feelings about the need to upgrade American medical research according to the European plan we read in Chapter 9, and who supported Harrison in his early career at about this same time (Chapter 17). Given the strength of his feelings, it is not surprising to learn that he arranged for Barker to spend six months in Leipzig. Barker was there during the spring and summer of 1895, first in the physiological laboratory of Ludwig, one of the famous four biophysicists (Chapter 3); unfortunately, Ludwig died soon after Barker arrived. He also attended lectures by His in embryology, Wundt in experimental psychology, and Flechsig on brain anatomy. In the laboratory he worked with von Frey, the pioneer in localization of skin sensations. It was a tremendous cast of leading characters in medical science and vividly exemplifies why young students were eager for the stimulation and inspiration such centers provided. In Barker's case, the immediate result is best described in his own words (Barker, 1942):

> On returning to Baltimore I brought with me the serial sections of the brain stem that Hewetson had cut and stained in Leipzig and used them in teaching

> the histology of the central nervous system to medical students. (Among these students was Miss Gertrude Stein, and I have often wondered whether my attempts to teach her the intricacies of the medulla oblongata had anything to do with the development of the strange literary forms with which she was later to perplex the world.) Flechsig's lectures in Leipzig had aroused my interest in the structure of the nervous system and the work of Golgi, Ramón y Cajal, and Nissl upon the cellular units of the nervous system including cell body, dendrites, axis cylinder and its collaterals, and the end arborizations led me to become a strong champion of the validity of the neurone doctrine as formulated by Waldeyer, despite the objections that had been raised to it by Held and Apáthy. . . . Encouraged by Dr. Mall, I decided to write a systematic account of the histology of the cerebrospinal and sympathetic nervous systems and of their motor, sensory, and association paths. Thanks to the help of an efficient secretary, Miss Eleanor Watts, it was possible to complete the writing of this in about one year [Barker, 1899]. . . . It was a book of 1122 pages and was profusely illustrated, including admirable drawings made by the artist, Mr. L. Schmidt, from Hewetson's serial sections of the brain stem, as well as many drawings by Mr. Max Broedel and Mr. H. Becker. I had thus the fine opportunity of entering the field of modern neurological histology in America, a field of description in which I am proud to count myself one of the pioneers. Though I have written a number of books since, I doubt if any one of them is of greater scientific worth than this volume on the neurone systems, for in it, for the first time, the conduction paths of the central and peripheral nervous system were comprehensively and systematically described from the standpoint of the neurone doctrine.

Barker succeeded Osler in 1905, and went on to a distinguished career in American medicine; he died in 1943.

In his book, Barker summarized the developments leading to the neuron theory and then gave an exhaustive account of the work of Cajal and others that had provided evidence in support of it in the 1890s. This began with a section on the external forms of neurons and their "axone collaterals," the latter termed variously "paraxons" (von Lenhossék), "cylindrodendrites" (Retzius), or "side fibrils" (Golgi). There followed a section on the internal structure of neurons, much influenced by the recent studies of Nissl on stainable masses (the "Nissl substance") in the neuronal cytoplasm. A section on the histogenesis of the neuron followed closely the work of His. Barker then reviewed the results of nerve transections showing the response of the "nerve units" to injury. A final long section dealt with the main centers and tracts of the brain.

Of most interest to us here are Barker's (1899) conclusions regarding the nerve cell as a unit. His views were unequivocal. Two examples will suffice. On the question of the functions of the dendrites, the best evidence is the olfactory pathway, where "the only possible path for the olfactory nerve impulses is from the terminals of the olfactory fibers in the glomeruli to the dendrites of the mitral cells."

From this and other evidence he supported fully the position of Cajal, van Gehuchten, and Kölliker, that dendrites have nervous functions. So sure was he that he felt the "onus of proof . . . lies with those who deny the nervous function, not with those who maintain it." He further observed:

> Now that the cell body of the neurone is known to possess nerve functions, the fact that the axon often comes off from a dendrite instead of from the cell body is further evidence of the . . . similarity of function of cell body and dendrites. . . . Further, if *anaxones* [cells that lack axons] are to be regarded as nerve cells . . . the dendrites must surely possess nerve functions.

We shall see the prescience of this last remark in Chapter 20.

With regard to the nerve cell as an independent unit, Barker considered Apáthy's work on neurofibrils at length, but discounted, rightly, the likelihood, and indeed, even the importance, of neurofibrils passing between nerve cells. The occasional presence of anastomoses was likened to the occasional occurrence of Siamese twins; neither anomaly negates the prevailing principle of independent units. This leads him to a discussion of the organization of organisms according to units of different grades of complexity.

> There may be units smaller than cells, and in all probability there are; there may be, and probably are, in the nervous system units other than those generally described, and it is important that we should find out all that there is to learn about them; but that the human body is made up largely of a mass of cells, and that the human nervous system is made up largely of great numbers of cell units, the so-called neurones, would seem to be facts too firmly established ever to be utterly overthrown.

Here indeed is a passionate affirmation of the new doctrine, indicating that, for most scientists, the quest that had begun in 1839 to bring the cell theory to the nervous system had ended successfully. That the nerve cell might harbor other kinds of "units" is hinted at; whatever Barker may have had in mind, it presaged the idea of hierarchical organization that was to emerge in the modern analysis of neuronal organization (see Chapter 20).

19
Confrontation in Stockholm

In October 1906, Golgi and Cajal were informed by telegraph that they had jointly been awarded the Nobel Prize for Physiology or Medicine for that year, "in recognition of their work on the anatomy of the nervous system," which had made them "the principal representatives and standard bearers of the modern science of neurology" (Golgi, Nobel Lectures, 1906: English translation, 1967).

The award had been urged by many in the preceding years. Cajal's predominant role in establishing the cellular basis of neural organization was widely recognized. Golgi's stain had made it all possible. Golgi's scientific contributions were not limited to this one technical innovation. In fact, his career following his studies with the "black reaction" in the 1870s had seen an astonishing series of major discoveries in different fields. As we have mentioned, the musculo-tendinous organs (now called the Golgi tendon organs) were described in 1880. Between 1884 and 1893 he turned his attention to the pathology of malaria and described, for the first time, the specific forms of the parasite associated with the later types of fever that characterize this disease. His work "transformed clinical ideas" on this terrible disease "and would alone have sufficed to make his name lasting" (Viets, 1926). Then, in 1898, by modifying slightly his silver staining methods, he was able to report the discovery of "a fine network hidden within cells" (Da Fano, 1926). This "internal apparatus" became known as the Golgi apparatus, or Golgi body. Later, the electronmicroscope showed that it is a system of flattened internal membranes, and it is now recognized as the essential machinery within the cell for manufacture and packaging of secretory products. These achievements are all the more amazing considering that Golgi also led a busy public life as rector of the University of Pavia and a senator in Rome.

Cajal and Golgi met for the first time in Stockholm in December to receive their awards. In the formal ceremony of presentation on December 10, Golgi was cited as "the pioneer of modern research into the nervous system," and Cajal was cited for having "given the study of the nervous system the form it has taken at the present day" (Golgi, Nobel Lectures, 1967). Public lectures by the recipients followed, Golgi's on the eleventh, Cajal's on the twelfth of December. These promised to be more than the usual recollections of past discoveries, for they juxtaposed the main proponents of two heretofore irreconcilable views of nervous organization, the one based on the network concept, the other on the neuron theory. Over the years there had been hints that Golgi might be softening his belief in continuity between nerve terminals. On the other hand, the recent claims of Apáthy and others for continuity by means of fine neurofilaments at cell junctions had again inflamed the subject. Would the two protagonists use this occasion to seek a resolution of these issues?

Golgi's Lecture: "The Neuron Doctrine—Theory and Facts"

Golgi (1967) begins his lecture by attacking the neuron doctrine head-on in the first sentence: ". . . this doctrine is generally recognized to be going out of favor." However, in the next sentence, he admits that "the majority of physiologists, anatomists and pathologists still support the neuron theory, and no clinician would think himself sufficiently up to date if he did not accept its ideas like articles of faith." He notes that "neuron" has come to stand for "nerve cell," and feels that this is not what Waldeyer intended.

The "neuron theory," he states, rests on three ideas: "(1) *The neuron is an embryological unit* . . . (2) *The neuron, even in its adult form, is one cell* . . . (3) *The neuron is a physiological unit.*" After some preliminary critical remarks, he takes up his objections to each of these ideas.

"*The neuron as an embryological unit, i.e., it is derived from one cell.*" Golgi acknowledges the "well-known and classical works of His," establishing nerve fibers as "direct emanations of neuroblasts, which [His] considers as independent units." However, citing the recent work on neurofibrils, he wonders if "we suppose they are independent only because we cannot prove that more intimate connections do exist." He notes that the recent studies claiming the multicellular origin of nerve fibers (Beard and others; see Chapter 17) are in opposition to the neuron theory, but he considers the evidence "hardly conclusive," citing studies from his own laboratory showing that regenerating fibers are from preexisting fibers. All in all, he concludes, "it is not possible to state with certainty that what we know of the origin of nerve cells has a well-proved fundamental value, and can be used to support the alleged embryological independence of the nerve cell." This seems an extremely negative position on the classical work of His, Cajal, and many others. In any case, most of these reservations were rendered moot by the decisive experiments of Harrison, which at the very moment of Golgi's lecture were underway (see Chapter 17).

"*The neuron is, in the adult state too, an independent cell unit.*" Golgi first defends his original division of nerve cells into two categories, "with long axons and short axons," and defends his attribution to them of motor and sensory functions, respectively, despite the criticisms that the two types are intermingled in most regions of the nervous system. The first category is motor because anterior horn cells in the spinal cord are indubitably motor, and most other long axon cells can be considered to bear some direct or indirect relation with them, and can therefore be thought of as motor or psychomotor. As for the second type, their role has to be understood within the context of a diffuse network:

> When the neuron theory made, by almost unanimous approval, its triumphant entrance on the scientific scene, I found myself unable to follow the current of opinion, because I was confronted by one concrete anatomical fact; this was the existence of the formation which I have called the diffuse nerve network. I attached much more importance to this network, which I did not hesitate to call a nerve organ, because the very manner in which it is composed clearly indicated its significance to me. In fact, although in various ways and to varying extent, every nerve element of the central nervous system contributes toward its formation.

Let us first consider the anatomical basis which Golgi advanced for the diffuse network; it consisted in his view of the following elements:

> (1) collateral fibrils which radiate from the nerve process of cells of the first type;
>
> (2) the assemblage of nerve processes of the second type breaking up in a highly complicated way;
>
> (3) collateral fibrils coming from nerve fibres of the first type to make direct contact with ganglion cells of the first type;
>
> (4) a large number of other nerve fibres which, like the nerve process of cells of the second type, gradually lose their individuality while dividing to become extremely thin filaments.
>
> As regards the importance I attached to this network, may I repeat again that I have always considered it as an organ playing a fundamental part in

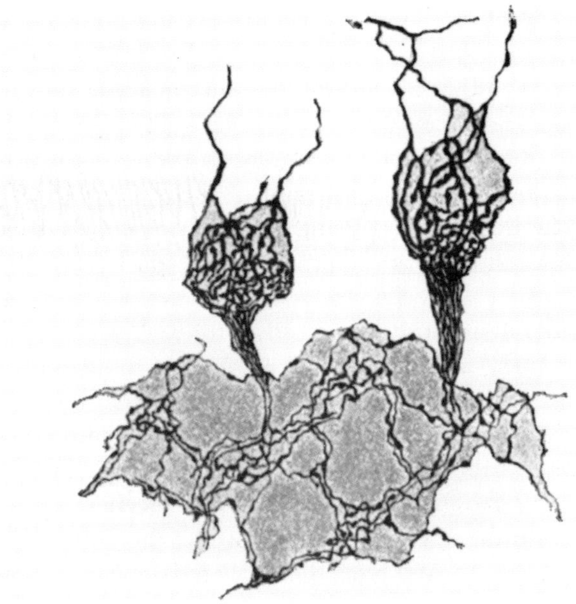

Fig. 37. Golgi's depiction of the ramifications of stellate cell axons passing around the Purkinje cell bodies to join a reticulum in the granule cell layer. (Golgi, 1967)

> the specific function of the nervous system and that I have, many times, said that I considered it as an entirely distinct anatomical entity and not as a simple hypothesis.
>
> I have demonstrated its existence in the chief areas of the nervous system, in the spinal cord, in the cerebellum, and in the cerebral cortex, realizing that it is a little modified from site to site.

Golgi's diagrams depicting his conception of the diffuse network are shown for the cerebellum in Figure 37 and for the dentate gyrus in Figure 38. With regard to the cerebellum, he states, "I have verified that the fibres coming from the nerve process of the cells of the molecular layer only pass near the cells of Purkinje to proceed into the rich and characteristic network existing in the granular layer."

Thus, Golgi's interpretation of the "descending fringes," what we now call "basket endings," was that they do not terminate on the Purkinje cell bodies and initial axon segment, as Cajal believed and as has been confirmed by modern research, but rather that these merely passed over the Purkinje cell bodies (as indicated in Figure 37) in order to enter a diffuse network of fibers in the granular layer where the true nervous activity took place. Similarly, in Figure 38, the granule cells of the dentate gyrus are considered to belong to the second type, their fine fibers (axons) subdivid-

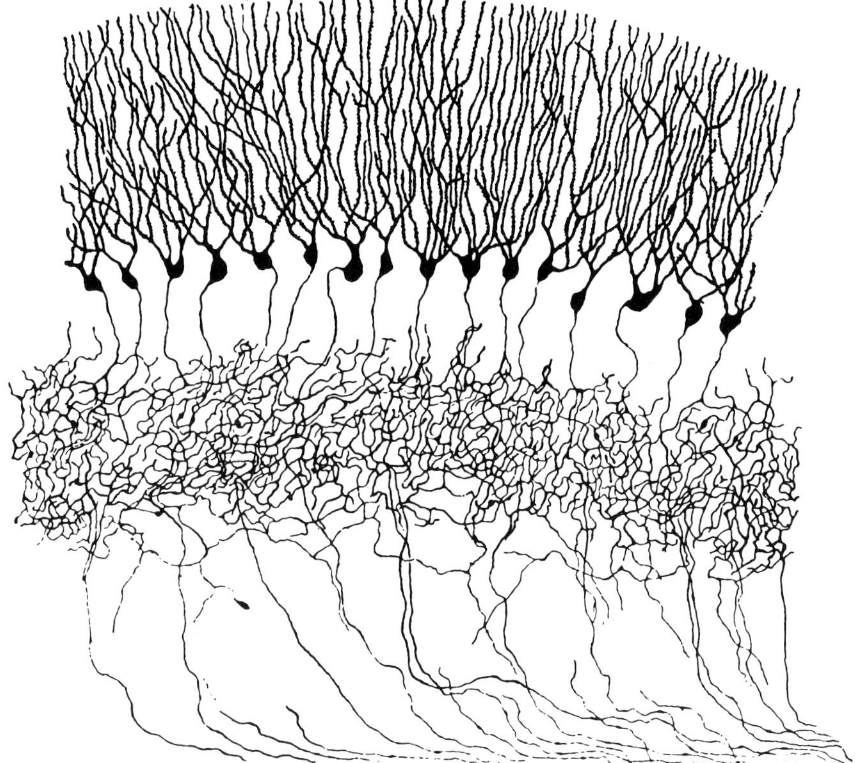

Fig. 38. Golgi's depiction of the reticulum formed by axon collaterals in the dentate gyrus. (Golgi, 1967)

ing beneath the cell body layer within a "reticular zone" where the input fibers also subdivide. Golgi notes that this reticular zone looks like a "*punkt-substanz*" ("dotted substance") when stained with ordinary methods.

Figure 38 gives probably the clearest view of Golgi's concept of his diffuse nerve reticulum. The reticulum is the "meeting place" for fibers of a given region and incoming fibers from other regions. Above, in the figure, the protoplasmic processes (dendrites) of the cells are depicted reaching out toward the surface of the dentate gyrus, exchanging nutrients (in Golgi's view) with the vascular supply to nourish the cell bodies and fibers. Unfortunately, crucially missing from Figure 38 is the fact that (1) the granule cell axons give rise to so-called mossy fibers, which carry the output of the dentate gyrus to the nearby hippocampus; (2) these axons give rise to collaterals that terminate locally on cells; and (3) there is a massive input by way of perforant fibers to the layer of the granule cell dendrites, with synaptic connections onto the spines of the granule cell dendrites. There is no explanation for why Golgi missed seeing the mossy and perforant fibers in his stained specimens. Some 15 years had passed since Cajal's first results challenged Golgi's results and interpretations, but apparently Golgi considered his early results definitive and did not feel it necessary to reexamine the question with new material.

With regard to the question of dendritic spines, whether they were reality or artifact, he comments:

> Above all there has been the question of the spines which the protoplasmic processes are provided with. A major functional role has been given to these spines and there are innumerable accounts in the literature which aim to show what modifications they undergo in varying states of activity, rest, sleep and of wakefulness. Now, if one considers that similar structures are found not only on protoplasmic processes but also on cells of the neuroglia and on the nerve process, it is not hard to imagine that, even disregarding any estimation of the worth of the experiments, I have never attached any final importance to this statement regarding protoplasmic processes as cellulipetal conductors.

The dendritic spine as a critically important anatomical structure has been fully confirmed by modern studies. Golgi's argument is an instance of how a structure may appear similar in quite different cell types, yet be adapted for quite different functions.

We turn next to Golgi's interpretation of the physiological significance of the diffuse network. First, with regard to the question of contact or continuity, he downplays the importance of this issue, since it seems likely that "contacts between fibrils" are more than sufficient for a nerve impulse to be transmitted from one to the other. He curiously cites Forel in favor of this idea. What is crucial in his opinion is that the network provides for the "anatomical and functional continuity" between nerve cells in all parts of the nervous system. By this means, there is "group action" of nerve cells within a region, as in the case of the network in the dentate gyrus (see Fig. 38); these connections speak in favor "of the whole dentate gyrus acting as a group and against any individual action of these cells." Furthermore, "this network is the organ by which both an anatomical and functional liaison is effected between different parts of the nervous system."

The neuron is a physiologically independent unit. Given this emphasis on diffuse network properties, it is not surprising that Golgi leaves little place for the individual nerve cell as an independent unit. Similarly, within the network, it is assumed that impulses can pass in any direction, so that the idea of "dynamic polarization," while it may apply to certain cells or fibers, is not a general necessity.

Golgi further considers whether the idea of the functionally independent neuron might gain support from the evidence for sharply demarcated functional areas in the cerebral cortex. However, he argues against the presence of sharp localization, as demonstrated in the well-known experiments of Hitzig and Fritsch (1870), Ferrier (1876), and many others of that period, in favor of territories that gradually merge with each other; here he seems also to be thinking about the capacities to recover from localized brain damage. He states that he has "come round to the idea that specific function is not associated with the characteristics of organization of centres, but rather with the specificity of peripheral organs destined to receive and transmit impulses." This is an early expression of the idea that differences in behavior are due to differences in peripheral organs rather than in central brain structures; modern research supports the roles of both.

Golgi ends by summarizing his stand as follows:

> The conclusion of this account of the neuron question, which has had to be rather an assembly of facts, brings me back to my starting-point, namely that no arguments, on which Waldeyer supported the theory of the individuality and independence of the neuron, will stand examination.
>
> We have seen, in fact, how we lack embryological data and how anatomical arguments, either individually or as a whole, do not offer any basis firm enough to uphold this doctrine. In fact, all the characteristics of nerve process, protoplasmic process and cell-body organization which we have examined seem to point in another direction.
>
> We find the same situation regarding the so-called physiological independence of the neuron. Just as we have said regarding the functional mechanism, far from being able to accept the idea of the individuality and independence of each nerve element, I have never had reason, up to now, to give up the concept which I have always stressed, that nerve cells, instead of working individually, act together, so that we must think that several groups of elements exercise a cumulative effect on the peripheral organs through whole bundles of fibers. It is understood that this concept implies another regarding the opposite action of sensory functions. However opposed it may seem to the popular tendency to individualize the elements, I cannot abandon the idea of a unitary action of the nervous system, without bothering if, by that, I approach old conceptions.

Summary

We have dealt with Golgi's lecture at some length, to consider the development of his work and to assess the strengths and weaknesses of the evidence and the concepts. With regard to his development, he was at this time 63; it was some 30 years since he had first glimpsed the "black reaction" in the flickering lamplight of his home-made laboratory. Many other endeavors, scientific and public, had intervened in his life. One gets the impression that his ideas had changed little from the extensive views on neural organization he had formulated in the 1870s and early 1880s (see

Chapter 8). Similarly, there seemed to be little development or reexamination of his own Golgi-stained material. Many inadequacies were apparent, yet he seemed unmindful of them, indeed, even more willing to overinterpret the material he did have.

The ideas, however, are a somewhat different matter. Important ideas do not necessarily stand on sound anatomical evidence, as we learned in considering the cell theory itself of Schleiden and Schwann (Chapter 2). Clearly, Golgi's ideas about the structure and function of individual neurons were in error. However, one could say in his defense that this was not for him the important question; the crucial problem was, rather, how does the nervous system function as a whole? At this level, what mattered was how the nerve cells provide for a system of extensive interaction so that consciousness and mental activity could emerge in a holistic manner. If we were to act as advocates of his position, we would say that he could not conceive how this holistic behavior could be the product of the individual actions of nerve cells acting independently, if "independence" was to have any real meaning. Instead, what was needed was a system providing the maximum opportunity for nerve cells and nerve fibers to function together in a coordinated manner.

Seen from this perspective, Golgi's idea of a nerve network appears as a valid attempt to deal with some of the holistic aspects of brain function. It took account of the fact that there often is considerable recovery of function following focal brain damage. It anticipated the gestalt psychologists, who, beginning around 1910, emphasized that we perceive things as wholes, not as sums of individual parts. It further anticipated the life-long work of Karl Lashley, who developed the idea (see Lashley, 1929) that learning (at least learning of a maze by rats) was correlated simply with the amount of brain tissue remaining after lesions of different extents. We know now that holistic functions of the mind are understandable in terms of distributed systems that unite different structures with different functions, all built up from individual neurons. Some of the network idea, in fact, is expressed in the computational neural nets developed in recent years to simulate brain functions (see Chapter 20). Thus, we may better appreciate that Golgi placed himself firmly in a tradition of viewing nervous function in a holistic manner.

Cajal's Lecture: "The Structure and Connections of Neurons"

Cajal (1967) was furious at Golgi for his "display of pride and self worship," for ignoring all of the work on the nerve cell that had occurred since Golgi's early discoveries (no mention even of Kölliker!), for the drawings that distorted the facts, for an ego that was "hermetically sealed . . . and impermeable to the incessant changes taking place in the intellectual environment."

> What a cruel irony of fate to pair, like Siamese Twins united by the shoulders, scientific adversaries of such contrasting character!

Cajal's lecture was largely a straightforward description of his work.

> From my researches as a whole, there derives a general conception which comprises the following propositions:
>
> 1. The nerve cells are morphological entities, neurons, to use the word brought into use by the authority of Professor Waldeyer. My celebrated colleague Professor Golgi has already demonstrated this property with respect to the dendritic or protoplasmic processes of the nerve cells; but at the beginning of our research there were only vague conjectures as regards the behaviour of the axon branches and collaterals. We applied Golgi's method, firstly in the cerebellum and then in the spinal cord, the cerebrum, the olfactory bulb, the optic lobe, the retina and so on of embryos and young animals, and our observations revealed, in my opinion, the terminal arrangement of the nerve fibres. These fibres, ramifying several times, always proceed towards the neuronal body, or towards the protoplasmic expansions around which arise plexuses or very tightly bound and rich nerve nests. The pericellular baskets and the climbing plexuses, and other morphological structures, whose form varies according to the nerve centres being studied, confirm that the nerve elements possess reciprocal relationships in *contiguity* but not in *continuity* It is confirmed also that those more or less intimate contacts are always established, not between the nerve arborizations alone, but between these ramifications on the one hand, and the body and protoplasmic processes on the other. A granular cement, or special conducting substance would serve to keep the neuron surfaces very intimately in contact.
>
> These facts, recognized in all the nerve centres with the aid of two very different methods (that of Golgi and that of Ehrlich), confirmed and notably developed by the research of Kölliker, von Lenhossék, Retzius, Van Gehuchten, Lugaro, Held, my brother, Athias, Edinger, and many others, imply three physiological postulates:
>
> (a) As nature, in order to assure and amplify the contacts, has created complicated systems of pericellular ramifications (systems which become incomprehensible within the hypothesis of continuity), it must be admitted that the nerve currents are transmitted from one element to the other as a consequence of a sort of induction or influence from a distance.
>
> (b) It must also be supposed that the cell bodies and the dendrites are, in the same way as the axis cylinders, conductive devices, as they represent the intermediary links between afferent nerve fibres and the afore-mentioned axons. This is what Bethe, Simarro, Donaggio, ourselves, etc. have confirmed quite recently by demonstrating, with the aid of neurofibrillar methods, a perfect structural concordance between the dendrites and the prolongation of the axon cylinder [Cajal here begins to adopt Kölliker's term "axon"].

(c) The examination of the movement of nervous impulses in the sensory organs such as the retina, the olfactory bulb, the sensory ganglia and the spinal cord, etc. proves not only that the protoplasmic expansions play a conducting role but even more that nervous movement in these prolongations is *towards the cell or axon,* while it is *away from the cell* in the axons. This formula, called the *dynamic polarization of neurons,* originated a long time ago by Van Gehuchten and us as an induction from numerous morphological facts, is not in contradiction with the new research on the constitution of nerve protoplasm. Indeed we will see that the neurofibrillar framework constitutes a continuous reticulum from the dendrites and the cell body to the axon and its peripheral termination.

During twenty-five years of continued work on nearly all the organs of the nervous system and on a large number of zoological species, I have never met a single observed fact contrary to these assertions, and yet I have used in my research, in addition to the usual processes of coloration, the chosen methods of Golgi, Cox, Ehrlich and lastly the neurofibrillar methods. Let us add that the same doctrine also arises out of the assemblage of observations of Kölliker, von Lenhossék, Van Gehuchten, my brother, Edinger, Lugaro, etc., on the nervous system of the vertebrates and from those very important observations of Retzius on the nervous system of the invertebrates.

Here we have Cajal at his best: the key facts stated succinctly, the main authors carefully acknowledged, the concepts spare and tied closely to the facts. Note that he gives credit to Golgi for demonstrating the dendrites as entities, whereas his own work clarified "the terminal arrangements of the nerve fibers (axons)." This perhaps was one of the things that most galled Golgi, for the axon collaterals were one of Golgi's main discoveries; his definitive explanation for their significance was contained in his diffuse nerve net, not in the terminal structures shown by Cajal.

In this summary statement there is in fact little new beyond the ideas set forth in Cajal's Croonian lecture 12 years previously, except for a more explicit statement of the "Law of Dynamic Polarization." The next part of his lecture presents examples of "parallel fibers." One new finding in Purkinje cells is that he has been able to see terminals of recurrent collaterals ending on the dendritic trunks of neighboring Purkinje cells. This confirms for him "that the recurrent collaterals serve to associate in a dynamic ensemble the neurons of the same kind from the same area of the grey matter." How far is it conceptually, we may ask, from the idea of "group action" mediated by Golgi's diffuse nerve net of axon collaterals and a "dynamic ensemble" of neurons interconnected by axon collaterals? (Cajal also had the idea that excitation could circulate through the axon collaterals and their connections to produce an "avalanche conduction," a further mechanism for bringing large populations of cells into coordinated activity: see Cajal, 1909, 1911). This part of the lecture on neuronal connections ends with consideration of centrifugal fibers that originate in the brain and supply the peripheral sensory pathways.

Cajal then takes up several new topics. First is the new evidence on the internal structure of the "nerve protoplasm," what we now call the organelles of the cytoplasm. He mentions the "basophilic bodies" of Nissl ("Nissl bodies"), and then turns his attention to the neurofibrils, especially the effects on them of crushing a nerve, emphasizing their dynamic state. He cannot deny the possibility of "some enigmatic system of filaments" making connections between neurons (as claimed by Apáthy and others) "as creepers attach to the trees of tropical forests." Such an "intermediary network" would be convenient for theorists, but "nature seems unaware of an intellectual need for convenience and unity, and very often takes delight in complication and diversity." It must be said that Cajal seems here to have been going out of his way to put down Golgi. Nowhere in his account of the nerve protoplasm does he mention Golgi's discovery of the internal reticulum.

The last part of the lecture deals with the attacks on the outgrowth theory of the nerve fiber. He cites extensive recent work by himself and others on the outgrowth of nerve fibers during regeneration and during embryonic development. He shows an illustration of primitive nerve cells (neuroblasts) sending out an axon capped by a "cone of development" ("growth cone") (see Fig. 30, Chapter 17). These views of primitive cells in the embryonic spinal cord, in sections stained with silver, are remarkably similar to the illustrations by Harrison of cell processes growing in tissue culture, published in the following year (Harrison, 1907, 1908; see Chapter 17). Cajal ends by saying that all the work he has cited supports "the doctrine of neurogenesis of His. . . . We mourn this scientist who, in the last years of a life so well filled [His died in 1904], suffered the injustice of seeing a phalanx of young experimenters treat his most elegant and original discoveries as errors."

Final Thoughts from the Classical Era

The ceremonies in Stockholm were of interest mostly as a dramatic occasion for summarizing and contrasting the contributions of Golgi and Cajal. In the fields of anatomy, physiology, psychology, and clinical neurology, the evidence for the nerve cell as an individual cellular unit seemed overwhelming and, as we have discussed, was widely regarded as the departure point for the modern development of these fields. The rearguard actions against the neuron doctrine sputtered along, however, fueled as long as definitive proof could not be obtained under the light microscope against any remote possibility of continuity or anastomoses between fine, unresolvable processes. Cajal never wavered in defending his cherished neuron against these snipers. In the year before his death, he published "Neuronismo o reticularismo?" ("Neuron or reticulum?") (Cajal, 1933), a restatement of all the facts and arguments. By then, however, the battle had long been won. The Golgi stain had fallen into disuse as anatomists moved on to other methods and problems. Most investigators wanted to avoid rehashing the old polemics.

For those who had fought the battle for the neuron, however, there would always be the memories of the difficult terrain, the formidable opponents, the scars and injuries. Perhaps Retzius expressed it best; in his Croonian lecture of 1908, he recalled:

> The difference between our knowledge then and that we possessed, for instance, in 1880, was prodigious. Yet, in reality, it was a mere handful of investigators, dwelling far apart from one another, who had accomplished this work. In some quarters, even among eminent anatomists, physiologists, and especially neurologists, the work and results of those investigators were long regarded with a certain suspicion; now and then that suspicion found expression in a rather startling form. I might, for instance, read to you letters which I received from celebrated histologists abroad, who were otherwise favourably disposed towards me and my work, conjuring me in the most serious and moving terms not to go on experimenting with that wretched Golgian method which only resulted in art effects, impure chrome-silver precipitations within the tissues, and were misleading and dangerous for real scientific inquiry. Pretty much the same verdict was pronounced, too, from a specially authoritative source upon the methylene method as we applied it. From the point of view of the history of science it may be of a certain interest to note that our labours by no means met with encouragement and recognition in all quarters.

20
Modern Revisions of the Neuron Doctrine

By the early part of this century the incorporation of the nerve cell into the cell theory was widely accepted in biology and the neurological sciences. Its importance was stated eloquently by Sherrington (1906) in the first sentence of his landmark book, *The Integrative Actions of the Nervous System*:

> Nowhere in physiology does the cell-theory reveal its presence more frequently in the very framework of the argument than at the present time in the study of nervous reactions.

With this degree of acceptance, interest in the neuron doctrine as a topic of discussion rapidly faded. This was partly because the conclusion seemed patent to most, and partly because the debate carried on around the issue of neurofibrillary continuity between neurons seemed acrid and sterile. In these circumstances, scientists generally avoid unpleasantness and get on with their work. That is exactly what happened in the first half of this century; interest turned to other types of cell stains and other kinds of issues. The Nissl stains, for example, which reveal the nuclei and parts of the cytoplasm of all neurons, became widely used to classify the cerebral cortex into numerous local areas on the basis of fine distinctions in the staining pattern of different cell layers. With the exception of a widely read and quoted chapter on Golgi-stained neurons and their postulated reverberatory circuits in the cerebral cortex by Lorente de Nó, which appeared in Fulton's *Physiology of the Nervous System* in 1938, the Golgi stain attracted little attention. Without it, the whole thrust of analysis of questions surrounding the neuron in the classical period faded. Cajal's defense of his doctrine in 1933 belonged more to the old era than the new.

What was needed, of course, in order to make any further progress on the unresolved issues, was the introduction of new methods. This began in the 1920s and 1930s, but was delayed by the Second World War of 1939–1945. However, by the early 1950s anatomists had acquired the electron-microscope for high-resolution analysis of cell structure, while physiologists had developed the microelectrode for intracellular analysis of the membrane mechanisms of nerve impulses and synaptic potentials, as well as for extracellular recordings of single cell activity for analysis of information processing in neural circuits. Together with the solving of the structure of DNA in 1953, these new methods opened the modern era of biological research. These tremendous changes recall the great advances in biology that had been made around the 1880s and, before that, around the 1840s.

To discuss the introduction of these modern methods would be to chronicle the rise of modern neuroscience, which is beyond our scope. Our aim in this chapter will therefore be to focus narrowly and briefly on those advances that had specific relevance to the neuron doctrine. We will organize the discussion around the four tenets originally put forward by Waldeyer: that the neuron is the anatomical, physiological, genetic, and metabolic unit of the nervous system. To what extent were these tenets supported, modified, or disproved by the early work of the modern era? Much of the theory stood the test, and has served well as the basis for the remarkable advances that have occurred in recent decades. However, some surprises occurred that had not been anticipated by the classical concepts. We will summarize the attempts that were made to deal with these, and finally indicate some future directions in which revisions are likely to be needed.

The Neuron as an Anatomical Unit

The light microscope lacks adequate magnification to visualize adequately the cell surface and resolve the issue of contact or continuity between neurons, to say nothing of visualizing all the other organelles that make up neurons and other cells of the body. What was needed was an entirely new type of microscope with much higher resolving power. The answer to this need was the electronmicroscope. Whereas the light microscope forms images using light waves, which limits the resolving power in most circumstances to the wave length of light (slightly less than one micron—one thousandth of a millimeter), the electronmicroscope, as its name implies, forms images by using beams of electrons, whose resolving power is about 10,000 times greater. The application to animal tissue encountered great difficulties in obtaining adequate fixation and staining of the tissue so that it would give clear images while withstanding the high intensity of the electron beams. These difficulties were most extreme with nervous tissue, but gradually the images furnished the long-awaited answers.

The Synapse

The most critical point of attack in assessing the question of continuity or contact between neurons was the synapse. The first problem in studying the synapse was how to identify it in single electronmicroscopic sections containing a jumble of the light and dark profiles of neuronal processes cut across at different angles. One strategy was to study the neuromuscular junction, where the difference between the nerve terminal and the muscle cell is marked. At central synapses, an important clue was the high density of mitochondria in most axon terminals. At these sites, there is a presumed physiological sequence of activity, such that the axon terminal is the *presynaptic* process, and the soma or dendrite that it contacts is the *postsynaptic* process.

At a variety of such sites, certain common features were found (Palade and Palay, 1954; Palay, 1956; 1958; de Robertis and Bennett, 1954; de Robertis, 1955, 1959; see Fig. 39): (1) pre- and postsynaptic process are each surrounded by a surface membrane that is everywhere continuous; (2) the apposed membranes are everywhere separated by a space, or cleft, of approximately 20 nanometers (20 millionths of a millimeter); (3) there is no evidence of fibrillary or other connections bridging this gap between the two processes; (4) the apposed membranes have an increased density; (5) in addition to mitochondria, the presynaptic terminal also contains numerous small vesicles, 20–60 nanometers in diameter, some of them forming clusters near the presynaptic membrane densities.

These findings were immediately interpreted as providing a definitive resolution of the old question of neuron versus reticulum. As one of the pioneers in this work, Sanford Palay (1956), observed:

> The absence of protoplasmic continuity across the contact surface between the two members of the synaptic apparatus is impressive confirmation of the neuron doctrine enunciated and defended by Ramón y Cajal during the early part of this century.

This same verdict was reached by another pioneer, Eduardo de Robertis (1959):

> The observation of a neat delimitation of both the pre- and postsynaptic cytoplasm confirms and extends to a submicroscopic level the concept of the

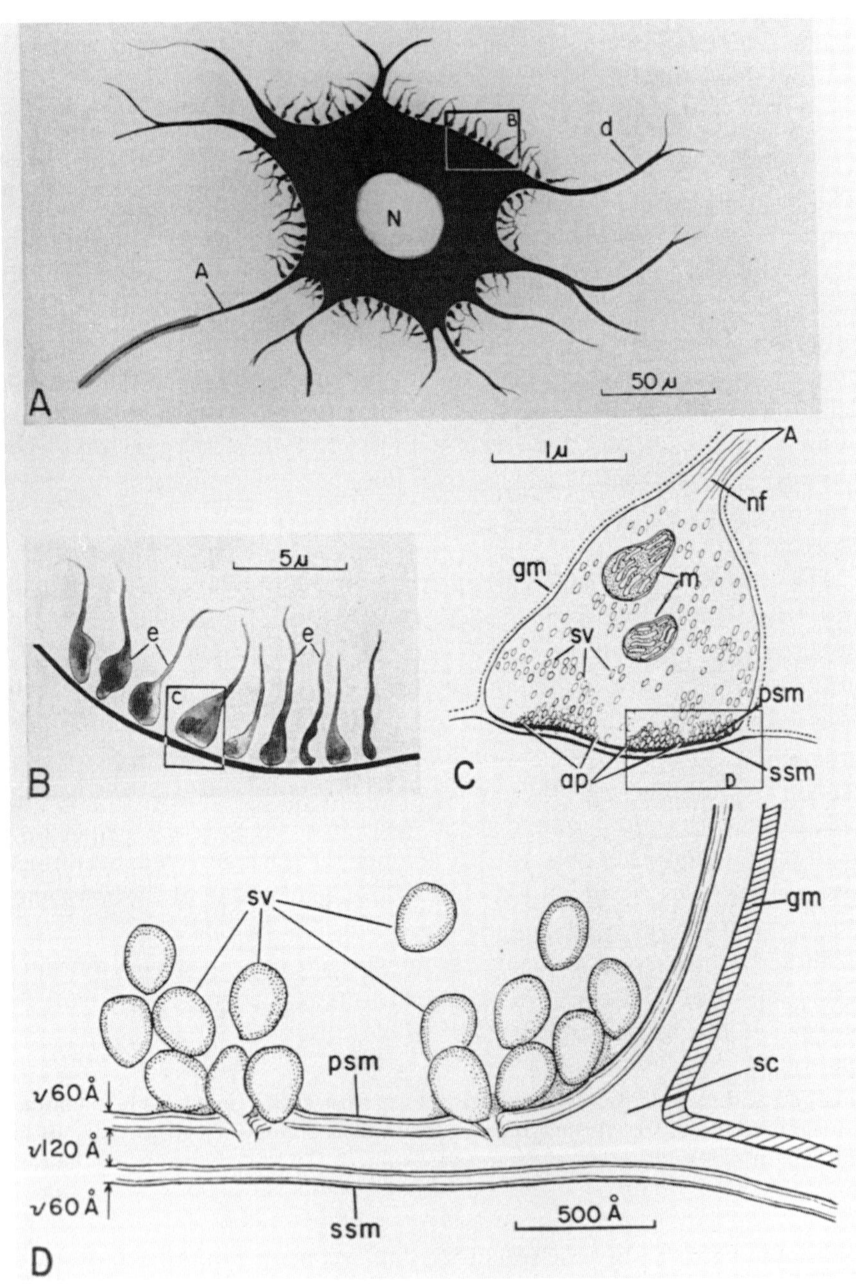

Fig. 39. "Diagram showing bouton-like synaptic junctions at different magnifications with the optical and electron microscope. (A) Illustrates a motoneuron as seen at medium power of the optical microscope. The nucleus (*N*), the axon (*A*), and the dendrites (*d*) are indicated. Numerous bouton-like endings make synaptic contact

> individuality of the nerve element which is implicit in the neuron doctrine of Cajal. The reticularist hypothesis, which still has its followers, cannot be maintained, even in those regions of the central nervous system called neuropiles, where most of the elements are of submicroscopic dimensions. The reticular appearance is the result of technical artifacts, plus the limited resolving power of the optical microscope to detect those structures and their boundaries. These facts indicate that for an exact interpretation all structures below 1 to 0.5 micrometers should be studied with the electron microscope.

Note that, in both these cases, the credit for the neuron doctrine is given to Cajal; the citations, in fact, were to his last writings on the subject in 1933.

These early electronmicroscopic studies of the synapse constitute one of the great discoveries in neuroscience. The directionality of the synaptic action was correctly deduced, as well as the probability that the small vesicles contain or are associated with transmitter or hormonal substances that can be released by fusion of the vesicles with the surface membrane, and the probable relation of these events to the newly discovered "quanta" of activity at a synapse (Fatt and Katz, 1952; see below). Much of modern neuroscience revolves around these structures and these actions (for overviews, see Kuffler et al., 1984; Kandel and Schwartz, 1985; Shepherd, 1988). A modern view of the morphology of a synapse is shown in Figure 40.

Electrical Synapses

These early studies seemed to resolve a long-standing debate (summarized in Forbes, 1939) over whether synaptic transmission occurs by means of the release of chemical transmitter substances or the spread of electric current. But just as the concept of the chemical synapse began to be formulated as a general principle for neuronal interconnection, physiological studies

---

with the surface of the pericaryon (axosomatic junctions) and of the dendrites (axodendritic junctions). Enclosure *B* is magnified ten times in B. (B) End feet (*e*), as seen at high magnification with the optical microscope. The afferent axons are enlarged at the endings. The presence of mitochrondria is indicated. Enclosure C is magnified about six times with the electronmicroscope in C. (C) Diagram of an end foot as observed with the electronmicroscope. Mitochondria (*m*), neuroprotofibrils (*nf*), and synaptic vesicles (*sv*) are shown within the ending. Three clusters of synaptic vesicles become attached to the presynaptic membrane (*psm*); these are probably active points (*ap*) of the synapse. Both the *psm* and the subsynaptic membrane (*ssm*) show higher electron density. The glial membrane is shown in dotted lines (*gm*). Enclosure *D* is magnified about twenty times in D. (D) Diagram of the synaptic membrane as observed with high-resolution electronmicroscopy (see description in the text). Some synaptic vesicles (*sv*) are seen attached to the *psm* and opening into the synaptic cleft (*sc*)." (From De Robertis, 1959)

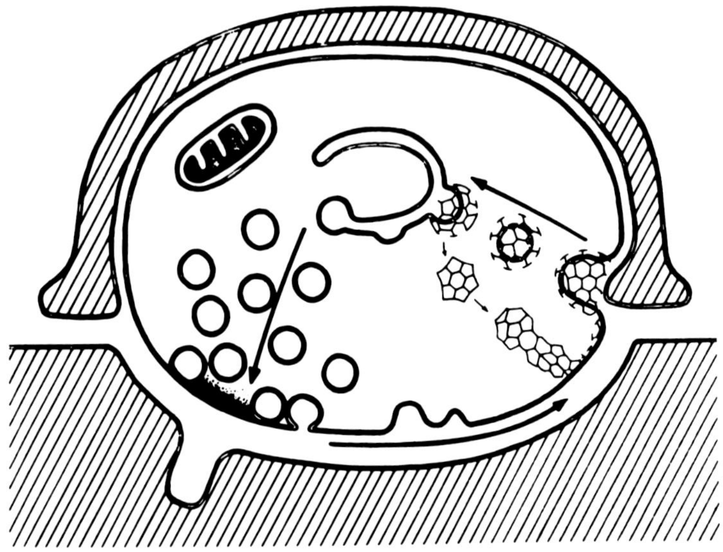

Fig. 40. Modern view of the neuromuscular junction, representing the main structures and sequence of events that take place at a typical synapse during release of vesicles and recycling of vesicle membranes. (From Heuser and Reese, 1973)

brought forth clear evidence for electrical synapses as well (Furshpan and Potter, 1959). At certain sites, electric current spreads directly from cell to cell through special junctions. The earliest electronmicroscopic studies of these sites showed specializations, including densification and apparent fusing of the apposed membranes, interdigitation of finger-like processes, and accumulation of intracellular filaments and membranous structures (Robertson, 1955). It took a great deal of subsequent electronmicroscopical work to show that in fact the membranes are separated by a narrow "gap" (Revel and Karnovsky, 1967), and that across this "gap junction" there is direct communication between two cells through pore-forming proteins that span the gap. A view of these junctions at the molecular level is shown in Figure 41.

Gap junctions have posed an interesting challenge, not only to the neuron doctrine, but to the cell theory in general. The channels that connect two cells have a diameter of approximately 20 Ångstrøms (20 ten billionths of a meter), sufficient to allow the passage not only of electric current and all the common ions (simple charged atoms such as Na+, K+, Ca(2+), and Cl−), but also many small molecules such as glucose. Gap junctions are found scattered in most organs of the body. They are believed to subserve a variety of general functions that play important roles in development, cell metabolism, and homeostasis, though proof of these roles is still

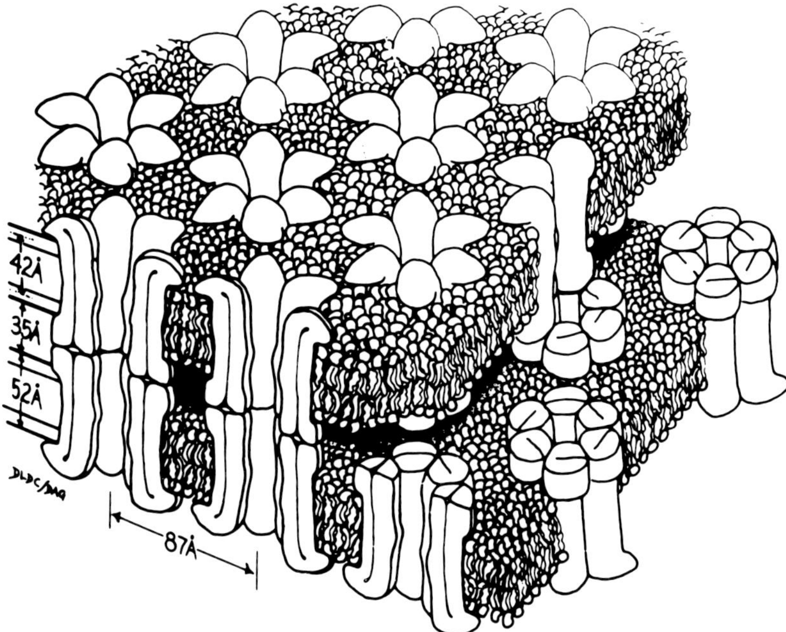

Fig. 41. Diagram summarizing the fine structural organization of a gap (electrical) junction. The two apposed membranes are shown, with channel proteins composed of six circularly arranged subunits forming bridges across them that allow for the passage of ions, small molecules, and electric current. (From Mackowski et al., 1977)

lacking. In the nervous system, the spread of electric current through electrical synapses can also mediate such functions as sequential spread of impulse activity from cell to cell, synchronization of activity in neighboring cells, or enhancement of signal-to-noise relations in sensory receptors (see Bennett et al., 1963).

The incompatibility of these findings with a strict interpretation of the cell theory was gradually realized. The implications are potentially profound, as pointed out by Werner Loewenstein (1981):

> The discovery of this form of intercellular communication has meant a sharp departure from classic cell theory. It is the coupled cell ensemble, and not the single cell, that is the functional compartmental unit for the smaller cytoplasmic molecules; the ensemble inside constitutes a largely uninterrupted interior milieu for somatic and genetic processes. This has wide implications for tissue regulation. . . .
>
> One may ask why it took so long to uncover this form of cellular communication. This sort of question, of course, comes up with any discovery, but here, I think, more sharply so because the opposite thought, cell unconnectivity, had rooted itself only 10 years before. The fact that it did take so long

> is a bouquet to cell theory and attests that not only in physics but also in biology (so dominated by serendipity) theory is the motor. Indeed cell theory has had few equals in influencing biological thought. Its grip has been such that in the 1940s and 1950s one was only too happy to extend the notion of the continuous pericellular diffusion barrier from a handful of special cell types to all tissues or to read such a barrier into a black line on electron micrographs. The facts reviewed here [on gap junctions] have modified cell theory in several ways regarding the smaller molecules of cells but not with respect to compartmentation of the macromolecules. For this, the cell continues to be the fundamental unit. There have been inklings of cell connectivity from time to time. There were many in the past century relating to a syncytial nature of tissues; those concerning nerve were snuffed out by Cajal's histology . . . , and those regarding heart and smooth muscle (these lingered the longest) were abandoned with the advent of electron microscopy.

The anatomical fact of these direct communications obviously means that neurons so connected are not completely separate anatomical entities. We shall discuss further the functional consequences of these anatomical connections, but first we must summarize the new information gained about the physiological properties of neurons.

The Neuron as a Physiological Unit

Electrical Activity of the Neuron

By 1950, the ability to introduce a microelectrode tip inside a nerve fiber or nerve cell had provided incontrovertible evidence that there is a resting potential across the cell membrane, and that electrical activity in nerves is due to changes in this potential. A great step forward occurred when Alan Hodgkin and Andrew Huxley (1952) provided a specific model for the generation of the impulse by sequential movements of Na and K ions through channels across the membrane. This model has served as the touchstone for all subsequent analyses of nervous activity.

Similar advances were made at about this time in understanding the nature of synaptic actions. At the neuromuscular junction, Fatt and Katz (1951) (see also Nastuk, 1953) obtained evidence for the "end plate potential" induced in the postsynaptic muscle membrane through release of acetylcholine by an impulse invading the presynaptic nerve terminals. Del Castillo and Katz (1954) then showed that this potential is due to simultaneous action of small quantal events linked to release of subunits, presumed by the anatomists to be equivalent to the vesicles. At central synapses, parallel experiments on motoneurons in the spinal cord provided evidence for "excitatory postsynaptic potentials" (EPSPs) due to stimulation of sensory nerves (Brock et al., 1952a), and "inhibitory postsynaptic potentials" (IPSPs) due to stimulation of inhibitory interneurons (Brock et al., 1952b; Coombs et al., 1955). These findings were soon confirmed and extended at a variety of synapses (see the crayfish stretch receptor: Eyzaguirre and Kuffler, 1955), establishing that excitatory and inhibitory synaptic actions are the main modes of communication between neurons. Although physiologists had recognized the importance of inhibition since the time of Sherrington, anatomists had been slow to read this property into their interpretations of connections between neurons; Cajal, for example, never invoked inhibition in his interpretations of neuronal circuits. However, it has come to be recognized as playing a role equally as important as excitation in neural systems.

Although these advances established the main modes of nervous activity, they did not by themselves reveal how that activity spreads within the neuron. This depends on the fact that electrical current spreads in a nerve fiber in a manner similar to the way current spreads in a submarine cable, through a low resistance core, shielded by the surface membrane that has a high resistance and capacitance. The similarity was recognized by the late nineteenth century, and in the work in the 1950s it was established that these cable-like "electrotonic" properties govern the spread of the impulse along an axon. Electric current spread in dendrites was much more difficult to analyze because of the complex branching structure of dendrites, but the methods of Wilfrid Rall (1959) provided the means for understanding how this occurs; with these methods, the way was open to analyzing and understanding the dominant role of dendrites in the integration of excitatory and inhibitory synaptic actions in the neuron.

Reassessment of the Concept of Dynamic Polarization

These new and dramatic findings forced a reappraisal of the neuron as a functional unit. Since the time of Cajal, it had been assumed that the flow of activity in the neuron, from dendrites and cell body through the axon, was by means of impulses similar to those that propagate through peripheral nerves; at synapses, it was imagined that the impulses somehow jumped from one neuron to the next (see Chapters 15, 18). The first direct recordings of the impulse by Gasser and Erlanger (1922) showed that the impulse is very brief, lasting only about one or a few milliseconds (thousands of a second). It was further found that the intensity of nervous reactions was signaled by the frequency of impulse firing (Adrian and Zotterman, 1926). In order to account for slow or long-lasting changes in nervous activity or behavior, it was postulated that repetitive impulse activity was sustained by self-reexcitatory reverberatory circuits (cf. Lorente de Nó, 1938).

By contrast, Sherrington conceived that the synapse had properties different from those of impulses (see Chapter 17), in particular, that it supported long-lasting changes in neuronal excitability. The discovery of the relatively slow (tens of milliseconds) potentials at the neuromuscular endplate, central synapses, and sensory receptors confirmed this idea, and revealed the essence of the mechanism: these junctional potentials involved simultaneous passive movements of Na and/or K ions in opposite directions across the postsynaptic membrane, in contrast to the impulse, which involved sequential movements of these ions in an explosive, regenerative, nonlinear relation to the membrane potential. By virtue of its regenerative property, the impulse was a threshold, "all-or-nothing" event, whereas the junctional potentials were graded in amplitude with the strength of input.

The neuron thus displayed not one, but two, types of activity. How could this be incorporated into the idea of the neuron acting as a functional unit? The resolution seemed to be found in a revision of the "Law of Dynamic Polarization," in which dendrites respond to their synaptic inputs not with an impulse, but with graded synaptic potentials that spread decrementally ("electrotonically") through the dendrites to the cell body and axon where impulses are generated. From this it was a small step to the inference that dendrites are the receptive "graded" response part of the neuron, and the axon is the transmissive "impulse-generating" part.

George Bishop, in a thought-provoking essay on the "Natural history of the nerve impulse" (1956), suggested this specific correlation between structure and function. It is a restatement of Cajal's concept of dynamic polarization, with the substitution of graded synaptic responses in dendrites in place of impulse flow. In Bishop's view "the chief and most characteristic function of nervous and other excitable tissues are performed by means of graded responses." He speculated that the impulse is a specialization, an "incidental expedient," that came along later in evolution to permit communication over longer axons so that brains could get bigger and more complicated.

The process of reassessment was carried forward in 1959 by Theodore Bullock in "Neuron doctrine and electrophysiology." He emphasized four new findings: (1) the nerve impulse is a special property confined to the axon; (2) there is a variety of local graded responses set up in dendrites that can remain local and subthreshold for impulse firing by that neuron; (3) these local responses may also affect other neurons directly by spread of electric current between them "without the intervention of nerve impulses"; and (4) labile and integrative processes such as these occur not only at synapses but can be located at several places in different parts of the neuron.

Bullock proposed that "these changes in viewpoint add up to a quiet but sweeping revolution," a phrase that very much captured the atmosphere of that exciting period when the physiology of the neuron was being studied directly for the first time. He concluded that "anatomically, the neuron doctrine has never been more firm," because the electronmicroscopic studies had proven the case against continuity between neurons (this was just before the discovery of gap junctions; see above). However, with regard to function, he felt there was a need for a "reappraisal," a need he stated eloquently in his conclusion:

> Physiologically . . . we have a new appreciation of the complexity-within-unity of the neuron. Like a person, it is truly a functional unit, but it is composed of parts of very different function. . . . The impulse is not the only form of nerve cell activity; excitation of one part of the neuron does not necessarily involve the whole neuron; many dendrites may not propagate impulses at all; and the synapse is not the only locus of selection, evaluation, fatigue and persistent change. Several forms of graded activity—for example, pacemaker, synaptic, and local potentials—each confined to a circumscribed region or repeating regions of the neuron, can separately or sequentially integrate arriving events, with the history and milieu, to determine output in the restricted region where spikes are initiated. The size, number, and distribution over the neuron of these functionally differentiated regions and the labile coupling functions between the successive processes that eventually determine what information is transferred to the next neuron provide an enormous range of possible complexity within this single cellular unit.

The Problem of Structure-Function Correlations

These two essays emphasized the difficulties in incorporating the new varieties of physiological properties into a simple model that would generalize to all neurons. These attempts introduced a new idea, that a given anatomical structure, as visualized in the Golgi stained neuron, has a given physiological property, specifically, that the axon may be defined as the impulse-generating part of the neuron, and that dendrites may be defined as the graded potential-generating part.

This formula seemed to apply neatly to many large neurons with long axons, such as the spinal motoneuron, but David Bodian recognized that there were problems in trying to make this correlation completely general. As an anatomist, he was aware of the old debate over the dorsal root ganglion cell. In his essay, "The generalized vertebrate neuron" (1962), he took issue with the common definition of dendrites as receptor structures that arise from the cell body and conduct synaptic activity toward it, pointing out that this definition could not apply to the dorsal root ganglion cell, "which has no synaptically activated dendrites associated with the cell body." He recalled that Cajal, in his final formulation of the "Law of Dynamic Polarization" in 1897 (see Chapter 15), deduced that the flow of activity may proceed directly from dendrites to axon, bypassing the cell body, as in the dorsal root ganglion cell (see Fig. 27) or other cells (see Fig. 28). Bodian further invoked Bishop's suggestion that the peripheral nerve endings of the "axons" of these cells were like dendrites, because they give decremental responses to sensory stimulation, which spread to the site where myelination begins to set up impulses. In this way, the dorsal root ganglion cell, despite the extreme differentiation of its peripheral dendrite into an axon-like myelinated process, and its unipolar cell body, could nonetheless be made to conform to Cajal's generalized functional model of a neuron because it had the three main parts: the graded response "dendrites" were the nerve endings of the peripheral "axon"; the transmission apparatus began at the most peripheral site of myelination and continued through the peripheral "axon" and central axon to the spinal cord; and the apparatus of emission was the axonal branches, or telodendria, in the spinal cord; the position of the cell body, attached to the nerve by its unipolar stalk, was incidental.

These aspects of the new findings were debated by some within the context of the neuron doctrine, but most workers ignored the finer points. As long as experimental analysis was restricted to large cells with long axons, such as the spinal motoneuron, the physiological properties of synaptic responses and impulse generation could be relatively easily assimilated within Cajal's concept of the dynamically polarized neuron. Thus, the common view was that axon terminals on dendrites and cell bodies set up either EPSPs or IPSPs; the excitatory depolarization and inhibitory hyperpolarization spread electrotonically to the cell body, where the algebraic summation of the two opposing effects controls the generation of impulses, which then propagate through the axon to the axon terminals, to activate the synapses onto the target neurons (see Eccles, 1957). The sequence, from input axons to dendrites and cell body to output from axon terminals, seemed like a neat and logical scheme for input-output operations, one that could apply to the wide range of shapes and sizes that different neurons display.

However, apart from the problems of correlating structure with function discussed earlier, the simple model for the neuron was encountering some other rude facts. For example, in most neurons the most obvious place for impulse generation to occur seemed to be at origin of the axon from the axon hillock. A careful test of this hypothesis in the large crayfish stretch receptor neuron showed that, instead, the impulse arises at some distance along the initial segment (Edwards and Ottoson, 1958). Evidence for sites of impulse generation in dendritic trees began to be uncovered (Eccles et al., 1958; Spencer and Kandel, 1961). Several instances of axo-axonal connections were found, that is, synapses by one type of axon onto another (e.g., the giant synapse of crayfish or squid), or one type of axon terminal onto another (e.g., crayfish muscle: Dudel and Kuffler, 1961; afferent fibers onto spinal motoneurons: Eccles et al., 1961). Axo-axonal synapses were certainly incompatible with the idea that the axon terminal is only an output structure, as presumed in the model of the polarized neuron, yet there was no doubt that the ability of one axon terminal to gate the effect of another terminal on a target neuron was a useful design feature for neural circuits.

Dendro-Dendritic Synapses

Despite these departures from classical ideas, they could still be viewed as exceptions that proved the rule. A more difficult problem was posed by neurons that lack axons, such as the granule cells of the olfactory bulb and amacrine cells of the retina. As long as the axon was regarded as the output part of the neuron, these anaxonal cells could never be covered by the "Law of Dynamic Polarization."

The solution to the problem of the olfactory granule cell came from physiological studies suggesting that granule cells function as inhibitory interneurons onto mitral cells (Phillips et al., 1963). An early computational study, using the methods of Rall, suggested that mitral cell dendrites synaptically excite the granule cells, and the excited granule cell dendrites then inhibit the mitral cell dendrites; anatomical studies then demonstrated reciprocal dendro-dendritic synapses between these two types of dendrite which could mediate these interactions (Rall et al., 1966; Rall and Shepherd, 1968). Parallel electronmicroscopical and electrophysiological studies in the retina provided evidence for analogous synaptic arrangements and interactions between amacrine cell dendrites and the processes of bipolar, ganglion, and other amacrine cells (Dowling and Boycott, 1966; Werblin and Dowling, 1968) (see Fig. 42). Various kinds of dendrodendritic synaptic arrangements were soon revealed in a number of other regions of the nervous system.

The new aspects of neuronal organization revealed by these studies included the following (Rall et al., 1966; Shepherd, 1974): (1) dendrites can be sites of synaptic output as well as synaptic inputs; (2) activation of output synapses from dendrites may occur through depolarization by local graded synaptic potentials or by active impulse spread; and (3) parts of a dendritic tree may serve as local subunits for synaptic input and output, functioning to some extent independently of other dendritic units and of impulse output through an axon (if an axon is present). These aspects greatly enlarged

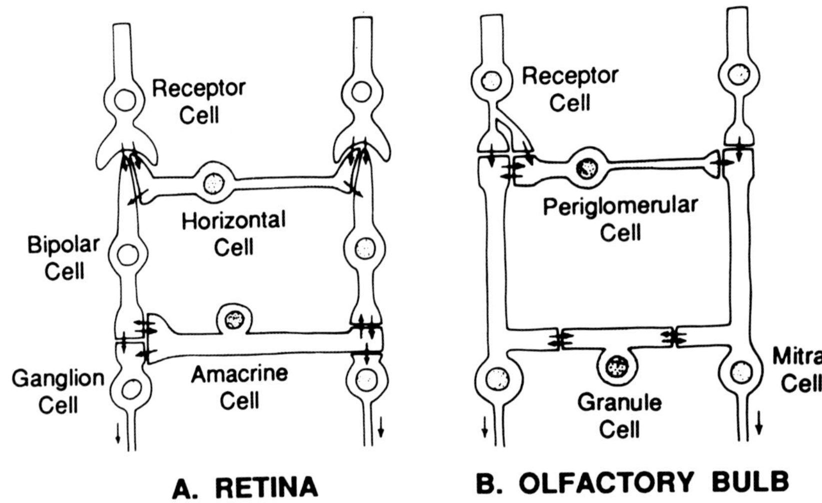

Fig. 42. Simplified diagrams summarizing the overall organization of the retina and the olfactory bulb as revealed by modern microscopical and electrophysiological studies. The arrows indicate the sites and directions of synaptic connections. The diagrams help to bring out the overall similarities in synaptic organization of these regions, and the complexity of synaptic connections. These diagrams may be compared with the diagrams of Cajal of the retina (Fig. 35) and olfactory bulb (Fig. 34). (See text). (From Shepherd, 1974)

the possible repertoire of input-output units contained in a single neuron, much as envisaged by Bullock, but now in terms of specific synaptic circuits. The new findings also proved that there is not a strict correlation between structure and function in the different parts of the neuron. Thus, similar structures may subserve different functions (e.g., dendrites may be presynaptic as well as postsynaptic; dendrites may support action potentials in addition to graded synaptic potentials); by the same token, different structures may support similar functions (e.g., recurrent inhibition may take place through axon collateral pathways or through dendro-dendritic pathways).

How could these new findings be reconciled with the classical view of the polarized neuron, and with the revisions reviewed above? A first step was to start with Bullock's idea of "complexity within unity" and recognize that the nervous system is built up of a hierarchy of levels of organization. It was proposed that, in a formal sense, at each level in the hierarchy, elementary neuronal structures interact to form the functional units that underly the next higher level of organization (Shepherd, 1972). In this hierarchy, the whole neuron does indeed function as a unit, but it defines only one level of organization; contained within it are several lower levels of functional subunits, and above it are several higher levels of multineuronal units (see below). The formation of these different levels is to a large extent an expression of the complexity of "local circuits" within each region (Rakic, 1976).

Seen from this perspective, the "Law of Dynamic Polarization" still expresses a correct concept about the overall flow of activity in most kinds of neurons at the level of the whole neuron. In particular, output neurons with long axons must receive synaptic inputs in their dendrites and somata and send synaptic outputs to target neurons in other regions through their long axons. However, within a region, and within a neuron, this overall constraint no longer applies, and synaptic inputs and outputs can occur at any point on a neuron (cf. Bodian, 1972). Moreover, there may, in addition, be any arbitrary combination of active, voltage-gated membrane properties to carry out one or more kind of physiological operation at that point (see Llinás, 1988). Hence, the emerging idea of "the neuron as a complex system."

What functions does this complexity subserve? For this, we need to introduce a new tenet to the neuron doctrine. We shall do this after considering the remaining two tenets of the traditional doctrine.

The Neuron as a Genetic Unit

The observation by Harrison of the outgrowth of nerve fibers from embryonic nerve cells appeared to settle once and for all that the nerve cell is the developmental, or genetic, unit of the nervous system. The fact that a neuron has a single nucleus containing the genetic material—DNA—that controls its development supports this idea.

Although this tenet thus appears to be on very firm ground, there are several interesting aspects to be considered. One is the fact that cells may merge during development. Thus, some axons in invertebrates are formed by end-to-end merging of component axonal segments, each containing its own nucleus. Skeletal muscles of vertebrates are multinucleated, reflecting the fact that a single mature fiber is formed by the complete merging of many immature myotubes. Thus, the cell theory itself must be qualified to encompass these kinds of innovations.

A more serious challenge to the genetic unity of the cell and the neuron has been the gap junction. As noted before, this type of junction allows direct exchange between cells of electric current, ions, and small molecules up to about 500 daltons. Since gap junctions are prevalent early in development, there has been much speculation that they allow for the exchange of small molecules that could have gene-regulating functions. The functions might modify regulation of cell differentiation and/or cell growth (cf. Loewenstein, 1981; Alberts et al., 1988). Thus, gene expression in a cell is under control of regulatory elements both within that cell and from surrounding cells. This would help to explain how gene expression is coordinated between neighboring cells.

In the explosion of work on the nervous system in recent years, studies of development have been one of the most active areas, as the full cycle of neuronal birth, proliferation, differentiation, migration, maturation, degeneration, and death has come under study. With respect to the critical step of forming connections, there has been a shift from the older view that this was primarily under the control of recognition factors between the pre- and postsynaptic elements, toward a view that stresses the importance of competitive interactions between ingrowing fibers for postsynaptic targets, that determine which connections will survive (cf. Easter et al., 1984). The final pattern of connections is thus the outcome of both genetic and environmental factors.

The Neuron as a Metabolic Unit

Modern cell biology is built on the general rule that DNA is transcribed in the nucleus to RNA, and that messenger RNA is then transported to the cytoplasm where it is translated into enzymes that carry out the metabolic functions of the cell. The genetic unity of the cell thus is closely associated with metabolic unity of the cell. Metabolic functions include the enzymatic synthesis and degradation of molecules used in a vast range of functions. In neurons, these molecules go into the construction of a variety of organelles, which include the internal cytoskeleton, which imparts to neurons their characteristic elaborate branching forms; internal membranes involved in synthesis of hormones and neurotransmitters; microtubules involved in transport within the dendrites and axons; and the synapse. Far from being static structures, axons and dendrites are like busy motorways and railways, constantly shuttling substances from their sites of manufacture in the cell to their retail outlets in the peripheral branches; there is now a variety of methods for using this transport to demonstrate neuronal connections (cf. Cowan et al., 1972). At the synapse, neurons must provide for a variety of external signal molecules (neurotransmitters and neurohormones) and a variety of internal signaling molecules (cyclic nucleotides, lipid derivatives, etc.).

Multineuronal Metabolic Units

The traditional concept of the neuron as a metabolic unit originated in Forel's deduction, from the early observations of Waller, that degeneration following injury to a nerve does not spread forward beyond the injured nerve endings (Chapter 9), and the further observation that the degeneration does not spread back beyond the cell bodies of the cells that give rise to the injured nerves (retrograde degeneration). The development of special methods for staining degenerating axon terminals opened the door to the modern analysis of neuronal connections (cf. Nauta, 1956). However, even in classical times it was recognized that "transynaptic atrophy" could occur (see Meyer, 1971). This implies that neurons exchange substances that are involved in the maintenance of metabolic functions of neighbors. A recent example, among many, is the finding that degeneration of olfactory nerve fibers causes down-regulation in the target neurons in the olfactory bulb of tyrosine hydroxylase, the enzyme that synthesizes the neurotransmitter dopamine (Baker et al., 1983). Many studies, in fact, have demonstrated transynaptic transport, that is, the transport of substances between neurons. Thus, amino acids injected into the eye are not only taken up by retinal ganglion cells and synthesized into protein that is then transported within the axon to the lateral geniculate nucleus, but some of the proteins are transferred to the target neurons in the lateral geniculate nucleus and transported through their axons to the usual receiving areas in the cerebral cortex (Wiesel et al., 1974). Although only a small percentage of protein is exchanged transynaptically, it nonetheless shows that the metabolic machinery of neurons is dependent on interactions across their cell membranes.

This argument is even more persuasive in the case of small molecules. As we have discussed before, gap junctions have a sufficient diameter of interconnecting channels to allow the exchange of molecules up to a size of about 20 Ångstrøms, which includes most molecules that are sources of energy metabolism (e.g., sugars), amino acids, nucleotides, or metabolic breakdown products, up to a molecular weight of approximately 500. This raises obvious questions about the metabolic unity of the cell for these substances. However, it remains true that gap junctions are not frequent between neurons in many regions of the nervous system; by contrast, they could play a much larger role in neuroglia, where gap junctions are much more common (cf. Peters et al., 1990). Even when they are present, their potency and directionality is likely to be closely regulated by a variety of means, as noted earlier.

Metabolic Subunits Within the Neuron

Thus far we have considered only the relations between neurons that make a single neuron a part of multineuronal metabolic units. By contrast, it is becoming clear that the neuron is not one homogeneous metabolic unit but rather is composed of distinct metabolic subunits. The most obvious subdivision is between the axon and the dendrite. Although these two types of structures share many aspects of cell structure and function, the singular character and, particularly, the great length of many axons, impose quite different metabolic demands. There are special properties and arrangements of microtubules within axons to provide for transport of vesicles and substances over these long hauls. Since the axon terminals are at such a great distance from the cell body, they must act as relatively independent structural, functional, and metabolic units in carrying out such functions as vesicle storage, transmitter uptake, and presynaptic autoregulation. Current studies on neurons grown in tissue culture, using the methods introduced by Harrison (Chapter 17), are aimed at identifying the molecular basis for the differentiation of axons from dendrites (cf. Dotti et al., 1988).

On the dendritic side, special interest has been focused on the spines that characterize the distal branches of so many types of neurons (see Fig. 43). The early electronmicroscopical studies fully confirmed Cajal's belief that these are real structures, showing that they are small outcroppings that are the sites of synaptic inputs (some spines are the sites of synaptic outputs as well; see above). There were early speculations that the high resistance of the spine neck would attenuate the spread of synaptic potentials from the spine, but it required the methods of Rall to describe how the spine neck may be important in controlling the spread of membrane potential changes into and out of the spine head, and how activity-dependent changes in that control might be a basis for learning (cf. Rall and Rinzel, 1971). By analogy, it was also realized that the narrow spine neck (0.05 to 0.2 micrometers in diameter) would also limit the diffusion and transport of substances, "through which long-term control over metabolic processes in the spine could be exerted" (Shepherd, 1974), thus creating a local microenvironment subject to maximal effect by local synaptic action. Supporting this notion of the spine as a metabolic unit is the fact that some spines show accumulations of ribosomes, where protein synthesis is carried out, at the spine neck origins (cf. Steward and Levy, 1982) or even within the spines. Mitochondria are also present at these sites to provide immediate supplies of metabolic energy. Such spines are the sites of synaptic inputs that are not only generally excitatory onto the postsynaptic neuron, but also display a range of activity-dependent synaptic and intrinsic membrane properties that are believed to underly learning and memory (reviewed in Brown and Zador, 1990). It therefore appears that spines provide a dendritic tree with a large population of microcompartments, each supporting the metabolic requirements of a semiindependent functional subunit within the whole neuron.

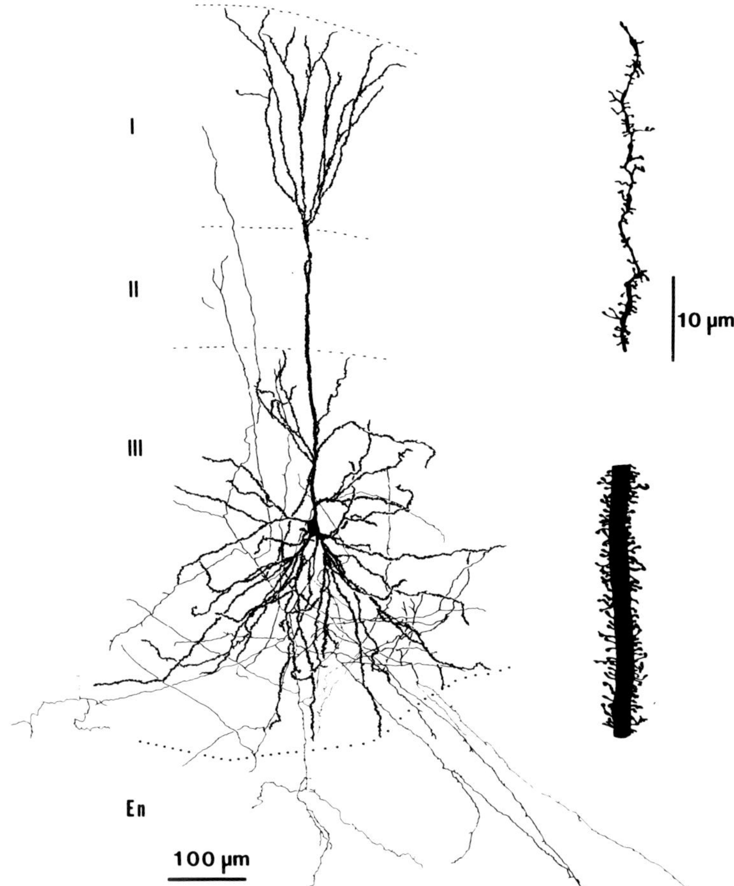

Fig. 43. Example of a cell injected intracellularly with a dye (lucifer yellow) and then visualized by reacting with an antiserum. This is a deep pyramidal cell in the olfactory cortex of a rat. The fine processes below are the axon and axon collaterals. On the right are shown proximal and distal segments of apical dendrite covered with dendritic spines. These modern methods have confirmed the basic patterns of neuronal branching shown by the Golgi method, while revealing new details of structure and interconnection. (From Tseng and Haberly, 1989)

Revising the Neuron Doctrine

We may conclude that much of the neuron doctrine has stood the test of time (see Peters et al., 1990, for a scholarly retrospective). This is the more remarkable in that over half a century passed, between the 1890s and 1950s, before the theory could be adequately tested. Since then, it has served well as the theoretical basis for the great advances in modern times in understanding the cellular basis of nervous function. In fact, one may fairly observe that most workers in neuroscience simply accept the idea that the neuron is the basic unit of the nervous system in all the ways contained in the four tenets, because it provides an adequate basis for planning and performing experiments on the nervous system and interpreting most of the results. Few theories in science have met such demanding tests over so many years with such obvious success.

Despite this impressive achievement, it is clear from this review that the forward surge of research over the past 40 years has revealed many aspects of cellular structure and function that were not predicted either for cells in general by the cell theory or nerve cells in particular by the neuron doctrine. An enlarged view that builds on the classical neuron doctrine and incorporates the new findings discussed here would want to include the following elements:

1. Neurons, like all cells, are formed by common cellular macromolecules and organelles, surrounded by a continuous surface membrane. Some neurons (and especially neuroglia) are connected directly with each other through gap (electrical) junctions. These allow, when appropriately gated, the intercellulular passage of electric current, ions, and small molecules that can mediate a variety of functional interactions.

2. In most neurons, dendrites receive synaptic inputs and axons carry impulse outputs, consistent with the classical idea of dynamic polarization. However, in many neurons, dendrites can also have synaptic outputs, and axons can also have inputs from other axons.

3. In most neurons, synaptic responses occur in dendrites and are graded in amplitude, whereas impulses occur in axons and have a voltage-gated, all-or-nothing character. However, dendrites may also contain voltage-gated sites, and some axons may not support all-or-nothing impulses.

4. It follows from points 1–3 that any point in a neuron may function as a local processing subunit, by means of gap junctions, synaptic inputs or outputs, voltage-gated properties, or local metabolic machinery, its interactions with other subunits dependent on the electrotonic coupling between them.

5. The local subunits of varying properties mean that there is not a fixed correlation of structure and function within the different parts of the neuron; axons and dendrites provide flexible substrates in which a variety of membrane channels and local organelles can be expressed that can support different types of physiological properties and functional operations.

6. The neuron remains a basic anatomical, physiological, genetic, and metabolic unit, as proposed in the classical doctrine. It is the first point of departure for analyzing and understanding the development and the func-

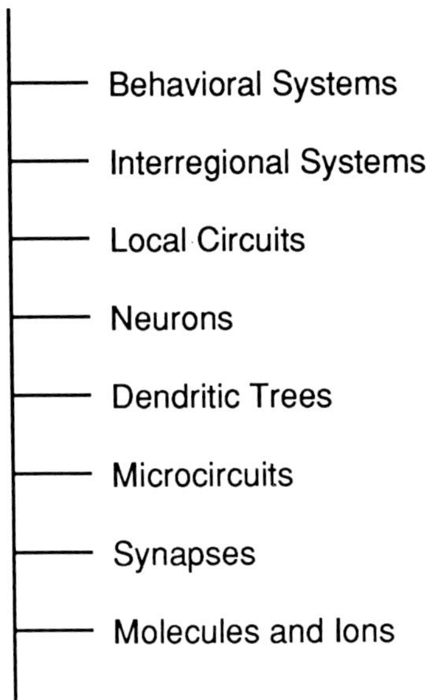

Fig. 44. Levels of organization in the nervous system. Each level represents a type of functional unit that forms the basis for the organization of the next higher level. Note that the neuron is only one type of functional unit, at a relatively intermediate level in the hierarchy. (From Shepherd and Koch, 1990)

tional organization of the nervous system, in health and disease. However, it is not the only unit; it contains several levels of local subunits, and is itself a part of larger multineuronal units. An understanding of the neuronal basis of nervous function depends on understanding the relations between these different levels of organization (Fig. 44).

Future Directions

Despite the 50 years of work that led to the classical neuron doctrine, the progress over the past 100 years, and the accelerated pace of recent research, our understanding of the neuron is still at an early stage. Perhaps the greatest legacy of the classical neuron doctrine in guiding work in the future will be its emphasis on the fact that the neuron shares in all the essential attributes and mechanisms of cells in general. It thus provides the appropriate framework within which to apply the armamentarium of modern molecular and cellular methods. That armamentarium has had an explosive growth in recent years, and it may be expected to continue to grow in the future. The essential principle contained in the neuron doctrine is that virtually everything we learn about molecular and cellular mechanisms in any type of cell of the body from the application of these methods is likely to deepen our understanding of similar or equivalent mechanisms in nerve cells; by the same token, advances in understanding of nerve cells will contribute to broad biological principles as well. We have gotten away from thinking of neurons as specialized only for transmitting rapid electrical signals, and now we see them as expressing the widest possible range of cellular properties. The genius of the classical neuron doctrine was the expression of this basic and very modern outlook, contained in the four tenets of structure, function, metabolism, and development.

Apart from expressing a rich inventory of common cellular properties, neurons do something that is very different from other cells of the body: they process information. It seems likely therefore that a major contribution of research in the future will be to add a fifth tenet: the neuron as a basic *information processing* unit in the nervous system. This idea originated in the paper of Warren McCulloch and Walter Pitts (1943); they postulated that neurons might be interconnected in ways that could generate logic operations, and pointed out the similarity to the logic circuits of a digital computer. The intervening years have seen this initiative extended by new fields of study that include information theory, cybernetics, artificial intelligence, and, most recently, parallel distributed processing and neural networks. An irony of this work, noted in Chapters 8 and 19 above, is that the present generation of neural networks represents a view of nervous organization that harkens back to that of Golgi: the view that the complex interconnectedness of networks is more important than the details of neuronal structure and function.

At present the precise relevance of much of this work to real nervous systems is unclear; certainly McCulloch and Pitts' neurons and neural network nodes are too simple to represent the characteristic branching patterns of neurons first described by Cajal and his coworkers in the classical era, much less the complex array of biochemical and physiological processes revealed by modern research. However, the merit of these simple networks is that for the first time they provide tools and concepts for analyzing how systems might process information in order to simulate such cognitive functions as image recognition, memory, and language. An exciting challenge for the future is to incorporate real neuron properties into these networks. This will be an important means toward the end of obtaining an understanding of the biological basis of human thought built on first principles, means and end, one feels, that would have won the approval of the pioneers of the neuron doctrine.

Comment on Sources

With regard to primary sources in the classical literature, I have in all but a few of the earliest and briefest extracts (as noted) located and studied the original documents or their contemporaneous translations. Relatively little of the classical literature on the work contributing to the neuron doctrine was translated into English at the time, nor has it become available since. Translations have therefore constituted a major undertaking for the present work. Translations from the German have been done by Grethe Shepherd and Carol Hightower; from the French by Grethe Shepherd, Lisbeth Shepherd, and myself; from the Spanish by Javier DeFelipe, Tali Zulman, and myself; from the Italian by Juliana Vanucchi; and from the Norwegian by Grethe Shepherd, Kirsten Shepherd, and myself. Contemporary translations of Golgi into German and Ramón y Cajal into French were the main means of communicating their results to the scientific world at large, and I have used these as well as contemporaneous translations into English where available. I have also drawn on translations by Clarke and O'Malley (1968) and other sources in several cases, and have modified them in some cases with subheadings and other minor changes for improved readability. Even when I have provided my own partial or complete translations, I have noted alternative translations of those documents that are available in the literature, in order to assist the reader, and in order to draw attention to these other documents. All translations from the literature are fully acknowledged in the text.

A major problem facing the translation of documents in the classical literature is the very fact that the terminology was in a state of development, and many of the terms were cumbersome and have been supplanted by modern forms. Chief among these is "axis cylinder" for what we now call the "axon," and "protoplasmic prolongation" for what we now call "dendrite." In keeping with the guideline to render translations of the documents that are as literal and accurate as possible, I have retained the original terms, but have added the modern terms in brackets [ ] wherever it seemed it would aid the reader. This convention is essential because much of the debate in the classical literature concerned the meaning of the classical terms; the debate would be meaningless if not rendered in its original language. In this way I hope to have preserved the historical integrity of the documents while making them more readily accessible to the modern reader. A further warning is that the literal nature of the translations means that the prose is neither more nor less turgid than the original; I have done my best to make for readability, but if the original was obscure, it was a historical fact.

It may be useful to indicate some more readily available background material for the present study. As noted in Chapter 1, a basic reference for several of the documents is the section on "The Neuron" in Clarke and O'Malley's massive work, *The Human Brain and Spinal Cord* (1968). Anyone studying the development of ideas about the neuron is deeply indebted to this fine book. The present volume differentiates itself in including a number of articles and translations not considered by Clarke and O'Malley; in including a substantial number of scientists not covered by them, such as Leydig, Freud, Nansen, van Gehuchten, Schafer, Retzius, and von Lenhossék; and in being written from a perspective of current issues. Particularly fine accounts of the development of studies of the neuron in the nineteenth century are to be found in Liddell's *The Discovery of Reflexes* (1960), Meyer's *Historical Aspects of Cerebral Anatomy* (1971), the series of deft biographical sketches in Haymaker's *The Founders of Neurology* (1953), and van der Loos' review "The history of the neuron" (1967).

Among the older literature, a particularly good place to start is the masterful overview in Barker's *The Nervous System and its Constituent Neurons* (1899). However, for the full flavor of the debate surrounding the issues at stake, nothing replaces the documents themselves. Among those in English, Kölliker (1853), Nansen (1887), Golgi (1906), and Retzius (1908) are especially insightful. From 1888 on Ramón y Cajal is the key figure in the story. For the English-speaking student, Cajal's Nobel Prize lecture (1906; translated in 1967) paired with Golgi; his final summing up of the neuron versus reticular debate (1933); and his autobiography, *Recollections of My Life* (1937; reprinted in 1989), convey vividly his intellectual depth and integrity, and his zest for life. The translation and commentary by Javier DeFelipe and E. G. Jones (1988) in *Cajal on the Cerebral Cortex,* and by Neeland and Larry Swanson in the very recent *New Ideas on the Structure of the Nervous*

System in Man and Vertebrates (Cajal, 1894/1991), are essential complements to the accounts in the present book.

Although the necessity for translation of most of the original papers places a burden on the English-speaking reader, it reflects a particularly attractive aspect of the work on the neuron doctrine, namely, the extent to which it embraced such a diversity of workers of different nationalities spread throughout Europe in the nineteenth century. Among the nationalities represented here were German, Austrian, Swiss, Czech, Spanish, Italian, Hungarian, Russian, Belgian, Danish, Swedish, Norwegian, French, and English. Americans became involved toward the turn of the century. To the present writer this diversity stands as an inspirational testimony to the international character of science.

References

Adrian, E. D., and Lucas, K. (1912). Summation of propagated disturbances in nerve and muscle. *J. Physiol. London* 44: 68.

Adrian, E. D., and Zotterman, Y. (1926). The impulses produced by sensory nerve endings. Part 2. The response of a single end-organ. *J. Physiol. London* 61: 151–171.

Alberts, B., Bray, D., Lewis, J., Raff, M., Roberts, K., and Watson, J. D. (1988). *Molecular Biology of the Cell.* New York: Garland.

Amacher, P. (1965). Freud's neurological education and its influence on psychoanalytic theory *Psychol. Issues* 4, Monograph 16: 1–95.

Apáthy, S. (1897). Das leitende Element des Nervensystems und seine topographischen Beziehungen zu den Zellen. *Mittheil. aus der zool. Station zu Neapel. Bd. xii, H. r,* pp. 495–748.

Baker, H., Kawano, T., Margolis, F. L., and Joh, T. H. (1983). Transneuronal regulation of tyrosine hydroxylase expression in olfactory bulb of mouse and rat. *J. Neurosci.* 3: 69–78.

Barker, L. F. (1899). *The Nervous System and its Constituent Neurons.* New York: D. Appleton and Company.

Barker, L. F. (1942). *Time and the Physician. The Autobiography of Lewellys F. Barker.* New York: Putnam.

Barker, L. F. (1943). Obituary notice. *South. Med. J.* 36: 657–658. *J. A. M. A.* 122: 889. *Can. M. A. J.* : 244. *Bull. Med. Lib. Assoc.* 31: 372–373.

Bartelmez, G. W. (1953). Johannes Evangelista Purkinje. In *The Founders of Neurology* (W. Haymaker, ed.). Springfield, Ill.: Charles C. Thomas. pp. 70–73.

Bell, C. (1811). *Idea of a New Anatomy of the Brain Submitted for the Observations of his Friends.* [London: Straham and Preston]; Reprinted *J. Anat. Physiol.* (1869) 3: 147–182; *Med. Class.* (1936) 1: 105–120; Gordon-Taylor and Walls (1958) pp. 218–231.

Bellonci, G. (1881). Contribuzione alla istologia del cervelletto. Accademia dei Lincei. Gennaio. pp. 45–49.

Bennett, M. V. L., Aljure, E., Nakajima, Y., and Pappas, G. D. (1963). Electrotonic junctions between teleost spinal neurons: electrophysiology and ultrastructure. *Science* 141: 262–264.

Bernfeld, S. (1944). Freud's earliest theories and the school of Helmholtz. *Psychoanal. Q.* 13: 341–362.

Bernfeld, S. (1947). An unknown autobiographical fragment by Freud. *Yearbook of Psychoanalysis* 3: 15–29.

Bernfeld, S. (1950). Freud's scientific beginnings. *Yearbook of Psychoanalysis* 6: 24–50.

Bernfeld, S. (1951). Sigmund Freud, M.D., 1882–1885. *Intl. J. Psycho-Analysis* 32: 204–217.

Bernstein, J. (1902). Untersuchungen zur Thermodynamik der biolektrischen Ströme. *Pflügers Arch* 92: 521–562.

Bichat, M.-F. X. (1801). *Anatomie Générale Appliquée à la Physiologie et à la Médecine.* Paris: Brosson, Gabon.

Bishop, G. H. (1956). Natural history of the nerve impulse. *Physiol. Rev.* 36: 376–399.

Bodian, D. (1962). The generalized vertebrate neuron. *Science* 137: 323–326.

Bodian, D. (1972). Synaptic diversity and characterization by electron microscopy. In *Structure and Function of Synapses* (G. D. Pappas and D. P. Purpura, eds.). New York: Raven. pp. 45–66.

Bowditch, H. P. (1871). Über die Eigentumlichkeiten der Reizbarkheit welche die Muskelfasern des Herzen zeigen. *Ber. sächs. Akad. Wiss., Math.-nat. Klasse* 23: 652–689.

Brock, L. G., Coombs, J. S., and Eccles, J. C. (1952a). The recording of potentials from motorneurones with an intracellular electrode. *J. Physiol. London* 117: 431–460.

Brock, L. G., Coombs, J. S., and Eccles, J. C. (1952b). The nature of the monosynaptic excitatory and inhibitory processes in the spinal cord. *Proc. R. Soc. London Series B* 140: 170–176.

Brown, T. H., and Zador, A. M. (1990). Hippocampus. In *The Synaptic Organization of the Brain* (G. M. Shepherd, ed.). Third edition. New York: Oxford University Press. pp. 346–388.

Brögger, W. C., and Rolfsen, N. (1896). *Fridtiof Nansen.* London: Longman's.

Brun, R. (1936). Sigmund Freud's Leistungen auf dem Gebiete der organische Neurologie. *Schw. Arch. f. Neur. u. Psychiat.* 37: 200–207.

Bucholz, R. (1863). Bemerkungen über den histologischen Bau des Centralnervensystems der Süsswassermollusken. *Arch. F. Anat. u. Phys.*

Bullock, T. H. (1959). Neuron doctrine and electrophysiology. *Science* 129: 997–1002.

Burdon Sanderson, J. (1911). Ludwig and modern physiology. In *John Burdon Sanderson* (by Lady Burdon Sanderson). London: Oxford University Press.

Byck, R. (ed.). (1974). *Cocaine Papers. Sigmund Freud.* New York: Meridian.

Bynum, W. F., and Heilbron, J. L. (1991) Eighteen ninety one and all that. *Nature* 349: 9–10.

Cajal, S. Ramón y. (1887). Notas de laboratorio: I. Textura de la fibra muscular de los mamiferos. *Boletin Medico Valenciano.* Junio.

Cajal, S. Ramón y. (1888a). Observations sur la texture des fibres musculaires des pattes et des ailes des insectes. *Int. J. Anat. Physiol.* 5: 205–232; 253–276.

Cajal, S. Ramón y (1888b). Estructura de los centros nerviosos de las aves. *Rev. trim.*

Histol. norm. patol. 1: 1–10. (Reprinted in *Trabajos escogidos,* tomo 1. Madrid: Jimenez y Molina. 1924. pp. 305–315)

Cajal, S. Ramón y (1888c). Estructura de la rétina de las aves. *Revista trim. de Histol. norm. patol.* 1: 11–32

Cajal, S. Ramón y (1888d). Sobre las fibras nerviosas de la capa molecular del cerebelo. *Rev. trim. Histol. norm. patol.* 1: 33–49.

Cajal, S. Ramón y (1888e). Estructura del cerebelo. *Gac. méd. Catalana* 11: 449–457.

Cajal, S. Ramón y (1889a). Contribución al estudio de la estructura de la médula espinal. *Rev. trim. Histol. norm. patol.* 1: 79–106.

Cajal, S. Ramón y (1889b). Sur la morphologie et les connexions des éléments de la rétine des oiseaux. *Anat. Anz.* 4: 111–121.

Cajal, S. Ramón y (1889c). Conexión general de los elementos nerviosos. *La Medicina Práctica* 2: 341–346. (Reprinted in *Trabajos escogidos,* tomo 1. Madrid: Jimenez y Molina. 1924. pp. 478–487)

Cajal, S. Ramón y (1890a). A quelle époque apparaisent les expansions des cellules nerveuses de la moëlle épinière du poulet? *Anat. Anz.* 5: 631–639.

Cajal, S. Ramón y (1890b). Sobre la existencia ce células nerviosas especiales en la primera capa de las circunvoluciones cerebrales. *Gac. méd. Catalana* 13: 737–739. (Republished 1924 in *Trabajos Escogidos* 1: 625–628. Madrid: Jimenez y Molina.)

Cajal, S. Ramón y (1891a). Pequeñas contribuciones al conocimiento del sistema nervioso. I: Estructura y conexiones de los ganglios simpáticos. II: Estructura fundamental de la corteza cerebral de los batracios, reptiles y aves. III: Estructura de la retina de los reptiles y batracios. IV: Estructura de la médula espinal de los reptiles. *Trabajos del Laboratorio Histológico de la Facultad de Medicina, Barcelona* : 1–56.

Cajal, S. Ramón y (1891b). Sur la structure de l'écorce cérébrale de quelques mammifères. *La Cellule* 7: 125–176.

Cajal, S. Ramón y (1892a). La rétine des vertébrés. *La Cellule* 9: 119–257.

Cajal, S. Ramón y (1892b). El nuevo concepto de la histología de los centros nerviosos. *Rev. Ciencias Méd.* 18: 457–476.

Cajal, S. Ramón y (1894a). The Croonian Lecture: La fine structure des centres nerveux. *Proc. R. Soc. London Series B* 55: 444–467.

Cajal, S. Ramón y (1894b). The minute structure of the nervous centres. *B. med. J.* 98: 141–140.

Cajal, S. Ramón y (1894c). *Les Nouvelles Ideés sur la Structure du Système Nerveux chez l'Homme et chez les Vertébrés.* Paris: Reinwald.

Cajal, S. Ramón y (1896). Nouvelles contributions à l'étude histologique de la rétine et à la question des anastomoses des prolongements protoplasmiques. *J. Anat. Physiol., Paris* 33: 481–543.

Cajal, S. Ramón y (1906). Les structures et les connexions des cellules nerveux. In *Les Prix Nobel 1904–1906.* Stockholm: Norstedt.

Cajal, S. Ramón y (1909, 1911). *Histologie du système nerveux de l'homme et des vertébrés.* (Translation by L. Azoulay). Paris: Maloine, 2 vols.

Cajal, S. Ramón y (1917). *Recuerdos de mi vida, Vol. 2 : Historia de mi labor científica.* Madrid: Moya.

Cajal, S. Ramón y (1928). *Degeneration and Regeneration of the Nervous System.* (Translated and edited by Raoul M. May). London: Oxford University Press.

Cajal, S. Ramón y (1933). ¿Neuronismo o Reticularismo? Las pruebas objetivas de la unidad anatómica de las células nerviosas. *Arch. Neurobiol. Madrid* 13: 1–144.

Cajal, S. Ramón y (1955). *Studies on the Cerebral Cortex (Limbic Structures).* (Translated by Lisbeth Kraft). London: Lloyd-Luke.

Cajal, S. Ramón y (1967). The structure and connexions of neurons. Nobel Lecture, December 12, 1906. In *Nobel Lectures. Physiology or Medicine 1901–21.* New York: Elsevier Publishing Company, pp. 220–253.

Cajal, S. Ramón y (1989). *Recollections of My Life.* (Translated by E. H. Craigie with the assistance of J. Cano). Philadelphia: American Philosophical Society (1937). Reprinted (1989) Cambridge, Mass.: MIT Press.

Cajal, S. Ramón y (1990). *New Ideas on the Structure of the Nervous System in Man and Vertebrates.* (English translation of *Les Nouvelles Idées sur la Structure des Centres Nerveux chez l'Homme et chez les Vertébrés* by N. Swanson and L. W. Swanson). Cambridge, Mass.: MIT Press.

Cannon, D. F. (1949). *Explorer of the Human Brain.* New York: Henry Schuman.

Carnoy, J. B. (1884). *Biologie cellulaire.* Fasc. 1. Lierre: van In. pp. 192–193, and Fig. 38.

Chorobski, J. (1936). Camillo Golgi. In *Neurological Biographies and Addresses.* London: Oxford University Press.

Clarke, E., and O'Malley, C. D. (1968). *The Human Brain and Spinal Cord.* Berkeley: University of California Press.

Coombs, J. S., Eccles, J. C., and Fatt, P. (1955a). The specific ionic conductances and the ionic movements across the motoneuronal membrane that produce the inhibitory post-synaptic potential. *J. Physiol. London* 130: 326–373.

Coombs, J. S., Eccles, J. C., and Fatt, P. (1955b). Excitatory synaptic action in motoneurones. *J. Physiol. London* 130: 374–395.

Courville, C. B. (1953). Santiago Ramón y Cajal. In *The Founders of Neurology* (W. Haymaker, ed.). Springfield, Ill.: Charles C. Thomas. pp. 74–76.

Cowan, W. M., Gottlieb, D. I., Hendrickson, A. E., Price, J. L., and Woolsey, T. A. (1972). The autodiographic demonstration of axonal connections in the central nervous system. *Brain Rev.* 37: 21–51.

Cranefield, P. F. (1957). Biophysics of 1847 and today. *J. Hist. Med. Allied Sci.* 12: 407–423.

Cranefield, P. F. (1966). The philosophical and cultural interests of the biophysics movement of 1847. *J. Hist. Med. Allied Sci.* 21: 1–7.

Da Fano, C. (1926). Camillo Golgi, 1843–1926. *J. Path. Bact.* 29: 500–514.

Darwin, C. A. (1859). *On the Origin of Species.* London: John Murray.

DeFelipe, J., and Jones, E. G. (1988). *Cajal on the Cerebral Cortex.* New York: Oxford University Press.

del Castillo, J., and Katz, B. (1954). Quantal components of the endplate potential. *J. Physiol. London* 124: 560–573.

De Robertis, E. (1959). Submicroscopic morphology of the synapse. *Int. Rev. Cytol.* 8: 61–96.

De Robertis, E., and Bennett, H. S. (1954). Submicroscopic vesicular component in the synapse. *Fed. Proc.* 13: 35.

De Robertis, E. (1955). Changes in the "synaptic vesicles" of the ventral acoustic ganglion after nerve section (An electron microscope study). *Anat. Record* 121:284–285.

Deiters, O. F. K. (1865). *Untersuchungen über Gehirn und Rückenmark des Menschen und der Säugetiere.* Braunschweig: Vieweg.

Derry, T. K. (1957) *A Short History of Norway.* London: Allen and Unwin.

Dietl (1876). Die Organizsation des Arthropodengehirns. *Zeitschr. f. wiss. Zool.* Bd. XXVII: 488–517.

Dotti, C. G., Sulllivan, C. A., and Banker, G. A. (1988). The establishment of polarity by hippocampal neurons in culture. *J. Neurosci.* 8: 1454–1468.

Dowling, J. E., and Boycott, B. B. (1966). Organization of the primate retina: electron microscopy. *Proc. R. Soc. London Series B* 166: 80–111.

du Bois-Reymond, E. (1843). Vorläufiger Abriss einer Untersuchung über den sogenannten Froschstrom und über die elektromotorischen Fische. [Poggendorffs] *Annln. Phys.* 58: 1–30.

du Bois-Reymond, E. (1848). *Untersuchungen über thierische Elektricität.* Berlin: Reimer.

Dudel, J., and Kuffler, S. W. (1961). Presynaptic inhibition at the crayfish neuromuscular junction. *J. Physiol. London* 155: 543–562.

Duval, M. (1895). Hypothèse sur la physiologie des centres nerveux: théorie histologique du sommeil. *Compt. Rend. Soc. Biol., Paris (series 10)* 2: 74–113.

Eccles, J. C. (1957). *The Physiology of Nerve Cells.* Baltimore: Johns Hopkins.

Easter, S. S., Purves, D., Rakic, P., and Spitzer, N. C. (1984). The changing view of neural specificity. *Science* 230: 507–511.

Eccles, J. C. (1959). The development of ideas on the synapse. In *The Historical Development of Physiological Thought* (C. Mac. Brooks and P. F. Cranefield, eds.). New York: Hafner. pp. 39–66.

Eccles, J. C., Eccles, R. M., and Magni, F. (1961). Central inhibitory action attributable to presynaptic depolarization produced by muscle afferent volleys. *J. Physiol. London* 159: 147–166.

Eccles, J. C., Libet, B., and Young, R. R. (1958). The behaviour of chromatolyzed motoneurons studied by intracellular recording. *J. Physiol. London* 143: 11–40.

Edwards, C., and Ottoson, D. O. (1958). The site of impulse initiation in a nerve cell of a crustacean stretch receptor. *J. Physiol. London* 143: 138–148.

Ehrenberg, C. G. (1833). Nothwendigkeit einer feineren mechanischen Zerlegung des Gehirns und der Nerven vor der chemischen, dargestellt aus Beobachtungen von C. G. Ehrenberg. [Poggendorffs] *Annln. Phys.* 28: 449–473.

Ehrlich, P. (1886). Über die Methylenblau-reaktion der lebenden Nervensubstanz. *Dtsch. med. Wochenschr.* 12: 49–52.

Eyzaguirre, C., and Kuffler, S. W. (1955). Processes of excitation in the dendrites and in the soma of single isolated sensory nerve cells of the lobster and crayfish. *J. Gen. Physiol.* 39: 87–119.

Fatt, P., and Katz, B. (1951). An analysis of the end-plate potential recorded with an intra-cellular electrode. *J. Physiol. London* 115: 320–270.

Fatt, P., and Katz, B. (1952). Spontaneous subthreshold activity at motor nerve endings. *J. Physiol. London* 117: 109–128.

Ferraro, A. (1953). Camillo Golgi. In *The Founders of Neurology* (W. Haymaker, ed.). Springfield, Ill.: Charles C. Thomas. pp. 41–45.

Ferrier, D. (1876). *The Functions of the Brain.* London: Smith, Elder.

Fick, H. (1921). Wilhelm von Waldeyer-Hartz. *Zentralblatt f.d. ges. Wiss. Anatomie* 56: 508–521.

Floegel. (1878). Ueber den einheitlichen Bau des Gehirns in den verschieden Insektenordnungen. *Zeitschr. f. wiss. Zool.* Rd. 30, Suppl. p. 556–592.

Florey, E. (1985). The zoological station at Naples and the neuron: personalities and encounters in a unique institution. *Biol. Bull.* (Suppl.) 168: 137–152.

Forbes, A. (1939). Problems of synaptic function. *J. Neurophysiol.* 2: 465–472.

Forel, A. (1887). Einige hirnanatomische Betrachtungen und Ergebnisse. *Arch. Psychiat. Berlin* 18: 162–198.

Forel, A. H. (1937). *Out of My Life and Work.* New York: Norton.

Forel, O. L. (1948). In memoriam Auguste Forel. *Schweiz. Med. Wochenschrift.* 79: 838–839.

Foster, M. (1897). *A Text-Book of Physiology.* Part III. London: Macmillan.

Freud, S. (1877). Über den Ursprung der hinteren Nervenwurzeln im Rückenmark von Ammocoetes (Petromyzon Planeri). *Sitz. Math.-Naturwiss. Classe Kais. Ak. Wiss.* 75: 15–27.

Freud, S. (1878). Über Spinalganglien und Rückenmark des Petromyzon. *Sitz. Math.-Naturwiss. Classe Kais. Ak. Wiss.* 78: 81–167.

Freud, S. (1882). Über den Bau der Nervenfasern und Nervenzellen beim Flusskrebs. *Sitz. Math.-Naturwiss. Classe Kais Ak. Wiss.* 85: 9–46.

Freud, S. (1884). Jahrbücher für Psychiatrie. In *The Life and Works of Sigmund Freud.* Vol. 1. E. Jones. (1953).

Freud, S. (1935/1952). *An Autobiographical Study.* New York: Norton.

Furshpan, E. J., and Potter, D. D. (1959). Transmission at the giant motor synapses of the crayfish. *J. Physiol. London* 145: 289–325.

Gad, J. (1884). *66te Versamml. deutsch. Naturf. Aertze* (quoted in Sherrington, 1906).

Gasser, H. S., and Erlanger, J. (1922). A study of the action currents of nerve with the cathode ray oscillograph. *Am. J. Physiol.* 62: 496–524.

Gay, P. (1988). *Freud. A Life for our Time.* New York: W. W. Norton.

Gerlach, J. von (1872a). Über die struktur der grauen Substanz des menschlichen Grosshirns. *Zentralbl. med. Wiss.* 10: 273–275.

Gerlach, J. von (1872b). Von der Rückenmark. In Stricker (1869–1872, II, 665–693); English translation, "The spinal cord," in Stricker (1870–1873, pp. 327–366).

Golgi, C. (1873). On the structure of the grey matter of the brain. (Translated by M. Santini). In *Golgi Centennial Symposium* (1975, M. Santini, ed.). New York: Raven. pp. 647–650.

Golgi, C. (1873). Sulla struttura della grigia del cervello. *Gazetta medica italiana Lombardia* 6: 244–246. (See *Opera Omnia,* 1903, Vol. 2, pp. 91–98. Milan: Hoepli.)

Golgi, C. (1874). Sulla fina anatomia del cervelletto umano. *Gazetta medica italiana Lombardia* 7: XXX-XXX.

Golgi, C. (1875). Sulla fina struttura dei bulbi olfattori. *Riv. sper. Freniatria Med. legal.* 1: 66–78.

Golgi, C. (1880). *Arch. ac. med., Tor.,* 4: 221–246.

Golgi, C. (1883). Chap. II. Continuation of the study of the minute anatomy of the central nervous system. Chap. III. Morphology and disposition of the nervous cells in the anterior, central, and superior-occipital convolutions. *Alienist and Neurologist* 4: 383–416.

Golgi, C. (1883a). Recherches sur l'histologie des centres nerveux. *Arch. ital. Biol.* 3: 285–317.

Golgi, C. (1884). Recherches sur l'histologie des centres nerveux. *Arch. ital. Biol.* 4: 92–123.

Golgi, C. (1885). Continuation of the study of the minute anatomy of the central nervous system. Chap. V. On the minute anatomy of the great foot of the hippocampus. *Alienist and Neurologist* 6: 307–324.

Golgi, C. (1886). *Sulla Fina Anatomia degli Organi Centrali del Sistema Nervoso*. Milano: Hoepli.

Golgi, C. (1886). Sur l'anatomie microscopique des organes centraux du système nerveux. *Arch. ital. Biol.* 7: 15–47.

Golgi, C. (1890). Ueber den Feineren Bau des Rückenmarkes. *Anat. Anz.* 5: 431–

Golgi, C. (1891). La rete nervosa diffusa degli organi centrali del sistema nervoso; suo significata fisiologico. Trans. in *Arch. ital. de biol., Turin* t. xv, pp. 434–463.

Golgi, C. (1894). *Untersuchungen über den feineren Bau des centralen und peripherischen Nervensytems*. (Translated by R. Teuscher). Jena: Fischer.

Golgi, C. (1903). *Opera Omnia*. Milano: Hoepli.

Golgi, C. (1906). La doctrine du neurone, théorie et faits. In *Les Prix Nobel 1904–1906*. Stockholm: Norstedt.

Golgi, C. (1967). The neuron doctrine—theory and facts. Nobel Lecture, December 11, 1906. In *Nobel Lectures Physiology or Medicine 1901–1921*. New York: Elsevier Publishing Company, pp. 189–217.

Hannover, A. (1844). *Recherches Microscopiques sur le Système Nerveux*. Paris.

Harrison, R. G. (1907). Observations on the living developing nerve fiber. *Anat. Rec.* 1: 116–118.

Harrison, R. G. (1908). Embryonic transplantation and the development of the nervous system. *Anat. Rec.* 2: 385–410.

Haymaker, W. (1953). *The Founders of Neurology*. Springfield, Ill.: Charles C. Thomas.

Held, H. (1897). Beiträge zur Structur der Nervenzellen und ihrer Fortsätze. *Zweite Abhandlung. Arch. Anat. Physiol. (Anat. Abt.)*. pp. 204–294.

Helle, K. B. (1987) The young Nansen in Bergen (1882–1887). In *The Nansen Symposium on New Concepts in Neuroscience*. (ed. K. B. Helle, O. D. Laerum, and H. Ursin). Bergen: Sigma Forlag, pp. 3–10.

Helmholtz, H. von (1842). *De fabrica systematis nervosi evertebratorum*. Berlin, Inaugural dissertation.

Helmholtz, H. von (1850). Vorläufiger Bericht über die Fortpflanzungsgeschwindigkeit der Nervereizung. *Arch. Anat. Physiol.* (Anat. Abt., Supplement-Bd.) pp. 71–73; translation in Dennis, W. (1948). *Readings in Psychology*. New York: Appleton-Century-Crofts, pp. 197–198.

Hermann, E. (1875). Das Central-Nervensystem von Hirudo medicinalis. *Gekr. Preisschr.* München.

Heuser, J. E., and Reese, T. S. (1973). Evidence for recycling of synaptic vesicle membrane during transmitter release at the frog neuromuscular junction. *J. Cell Biol.* 57: 315–344.

His, W. (1865). *Die Haute ünd Hohlen des Körpers*. Basel: Schweighauser.

His, W. (1880–1885). *Anatomie menschlicher Embryonen*. Three volumes. Leipzig: Vogel.

His, W. (1886). Zur Geschichte des menschlichen Rückenmarkes und der Nervenwurzeln. *Abhandl. Math. -Phys. Class. Königl. säch. Gesellsch. Wiss., Leipzig* 13: 147–209, 477–513.

His, W. (1889). Die Neuroblasten und deren Entstehung im embryonalen Marke. *Abhandl. Math. -Phys. Class. Königl. säch. Gesellsch. Wiss., Leipzig* 15: 313–372.

His, W. (1890). Histogenese und Zusammenhang der Nervenelemente. *Abh. Internat. Med. Congress, Berlin, Anat. section* 7 August 1890. (Published in *Arch. Anat. Entwickl. Suppl.*, pp. 95–117)

Hitzig, E., and Fritsch, G. T. (1870). Über die elektrische Erregbarkeit des Grosshirns. *Arch. Anat. Physiol.* pp. 300–322; English translation in Bonin (1960) pp. 73–96; and H. Wilkins, "Neurosurgical classics XII," *J. Neurosurg.*, (1963) 20: 904–916.

Hodgkin, A. L., and Huxley, A. F. (1952). A quantitative description of membrane current and its application to conduction and excitation in nerve. *J. Physiol. London* 117: 500–544.

Høyer, L. N. (1957). *Nansen. A Family Portrait.* New York: Longman's.

Huxley, A. F. (1977). Looking back on muscle. In *The Pursuit of Nature: Informal Essays on the History of Physiology.* New York: Cambridge University Press. pp. 23–64.

Huzella, T. (1937/38). Michael von Lenhossék. *Anat. Anz.* 85: 168–187.

James, W. (1880). *Bost. Soc. Natural History.* (In Sherrington, C. S., *The Integrative Action of the Nervous System,* New Haven: Yale University Press, 1906).

Jansen, J. K. S. (1982/1987). Fridtiof Nansen og hierneforskningen ved sluten av forrige århundre. *Fridtiof Nansen Minneforelesninger* 17: 1–24 (Reprinted in English translation in *The Nansen Symposium on New Concepts in Neuroscience.* (K. B. Helle, O. D. Laerum, and H. Ursin, eds.) London: Sigma Forlag, pp. 11–30.

Jelliffe, S. E. (1937). Sigmund Freud as a neurologist. Some notes on his earlier neurobiological and clinical neurological studies. *J. Nerv. Ment. Dis.* 85: 696–711.

John, H. J. (1959). *Jan Evangelista Purkyne, Czech Scientist and Patriot.* Philadelphia: American Philosophical Society.

Jones, E. (1953). *The Life and Works of Sigmund Freud. Vol. 1.* New York: Basic Books.

Kandel, E. R., and Schwartz, J. S. (1985). *Principles of Neural Science.* New York: Elsevier.

Klein, E. (1878). Observations on the structure of cells and nuclei. I. *Quart. J. micr. Sci N.S.* 18: 315–339.

Kölliker, A. (1844). Die Selbständigkeit and Abhängigkeit des sympathischen Nervensystems. Zurich.

Kölliker, A. von (1849). Neurologische Bemerkungen. *Z. wiss. Zool.* 1: 135–163.

Kölliker, A (1852). *Handbuch der Gewebelehre des Menschen.* Leipzig: Engelmann.

Kölliker, A. (1853). *Manual of Human Histology.* (Translated by G. Busk and T. Huxley). London: Sydenham Society.

Kölliker, A. (1867). *Handbuch der Gewebelehre des Menschen,* 5th Edition. Leipzig: Engelmann.

Kölliker, A. von (1887). Die Untersuchungen von Golgi über den feineren Bau des centralen Nervensystems. *Anat. Anz.* 2: 480–483.

Kölliker, A. (1888). Zur Kenntnis der quergestreiften Musckelfasern. *Z. wiss. Zool.* 47: 689–710.

Kölliker, A. (1890a). Zur feineren Anatomie des centralen Nervensystems. Erster Beitrag. Das Kleinhirn. *Z. wiss. Zool.* 49: 663–689.

Kölliker, A. (1890b). Zur feineren Anatomie des centralen Nervensystems. Zweiter Beitrag. Das Rückenmark. *Z. wiss. Zool.* 51: 1–54.

Kölliker, A. (1896). *Handbuch der Gewebelehre des Menschen, 6th ed., Vol. 2: Nervensystems des Menschen und der Thiere.* Leipzig: Engelmann.

Kölliker, A. von (1905). Obituary. *Lancet* 83: 1514. *Br. Med. J.* Suppl. II: 1375–1377.

Környey, S. (1937). Michel von Lenhossék. *Arch. Neurol. Psychiat.* 38: 140–142.

Krieger, K. R. (1880). Ueber das Centralnervensystem des Flusskrebses. *Zeitschr. f. wiss. Zool.* Bd. 33, p. 527–594.

Kuffler, S. W., Nicholls, J. G., and Martin, A. R. (1984). *From Neuron to Brain.* Sunderland: Sinauer Associates, Inc.

Kuhlenbeck, H. (1953). August Forel. In *The Founders of Neurology* (W. Haymaker, ed.). Springfield, Ill.: Charles C. Thomas. pp. 35–37.

Kühne, W. (1862). *Über die peripherischen Endorgane der motorischen Nerven.* Leipzig: Engelmann.

Kühne, W. (1869). Nerv und Muskelfaser. In Stricker (1869–1872, I, 147–169); English translation, "The mode of termination of nerve fibre in muscle," in Stricker (1870–1873, I, 202–234).

Kühne, W. (1888). On the origin and the causation of vital movement (Über die Enstehung der vitalen Bewegung). *Proc. R. Soc. London Series B,* 44: 427–447.

Lang, A. (1881). Untersuchung etc. II. Ueber das Nervensystem der Trematoden. *Mitth zool. Stat. Neapel.* Bd. 2, p. 28–52.

Larsell, O. (1953). Gustaf Magnus Retzius. In *The Founders of Neurology* (W. Haymaker, ed.). Springfield, Ill.: Charles C. Thomas. pp. 83–86.

Lashley, K. S. (1929). *Brain Mechanisms and Intelligence: A Quantitative Study of Injuries to the Brain.* Chicago: University of Chicago Press.

Leeuwenhoek, A. van (1674). More Observations from Mr. Leeuwenhoek, in a letter of Sept. 7, 1674, sent to the Publisher. *Phil. Trans. R. Soc.* 9: 178–182.

Leeuwenhoek, A. van (1719). *Epistolae physiologicae super compluribus naturae arcanis.* Delft: Beman.

Leeuwenhoek, A. van (1817). *Antony van Leeuwenhoek.* The selected works by Samuel Hoole. London: Philanthropic Society. Vol. II, 303–306, contains an inaccurate and incomplete translation of the letter of 2 March 1717.

Leydig. (1857). *Lehrbuch der Histologie des Menschen und der Thiere.* Frankfurt: Verlag von Meidinger Sohn & Comp.

Leydig, F. (1864). *Vom Baue des thierischen Körpers.*

Liddell. (1960). *The Discovery of Reflexes.* Oxford: Clarendon Press.

Llinás, R. R. (1988) The intrinsic electrophysiological properties of mammalian neurons: insights into central nervous system function. *Science* 242: 1654–1664.

Locy, W. A. (1908). *Biology and its Makers.* New York: Henry Holt.

Loewenstein, W. R. (1981). Junctional intercellular communication: the cell-to-cell membrane channel. *Physiol. Rev.* 61: 829–913.

Lorente de Nó, R. (1938). The cerebral cortex: architecture, intracortical connections and motor projections. In *Physiology of the Nervous System* (by J. F. Fulton). London: Oxford University Press, pp. 291–339.

Mackowski, L. D., Casper, L. D., Phillips, W. C., and Goodenough, D. A. (1977). Gap junction structure. II. Analysis of the x-ray diffraction data. *J. Cell Biol.* 74: 629–645.

Magendie, F. J. (1822). Experience sur les fonctions des racine des nerfs rachidiens. *J. Physiol. exp. path., Paris* 2: 276–279.

Magendie, F. J. (1823). Sur le siège du mouvement et du sentiment dans la moelle épinière. *J. Physiol. exp. path., Paris* 3: 153–157.

Magini, G. (1887). Nevroglia e cellule nervose cerebrali nei feti. *Atti. 12 Congress. Med. Ital., Pavia.* 1: 281–291. (Also appeared as: Sur la névroglie et les cellules nerveuses cérébrales chez les foetus. *Arch. ital. Biol.* 11: 59–60 [1888].)

Maienshein, J. (1985). Agassiz, Hyatt, Whitman, and the birth of the Marine Biological Laboratory. *Biol. Bull.* (Suppl.) 168: 26–34.

Mall, F. P. (1905). Wilhelm His, his relations to institutions of learning. *Am. J. Anat.* 4: 139–161.

Matteucci, C. (1840). *Essai sur les phénomènes electriques des animaux.* Paris: Carillian, Goeury & Dalmont.

McCulloch, W., and Pitts, W. (1943). A logical calculus of the ideas immanent in nervous activity. *Bull. Math. Biophys.* 5: 115–133.

Melland, B. (1885). A simplified view of the histology of the striped muscle fibre. *Q. J. micr. Sci.* 25: 371–390.

Meyer, A. (1971). *Historical Aspects of Cerebral Anatomy.* New York: Oxford University Press.

Meyer née Bjerrum, K. (1932). Hans Christian Ørsted. (1777–1851). In *Prominent Danish Scientists* (ed. V. Meisen). Copenhagen: Munksgaard, pp. 89–93.

Muller, K. J., Nicholls, J. G., and Stent, G. S. (eds.) (1981). *The Neurobiology of the Leech.* New York: Cold Spring Harbor Press.

Müller, J. (1835). *Handbuch der Physiologie des Menschen für Vorlesungen,* I. 2d ed. Coblenz: Hölscher.

Nansen, F. (1887). *The Structure and Combination of the Histological Elements of the Central Nervous System.* Bergen: Bergens Mus. Aarsberetning.

Nastuk, W. L. (1953). Membrane potential changes at a single muscle end-plate produced by transitory application of acetylcholine with an electrically controlled microjet. *Fed. Proc.* 12: 102.

Nauta, W. J. H. (1956). An experimental study of the fornix system in the rat. *J. Comp. Neurol.* 104: 247–272.

Nauta, W. J. H., and Feirtag, M. (1986). *Fundamental Neuroanatomy.* New York: Freeman.

Newton, E. T. (1879). On the brain of the cockroach, Blatta orientalis. *Q. journ. micr. science London.* Vol. 19, p. 340–356.

Nicholas, C. (1959). Ross Granville Harrison. *Anat. Rec.* 137: 160–162.

Nissl, F. (1903). *Die Neuronenlehre und ihre Anhängen.* Jena: Gustav Fischer Verlag. 478 p. (Floren).

Nobili, L. (1825). Über einen neuen Galvanometer. *J. Chem. Phys., Nüremburg* 45: 249–254.

Oppenheimer, J. M. (1966). Ross Harrison's contribution to experimental embryology. *Bull. Hist. Med.* 40: 525–543.

Oppenheimer, J. (1972). Ross Granville Harrison. *Dict. Sci. Biog.* 6: 131–135.

Palade, G. E., and Palay, S. L. (1954). Electron microscope observations of interneuronal and neuromuscular synapses. *Anat. Rec.* 118: 335–336.

Palay, S. L. (1956). Synapses in the central nervous system. *J. Biophysic. and Biochem. Cytol.* Suppl. 2: 193–201.

Palay, S. L. (1958). The morphology of synapses in the central nervous system. *Exp. Cell Res., Suppl. 5*: 275–293.

Papez, J. W. (1953a). Arthur van Gehuchten. In *The Founders of Neurology* (W. Haymaker, ed.). Springfield, Ill.: Charles C. Thomas, pp. 38–40.

Papez, J. W. (1953b). Robert Remak. In *The Founders of Neurology* (W. Haymaker, ed.). Springfield, Ill.: Charles C. Thomas, pp. 80–82.}

Papez, J. W. (1953c). Theodor Meynert. In *The Founders of Neurology* (W. Haymaker, ed.). Springfield, Ill.: Charles C. Thomas, pp. 64–67.

Penfield, W. (1926). The career of Ramón y Cajal. *Arch. Neurol. Psychiat.* 26: 212–220.

Peters, A., Palay, S. L., and Webster, H. De F. (1976). *The Fine Structure of the Nervous System.* New York: Harper & Row. (3rd edition, 1990).

Phillips, C. G., Powell, T. P. S., and Shepherd, G. M. (1963). Responses of mitral cells to stimulation of the lateral olfactory tract in the rabbit. *J. Physiol. London* 168: 89–100.

Piccolino, M. (1988). Cajal and the retina: a 100-year retrospective. *Trends Neurosci.* 11: 521–525.

Purkyně [Purkinje], Society (1937). *In memoriam: Joh. Ev. Purkyně 1787–1937.* Prague: Purkyně Society.

Purkyně [Purkinje], J. E. (1838). *Bericht über die Versammlung deutscher Naturforscher und Ärzte in Prag im September, 1837.* Prague. Pt. 3, sec. 5, A. Anatomisch-phisiologische Verhandlungen, pp. 177–180. This report of the paper read by Purkyně on 23 September 1837 has been reprinted in his *Opera Selecta,* Prague, pp. 111–114.

Rabl-Rückhard, H. (1890). Sind die Ganglienzellen amöboid? Eine Hypothese zur Mechanik psychischer Vorgänge. *Neurol. Centralbl., Leipz.,* Bd. ix, p. 199.

Rakic, P. (ed.) (1975). Local circuit neurons. *NRP Bull.* 3: 291–446.

Rall, W. (1959). Branching dendritic trees and motoneuron membrane resistivity. *Expt. Neurol.* 1: 491–527.

Rall, W., and Rinzel, J. (1971). Dendritic spines and synaptic potency explored theoretically. *Proc. IUPS XXV Intl. Congress* IX: 466.

Rall, W., and Shepherd, G. M. (1968). Theoretical reconstruction of field potentials and dendrodendritic synaptic interactions in olfactory bulb. *J. Neurophysiol.* 31: 884–915.

Rall, W., Shepherd, G. M., Reese, T. S., and Brightman, M. W. (1966). Dendrodendritic synaptic pathway for inhibition in the olfactory bulb. *Exptl. Neurol.* 14: 44–56.

Rasmussen, A. T. (1953). Wilhelm His. In *The Founders of Neurology* (W. Haymaker, ed.). Springfield, Ill.: Charles C. Thomas. pp. 49–51.

Remak, R. (1836). Verläufige Mittheilung mikroscopischer Beobachtungen über den innern Bau der Cerebrospinalnerven und über die Entwicklung ihrer Formelemente. *Arch. Anat. Physiol.* 145–161.

Remak, R. (1837). Weitere mikroscopische Beobachtungen über die Primitivfasern des Nervensystems der Wirbelthiere. [Froriep's] *Neue Notizen* 3: cols. 35–40.

Remak, R. (1838). *Observationes anatomicae et microscopicae de systematis nervosi structura.* Berlin: Reimer.

Remak, R. (1844). Neurologische Erläuterungen. *Arch. Anat. Physiol.* 463–472.

Remak, R. (1855). Über den Bau der grauen Säulen im Rückenmark der Säugethiere. *Deutsche Klinik* 7: 295.

Retzius, G. (1881). Über die peripherische Endigungsweise des Gehörnerven. *Biol Unters.* I: 51, Tafel VI.

Retzius, G. (1890). Zur Kenntnis des Nervensystems der Crustaceen. *Biol. Unters., Neue Folge* 1: 1–99.

Retzius, G. (1890–1920). *Biologisches Untersuchungen von Gustav Retzius, Neue Folge,* Vols. 1–19. Stockholm: Samson and Wallin.

Retzius, G. (1891). Ueber den Bau der Oberflächenschicht der Grosshirnrinde beim Menschen und bei den Säugethieren. *Biol. Unters., Neue Folge* 3: 90–102.

Retzius, G. (1892a). Die nervösen Elemente der Kleinhirnrinde. *Biol. Unters., Neue Folge* 3: 17–24.

Retzius, G. (1892b). Die Endigungsweise der Riechnerven. *Biol. Unters., Neue Folge* 3: 25–28.

Retzius, G. (1896). Fridtiof Nansen as a biologist. In *Fridtiof Nansen* (by W.C. Brögger and N. Rolfsen). London: Longmans, pp. 112–122.

Retzius, G. (1908). The principles of the minute structure of the nervous system as revealed by recent investigations. *Proc. R. Soc. London Series B:* 414–443.

Revel, J. P., and Karnovsky, M. J. (1967). Hexagonal array of subunits in intercellular junctions of the mouse heart and liver. *J. Cell Biol.* 33: C7.

Robertson, J. D. (1955). Recent electron microscope observations on the ultrastructure of the crayfish median-to-motor giant synapse. *Exp. Cell Res.* 8: 226–229.

Santini, M. (1975). *Golgi Centennial Symposium: Perspectives in Neurobiology.* New York: Raven.

Schafer, E. A. (1893). The nerve cell considered as the basis of neurology. *Brain.*

Schwann, T. (1839). *Mikroskopische Untersuchungen über die Uebereinstimmung in der Struktur und dem Wachsthum der Thiere und Pflanzen.* Berlin: G. E. Reimer. (English translation by H. Smith; New York: Kraus Reprint Co., 1845, reprinted 1969).

Shepherd, G. M. (1972). The neuron doctrine: a revision of functional concepts. *Yale J. Biol. Med.* 45: 584–599.

Shepherd, G. M. (1974). *The Synaptic Organization of the Brain.* New York: Oxford University Press. (3rd edition, 1990).

Shepherd, G. M. (1988). *Neurobiology.* 2nd Edition. New York: Oxford University Press.

Shepherd, G. M., and Greer, C. A. (1988). The dendritic spine: Adaptations of structure and function for different types of synaptic integration. In *Intrinsic Determinants of Neuronal Form and Function* (R. Lassek, ed.). New York: Alan R. Liss, pp. 245–262.

Shepherd, G. M., and Koch, C. (1990). Introduction to synaptic circuits. In *The Synaptic Organization of the Brain.* G. M. Shepherd (ed.) New York: Oxford University Press, pp. 3–31.

Sherrington, C. S. (1906). *The Integrative Action of the Nervous System.* New Haven: Yale University Press.

Sherrington, C. S. (1935a). Santiago Ramón y Cajal 1852–1934. *Obit Not. R. Soc.* no. 4, pp. 425–441.

Sherrington, C. S. (1935b). Sir Edward Sharpey-Schafer and his contribution to neurology. *Edinburgh Med. J.* 42: 393–406.

Sherrington, C. S. (1935c). Sir Edward Sharpey-Schafer. *Q. J. Exp. Physiol.* 25: 98–104.

Singer, C. (1950). *A History of Biology.* New York: Henry Schuman.

Spencer, W. A., and Kandel, E. R. (1961). Electrophysiology of hippocampal neurons. IV. Fast prepotentials. *J. Neurophysiol.* 24: 272–285.

Steward, O., and Levy, W. B. (1982). Preferential localization of polyribosomes under the base of dendritic spines in granule cells of the dentate gyrus. *J. Neurosci.* 2: 284–291.

Taylor, D. W. (1975). Edward Albert Sharpey-Schafer. *Dict. Sci. Biog.* 12: 355–357.

Tello, J. F. (1935). *Cajal y su labor histológica.* Madrid: Universidad Central.

Temkin, O. (1946). Materialism in French and German physiology of the early nineteenth century. *Bull. Hist. Med.* 20: 322–327.

Tseng, G.-F., and Haberly, L. B. (1989). Deep neurons in piriform cortex. I. Morphology and synaptically evoked responses including a unique high amplitude paired shock facilitation. *J. Neurophysiol.* 62: 369–385.

Valentin, G. G. (1836). Über den Verlauf und die letzten Ende der Nerven. *Nova Acta Phys. -Med. Acad. Leopoldina, Breslau* 18: 51–240.

van der Loos, H. (1967). The history of the neuron. In *The Neuron* (H. Hydén, ed.). Amsterdam: Elsevier, pp. 1–47.

van Gehuchten, A. (1886). Étude sur la structure intime de la cellule musculaire striée. *La Cellule* 2: 289–453 + I–V.

van Gehuchten, A. (1888). Étude sur la structure intime de la cellule musculaire striée chez les vertébrés. *La Cellule* 4: 245–316 + I–II.

van Gehuchten, A. (1891a). La structure des centres nerveux: La moelle épinière et le cervelet. *La Cellule* 7: 79–122.

van Gehuchten, A. (1891b). Le bulbe olfactif chez quelques mammifères. *La Cellule* 7: 203–200.

van Gehuchten, A. (1900). *Anatomie du Système Nerveux de l'Homme. Third Edition.* Louvain: Uystpruyst-Dieudonné.

Vecsey, G. (1990). Soccer's little big man. *N.Y. Times Magazine.* May 27, VI, 24–32.

Viets, H. R. (1926). Camillo Golgi. *Arch. Neurol. Psychiat.* 15: 623–627.

Virchow, R. (1858). *Die Cellularpathologie.* Berlin: Hirschwald. (English translation in 1860 by Chance). *Cellular Pathology.* London: Churchill.

von Bechterew, W. (1895). Die Lehre von den Neuronen und die Entladungstheorie. Neurologisches Centralblatt 15: 50–111.

von Bonin, G. (1953). Rudolf Albert von Kölliker. In *The Founders of Neurology* (W. Haymaker, ed.). Springfield, Ill.: Charles C. Thomas, pp. 52–54.

von Lenhossék, M. (1895). *Der feinere Bau des Nervensystems im Lichte neuester Forschungen.* Berlin: Fischer.

Wagner, R. (1847). Neue Untersuchungen über den Bau und die Endigung der Nerven und die Struktur der Ganglienzellen. *Icones Physiologicae Suppl. Leipzig.*

Waldeyer, W. (1863). Untersuchungen über den Ursprung und den Verlauf der Axencylinders bei Wirbellosen und Wirbelthieren. *Zeits. f. rationelle Medizin* 20.

Waldeyer, W. (1921). Obituary. *J. A. M. A.* 76: 669.

Waldeyer-Hartz, H. W. G. von (1891). Über einige neuere Forschungen im Gebiete der Anatomie des Centralnervensystems. *Deutsch. med. Wschr.* 17: 1213–1218, 1244–1246, 1267–1269, 1287–1289, 1331–1332, 1352–1356.

Waller, A. V. (1850). Experiments on the section of the glossopharyngeal and hypoglossal nerves of the frog, and observations of the alterations produced thereby in the structure of their primitive fibres. *Phil. Trans. R. Soc.* 140: 423–429.

Waller, A. V. (1852). Examen des alterations qui ont lieu dans les filets d'origine du nerf pneumogastrique et des nerfs rachidiens, par suite de la section de ces nerfs au-dessus de leurs ganglions. *C. r. hebd. Acad. Sci., Paris* 34: 842–847.

Werblin, F. S., and Dowling, J. E. (1968). Organization of the retina of the mudpuppy, Necturus maculosus. II. Intracellular recording. *J. Neurophysiol.* 32: 339–355.

Wiesel, T. N., Hubel, D. H., and Lam, D. M. K. (1974). Autoradiographic demonstration of ocular-dominance columns in the monkey striate cortex by means of transneuronal transport. *Brain Res.* 79: 273–279.

Wilson, E. O. (1975). *Sociobiology.* Cambridge, Mass.: Harvard University Press.

Wilson, J. W. (1944). Cellular tissue and the dawn of the cell theory. *ISIS* 35: 168–173.

Wilson, J. W. (1947). Virchow's contribution to the cell theory. *J. Hist. Med. Allied Sci.* 2: 163–178.

INDEX